Leg Ulcer Management

Christine Moffatt CBE PhD
Professor of Nurs

and Nur

Ruth Martin B. , RN (adult)
Leg Specialist Nurse
Wandsworth Teaching Primary Care Trust

Rachael Smithdale RGN Undergraduate Dip.
Healthcare Practice
Leg Ulcer Specialist Nurse
Wandsworth Teaching Primary Care Trust

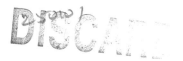

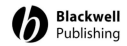

Blackwell
Publishing

Blackwell Publishing Ltd, 9600 Garsington Road, Oxford OX4 2DQ, UK
Tel: +44 (0)1865 776868
Blackwell Publishing Inc., 350 Main Street, Malden, MA 02148-5020, USA
Tel: +1 781 388 8250
Blackwell Publishing Asia Pty Ltd, 550 Swanston Street, Carlton, Victoria
3053, Australia
Tel: +61 (0)3 8359 1011

The right of the Authors to be identified as the Authors of this Work has been asserted in accordance with the Copyright, Designs and Patents Act 1988.

First published 2007 by Blackwell Publishing Ltd

ISBN: 978-1-4051-3476-7

Library of Congress Cataloging-in-Publication Data
Moffatt, Christine J.
Leg ulcer management / Christine Moffatt, Ruth Martin, Rachael
Smithdale.
p. ; cm.
Includes bibliographical references and index.
ISBN-13: 978-1-4051-3476-7 (pbk. : alk. paper)
ISBN-10: 1-4051-3476-3 (pbk. : alk. paper)
1. Leg–Ulcers–Nursing. I. Martin, Ruth, 1974– . II. Smithdale,
Rachael. III. Title.
[DNLM: 1. Leg Ulcer–nursing–Great Britain. 2. Delivery of Health Care,
Integrated–organization & administration–Great Britain. 3. Evidence-Based
Medicine–Great Britain. 4. Leg Ulcer–therapy–Great Britain. 5. Patient
Care Team–organization & administration–Great Britain. WY 154.5 M695L
2007]
RC951.L4443 2007
362.196′545–dc22
2006027509

A catalogue record for this title is available from the British Library

Set in 9/11 pt Palatino
by SNP Best-set Typesetter Ltd., Hong Kong
Printed and bound in Singapore
by Fabulous Printers Pte Ltd

For further information on Blackwell Publishing, visit our website:
www.blackwellnursing.com

Contents

Contents

Contents

Contents

DEDICATION

This book is dedicated to all the patients who have been treated in the Wandsworth leg ulcer service. They have taught us so much about leg ulceration and the impact it has on their lives. We have faithfully tried to portray their concerns within this book. We thank them for being willing to share their experiences with us over the years.

ACKNOWLEDGEMENTS

There are many people we would like to thank for helping us produce this book. In addition to our patients, we would like to thank our families for their patience during the production of this book. Particular thanks go to Neil and Peter for their wonderful artwork and to Susie for checking and formatting the book. We would also like to thank all those within the multi-disciplinary team who work with us, particularly Professor Peter Mortimer who provides us with such wise clinical counsel and support.

Ruth and Rachael would like to thank Christine for her mentorship and for giving them the opportunity to write this book.

Preface

This book is written by a team of specialist nurses who have responsibility for an integrated leg ulcer service in Wandsworth, South West London, UK. Over the last fifteen years this service has evolved and much has been learnt about the challenges of providing and sustaining high-quality care across a range of community and hospital boundaries within an ever-changing health service.

This book aims to provide clear clinical advice on the management of patients with leg ulceration within a model of care that integrates community and specialist care. The current evidence-base for treatment decisions is summarised and presented throughout. Many aspects of care have not been subject to research, and in these cases expert clinical advice is provided. Case studies are used throughout to illustrate the types of problems experienced in the practice setting.

Since the 1980s there has been a proliferation in the number of tissue viability and leg ulcer specialists. The book also aims to address the problems encountered by specialist nurses who are supporting leg ulcer care in the community provided by community and practice nurses. The model and clinical pathway presented in this book has proved to be effective in reducing the prevalence of leg ulceration and in delivering high-quality care that can easily be adopted in other areas of the country and healthcare settings.

One of the main problems in leg ulcer management is ensuring that a correct diagnosis is made. Too often the recording of the ankle to brachial pressure index (ABPI) is used as a substitute for correct assessment. The model presented in this book attempts to ensure that a correct diagnosis is made for all patients, and requires specialist intervention if there is any uncertainty. Formal mechanisms and time frames for evaluation have been used to prevent patients continuing for long periods without specialist advice being sought.

The nursing care of patients with leg ulceration requires an appreciation of the wide variety of problems that surround patients with this condition. Issues such as the psychological status of the patient and poor symptom control are frequently neglected when a medical model of care is adopted. In this book we have attempted to redress these issues, placing equal importance on these and the more traditional aspects such as choice of dressings and use of compression therapy. Since the 1980s, the focus has been on complete healing as the only outcome of care, at the expense of other outcomes such as control of pain and sleep disturbance that may be overwhelming for the patient and lead to a very poor quality of life.

While there is little doubt that nursing has played a major part in improving the care for patients with leg ulceration, this book clearly supports the requirement for an effective multi-disciplinary team to support services.

Many nurses are appointed to specialist nursing posts and are faced with the huge task of developing and evaluating their service. Many have had little preparation for this demanding and diverse role and frequently feel isolated and overwhelmed. We hope this resource will be useful for these practitioners.

Part I
A Model of Leg Ulcer Care

Patients, when faced with a leg ulcer for the first time, hope to receive treatment from a healthcare professional equipped with the skills, knowledge and resources to manage their wound. Sadly, the literature suggests that this hope often fails to be realised, and that many patients experience long periods of ineffective care.

Since the 1980s huge advances have been made in the field of leg ulcer management. A wealth of research together with best practice guidelines now informs our understanding. International experts continue to collate current knowledge and expertise and produce consensus position documents on the various aspects of leg ulcer care. Our understanding of compression bandaging systems continues to develop, and there is now a wide range of bandaging and dressing options available on the National Health Service (NHS) drug tariff.

The simple existence of these resources, guidelines and research studies, however, is not sufficient to guarantee benefit to patients. The transfer of knowledge from a set of best practice documents to actual patient experience requires the establishment of healthcare structures dedicated to ensuring their success. These structures should focus on equipping practitioners with the necessary skills and current knowledge, as well as providing them with the clinical support to manage complex or unusual ulcer aetiologies.

Part I of this book examines the ingredients necessary for the establishment of such a structure. Aimed particularly at managers, tissue viability nurses and leg ulcer specialist nurses looking to set up a leg ulcer service in their area, it draws extensively from the literature as well as the authors' own experience of developing and running one of Europe's most successful leg ulcer services

– the Wandsworth Primary Care Trust (PCT) leg ulcer service. Using a multi-faceted internationally celebrated model of care, Wandsworth has achieved a prevalence of leg ulceration one-third that of the national average and the lowest on record in Europe. The development of this service has, and continues to be, both exciting and challenging, and it is hoped that by sharing some of the lessons learnt, other areas of the country and other healthcare settings can also benefit.

A Leg Ulcer Service Model

LEARNING OBJECTIVES

Nurses involved in leg ulcer management should be able to demonstrate:

❏ An understanding of the way leg ulcer services have developed since the 1980s.

❏ An understanding of the importance of using evidence-based guidelines in venous ulcer management.

❏ An understanding of the patient journey within an effective leg ulcer service that involves specialist and community care.

❏ The ability to describe the benefits of the model of care depicted within this chapter.

❏ An understanding of how this service has reduced the prevalence of leg ulceration within this area of London.

❏ An understanding of the principles of providing education within a leg ulcer service.

INTRODUCTION

Studies suggest that, historically, leg ulcer service provision has been commonly regarded as being of low status and profile, with wide variations in standards of practice and co-ordination between care settings. The majority of leg ulcer patients have tended to be managed almost solely in the community, with only a small percentage of patients being treated jointly by the primary care team and outpatient departments (Callum et al., 1985). Wound care has traditionally been considered a nursing role, and leg ulceration is no exception. Most doctors lack sufficient involvement in leg ulcer management to develop expertise or adequately evaluate outcomes of care (Callum et al., 1987), and the responsibility for assessment, diagnosis and management decisions has remained largely with community nursing services. Poor recognition by health services of the complexity of leg ulceration and the need for a co-ordinated approach has frequently led to a lack of adequate clinical assessment and diagnosis, resulting in long periods of ineffective or inappropriate treatment (Cornwall et al., 1986). Not only does this represent a huge waste of healthcare resources, with an estimated annual cost for individual health authorities somewhere in the range of £0.9 m to £2.1 m (Carr et al., 1999), it also perpetuates the suffering experienced by patients, and a sense of frustration and lack of reward felt by their carers.

Since the 1980s, the profile of leg ulcer service provision has begun to change. There is now widespread recognition that leg ulceration is a complex disease process, often caused by a number of underlying pathologies. Nurses remain the main care providers for this group of patients. They continue to develop their expertise in this field, to be at the forefront of developments to create an evidence-based approach to leg ulcer care and to raise the profile of leg ulceration as a substantial health problem that has a significant impact on patients' quality of life.

A wealth of research now underpins care. National (RCN, 1998; SIGN, 1998) and international groups (International Leg Ulcer Advisory Board and the European Wound Management Association) have produced consensus documents and best practice guidelines for leg ulcer care in order to raise standards and reduce variations in practice.

No single model of care is appropriate to the needs and resources in every area. However, an examination of the literature suggests success depends greatly on the support of healthcare trusts to make provision for the development of an evidence-based service. This service has to be responsive to the needs of its population, and to span the boundary between primary and secondary care (Bosanquet et al., 1993; Schofield et al., 2000; Moffatt et al., 2004a).

This chapter describes the evolving model of care used in the authors' own area of clinical practice. It considers:

- The principles underpinning the leg ulcer service model.
- The effects of the model on standards of care and leg ulcer prevalence.
- How the model has developed over the course of time in response to research findings, observations in practice and changes within the healthcare setting.

4

It is hoped that areas that have not yet adopted an integrated leg ulcer service model can learn from the authors' experience and use it to drive forward change.

THE WANDSWORTH LEG ULCER SERVICE MODEL

There has been a dedicated leg ulcer service in the Wandsworth borough of Southwest London since the 1990s. It is based on the internationally acclaimed Riverside model established in West London in the 1980s (Moffatt et al., 1992).

Outline of the Wandsworth population

- Population of 260 380
- 22% of the population from ethnic minority groups
- 36.5% of population living alone
- High level of deprivation
- 13.4% of residents with long-term illness

(Census, 2001)

BASIC PRINCIPLES OF THE SERVICE

The service was, and still is, underpinned by a number of key factors:

- In the UK, the majority of patients with leg ulceration received the bulk of their care from nurses in the primary care setting, either in their homes or at a health centre/surgery.
- It sought to ensure that all patients received standardised evidence-based treatment, irrespective of where their care was delivered.
- It acknowledged that many patients with leg ulceration had numerous complex problems.
- Specialist advice and support was available within the community and through a dedicated hospital specialist clinic.
- A continuous process of training was required to ensure that standards of care were maintained.
- Ongoing service planning and evaluation were required to ensure that the service met the needs of the patients in a clinically cost-effective manner.

The patient journey

The majority of patients were treated by the community and primary care nursing services, with support from the community leg ulcer team as and when required. Further expert assessment was available from an integrated leg ulcer specialist assessment clinic based in the acute trust setting, which, in addition, provided access to the broader multi-disciplinary team (Fig. 1.1).

The following outlines the patient's journey, from initial care to a major service evaluation. Some elements have changed since the introduction of the Wandsworth model, reasons for which are discussed later in this chapter; essentially, however, many aspects remain the same.

First point of call

Most patients' first point of call was to their GP or practice nurse. Depending upon the patient's ability to attend regular clinic

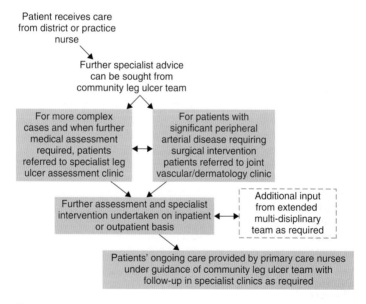

Fig. 1.1 The patient journey.

appointments, care was either provided at home by the district nursing (DN) team or in one of many community clinics in operation across the trust. These were previously run by a treatment-room nurse, often with other members of the DN team. The patient was assessed using a purpose-designed, leg ulcer assessment tool that included the Ankle Brachial Pressure Index. A treatment plan was then formulated based on the most likely cause of the ulcer.

Ensuring best practice

All DN teams and treatment room nurses had access to comprehensive guidelines, based on best practice (Fletcher et al., 1997; RCN, 1998; SIGN, 1998) written by the community-based leg ulcer specialist nurse. In addition, training in leg ulcer assessment and management was also provided. The combination of provision of guidelines and training has always been integral to the success of the model.

Specialist support

Community nurses received specialised support from a leg ulcer team. The team was made up of nursing and medical staff, with advanced training and experience in leg ulcer management in both primary and secondary care settings. Patients could be referred in the first instance to be seen jointly by one of the specialists and support nurses (based in the Wandsworth locality) in the primary care setting (wherever the patient usually received their care), where further assessment and treatment recommendations could take place. For those patients not responding to recommended changes of treatment, or who were identified as having more chronic or complex ulceration and when further specialist medical or surgical assessment or treatment was required, referral on to the specialist leg ulcer clinic or a joint dermatology/vascular clinic could be arranged by the community leg ulcer team. Other external and internal referrals were also made to the clinic. The majority of external referrals came from surrounding areas where there was no community-based leg ulcer specialist nurse.

Specialist clinics

The specialist leg ulcer clinic is a nurse-led clinic operating within a dermatology department. Led by a nurse consultant and staffed by the community leg ulcer team with access to a consultant dermatologist, it provides the facility for further specialist leg ulcer assessment and treatment of complex multi-factorial ulcers. Many patients present to this clinic with issues related to chronic pain and oedema, or rarer ulcer aetiologies due to inflammatory and autoimmune disorders and malignancy.

Patients with arterial or venous complications would previously have been referred to the joint dermatology/vascular clinic. This clinic was run within the vascular department and operated by the consultant dermatologist, a vascular surgeon and the community specialist and support nurses.

Communication between acute and primary care

Any patients referred to either of these clinics were given a hand-written letter to take home for their usual carers, ensuring rapid communication relating to suggested changes to treatment and plans for further assessment and intervention. The community specialist and support nurses followed up patients either within the clinics or in the community.

Benefits offered by the model

This means of service provision offered numerous benefits, including:

- Opportunities to monitor standards of care across a trust. In addition, as the specialist leg ulcer clinic acted as a tertiary centre, the standards in surrounding areas could also be gauged. Ensured that the treatment the practitioners were providing was in accordance with the best available evidence.
- Provided opportunities for one-to-one teaching sessions and an occasion for staff to put prior learning into practice.
- The clinic setting offered a rich learning experience for a range of participants from trainee doctors and nurses, post-graduate students, researchers and foreign visitors.
- Ensured appropriate referrals were taking place.
- The combination of primary and acute care staff ensured the most practical and appropriate treatment decisions were made.

- Continuity of care between the acute and primary care settings was maintained.
- Acted as a support system for patients and their carers.
- Supplied the community leg ulcer team nurses with expert clinical supervision.

Evaluation of the Wandsworth model and its impact on prevalence

A project to assess the impact of the leg ulcer service on prevalence levels within the Wandsworth locality was undertaken by Moffatt et al. (2004a).

Over a four-week period patients with leg ulceration were identified from relevant services and healthcare professionals throughout the area. The areas targeted included:

- All district and practice nurses
- All GPs
- Designated hospital wards and departments (medical, surgical, care of the elderly, dermatology, podiatry and vascular)
- Nursing homes
- Day care centres
- Other specialist services

Those patients identified were then interviewed and assessed to gather demographic data and information regarding their physical and psychological status. Ulcer aetiologies were diagnosed by clinical and non-invasive vascular (arterial and venous) assessments.

The project results differed considerably from studies undertaken in the 1980s when leg ulcer care was provided in a less standardised fashion and compression therapy rarely used (Table 1.1 contains a breakdown of the findings). Estimates of the prevalence of leg ulceration in the UK at the time were quoted around 1.48/1000 (Callum et al., 1985) and 1.79/1000 (Cornwall et al., 1986). However, the prevalence rates in Wandsworth were found to be less than one-third of previous studies at 0.45/1000 (Moffatt et al., 2004a).

The Wandsworth population presented with a range of aetiologies. However, there were two predominant groups: those identified with uncomplicated venous disease (43%) and those

Table 1.1 Findings of prevalence study to assess the impact of the Wandsworth leg ulcer service.

Demographics	Ulcer history
• 113 people identified	• 25 patients (22%) had bilateral ulceration
• 72 (64%) were female	• 55% had had their ulcer for over 1 year, 34% over 18 months (the range was 1 month to 12 years)
• Age ranged from 31 to 94 years (mean age 75)	
• Only six (5%) patients were receiving care in a hospital or residential setting	• Ulcer size ranged from $0.5\,cm^2$ to $171\,cm^2$ (mean size $4\,cm^2$)
• Over 70% had been previously referred for further specialist advice	• Over 60% of patients had had at least two episodes of ulceration
• 95 (84%) were classified as White British, 17 (15%) Black and 1 Asian	• Ages for the first episode of ulceration ranged from 10 to 94 years (mean age 67 years)

with more complex multi-factorial ulceration (35%). For those patients with multi-factorial ulceration, venous disease was still largely present as a major contributing factor, but it was complicated by other underlying conditions such as peripheral arterial disease, diabetes, lymphoedema and rheumatoid arthritis. Such a significant proportion of patients being identified with multi-factorial ulceration may relate to improvements in assessment compared to previous studies. However, it may also be a reflection of the increasing age of the patient group and improvements in the care and management of other chronic diseases.

Prior to setting up the leg ulcer service, prevalence levels in Wandsworth had been well above the national average, as evidenced by a previous audit. Results of the project demonstrated the effectiveness of the model in significantly reducing prevalence. While there may be many achievements a service could aim to meet, a general reduction in the number of people with active ulceration is incredibly important in terms of both human and financial costs. The study also helped to identify the increasing challenges that nurses and leg ulcer teams are required to meet in order to effectively manage patients with numerous complex aetiologies.

DEVELOPMENT OF THE LEG ULCER SERVICE

Several changes within the locality and the leg ulcer team have taken place since the prevalence study was undertaken. These include the:

- Trust going through several organisational and boundary transformations.
- Community-based leg ulcer team now consists of two specialist nurses, but no support nurse.
- Cessation of the community leg ulcer clinics with greater provision of leg ulcer care by practice nurses.
- Merging of the hospital-based leg ulcer clinics.

These changes, particularly in the primary care setting, had a significant impact on keeping the service from more proactively working to keep prevalence levels low; it left the team with some significant challenges, including:

- An increased area/population but reduced team size.
- A greater demand for training and need for equipment (e.g. hand-held Dopplers) for practice nurses.
- The need to update and increase the distribution of written guidelines.
- Less direct access to a vascular team.

The combination of leg ulcer care moving away from community clinics to more care from practice nurses, and the merger of Wandsworth PCT with one of its neighbouring boroughs where there was no similar leg ulcer service up and running, put the leg ulcer team under considerable strain in terms of maintaining and ensuring that all patients received the same level of care as most were receiving in the Wandsworth area. While one-to-one visits has always been an important means of sharing best practice, the team were now dealing with much greater numbers of practitioners and patients. Therefore, it was far more economical to significantly increase the provision of group training.

PROVISION OF LEG ULCER TRAINING

The training provided for the Trust by the community leg ulcer nurses remains in a continual state of transformation and metamorphosis, based on evaluations by attendees, observations in practice and developments in leg ulcer care. The changes are not always necessarily big ones, but subtle improvements are continually made to ensure that attendees go away with a good understanding of the fundamentals of assessment and management.

A regular comment made during most evaluations of leg ulcer courses was, and still is, 'It needs to be longer'. Prior to the epidemiology study the training sessions were made up of three half-day sessions, this progressed to two full days and is now three full days, with attendees saying it could be longer still.

Using a combination of both theory and practical sessions, the predominant angle on successful leg ulcer management is all about getting the assessment right, so this consumes nearly 50% of the course content (including Doppler assessment). Compression therapy is the other major topic, followed by other related issues such as infection, pain management and dressing choice. Case studies are employed to help apply learning to practice and tie assessment and management issues together. It is true the training could be longer, but getting such a substantial amount of time off work is difficult for many. However, several universities offer extended modules for those who are really interested in learning more about wound management and leg ulcers. More importantly, it is not expected that any learning should end just because a course is completed. Joint visits with the community and primary care nurses ensure that learning can continue out in the field.

In response to course evaluations, revision sessions on Doppler ultrasound, compression therapy and wound bed preparation were introduced. These sessions were deliberately kept very short 'bite size' in the hopes of attracting those practitioners who feel they have already 'done' leg ulcers and really do just need an update. Considering the number of requests for update sessions, attendance was very variable. So changes were made to improve the uptake of this training opportunity – selling it as a one-day event opposed to drop-in sessions, as nurses comment that it is easier to take a full day away for study rather than just a few hours, possibly because patient work can be somewhat unpredictable.

ADDITIONAL CHANGES TO PRACTICE

While training has been one of the key elements in improving standards across the trust, the community leg ulcer team has striven to improve efficiency and meet challenges through:

- **The introduction of a more formalised referral process to the specialist team.** Referrals must now be put in writing, detailing the patient's past medical history and results of their initial assessment, treatments in use and why the patient is being referred. This process has helped with screening and prioritising referrals, and enables more initial advice to be given over the phone.
- **Improved links with a vascular nurse consultant.** Direct liaison with the vascular nurse means that referrals to the vascular department can be streamlined to the appropriate clinics and for investigations, within appropriate time frames, for both venous and arterial leg ulcer related problems and with equal importance.
- **Improvements to the leg ulcer assessment documentation format.** Creating a user-friendly assessment tool that makes diagnosis easier and ensures a high standard of record keeping, which practitioners will be more inclined to use, will ensure standardisation of treatment wherever a patient seeks treatment across the trust. While a paper-tool is not the ideal for practice nurses, they have been advised to (at the very least) use the tool as a prompt or to complete it in full and scan it into their clients' electronic files.
- **Audits.** An audit was undertaken to assess the availability of hand-held Dopplers and staff trained to use them to measure the ankle brachial pressure index in GP surgeries. This enabled the team to secure funding to purchase the necessary equipment on the grounds of equality of service provision for patients. Once practice nurses confirmed their previous training or attended an in-house training session provided by the leg ulcer team, Dopplers were made available to all GP surgeries.

REFLECTIONS ON CURRENT PRACTICE

The work of the leg ulcer team continues to be an ongoing and evolving process, since there is always room for improvement. Monitoring standards across the Trust in order to meet the changing needs of both patients and staff takes place through:

- Joint visits
- Evaluation of referrals
- Formal audit

Joint visits with patients and their nurses remain one of the major functions of the day-to-day running of the service. The benefits of such visits are indispensable, especially in terms of sharing information and giving practitioners a real opportunity to put learning into practice; in addition, they often prove to be very enlightening. However, the amount of time such work consumes, in particular the additional travelling time, requires regular review to optimise the impact of the service.

The number of referrals, where they do or do not come from and the information contained within them, also provides valuable insights. Certainly, use of the service is somewhat sporadic across the Trust, suggesting potential areas of inequality for some patients. Of course, there may be many reasons for this, including:

- Individual practitioners may feel more confident regarding their knowledge of leg ulcer assessment and management than others.
- Practice nurses on temporary placements or locum GPs may be unaware of the service.
- Differences in caseloads.

There have been many changes to the service: in particular, significantly increased in-house training opportunities and ongoing efforts to continually raise the profile of the leg ulcer team. Despite this, it was still apparent that inconsistencies in practice were causing some concern in regards to patient care and the standard of nursing practice, and this was confirmed with a more formal audit.

Some examples of the issues arising

- Poor referrals demonstrating a lack of awareness in identifying the underlying aetiology: 'I have tried every dressing possible but the wound will still not heal.'
- Treatment such as compression bandaging in use for several months where there is no identified venous disease and the ulcers are deteriorating. Unfortunately, the assumption still exists that a good ABPI reading means the ulcer is venous.

Continued

- Rarer ulcer types are not being identified and referred on to appropriate medical/surgical teams. Nurses get caught up worrying about finding time to do the dressing without investing time in assessment or thinking about how to involve another practitioner in the process.
- High compression is still being instigated without formal assessment.

Addressing the issues

While written guidelines remained available to most DN teams within the Trust they were in need of updating as well as being further distributed and implemented. This required a critical review of the literature, including current recommendations based on the National Leg Ulcer Guidelines in addition to new international guidance on compression therapy (Marston & Vowden, 2003) and wound bed preparation (Moffatt et al., 2004b) plus findings from the epidemiology study (Moffatt et al., 2004a). It was important to ensure that all this information was considered in developing any new local guidelines. Work on updating the local guidelines had begun but was proving a difficult process and was resulting in an even lengthier document than the original.

Community nurses are involved with many patients who have many different social and health related problems, and keeping up to date in terms of best practice is rarely an easy task. To ensure that the majority of patients received the best possible care it was important to:

- Simplify the evidence
- Keep it relevant to the local population
- Make it easier to access
- Ensure it was easy to follow
- Make it available to all

THE NEW CARE PATHWAY

In 2003 the Leg Ulcer International Advisory Board developed a treatment pathway (Marston & Vowden, 2003) for decision-making in compression therapy and for the appropriate referral of patients. Its beauty is in its simplicity and yet it is detailed in its treatment options, particularly in regards to mixed disease and the importance of oedema control.

These qualities were key to Wandsworth's requirements, so permission was sought and the Leg Ulcer Advisory Board's recommended pathway was used to form the basis of the new Wandsworth tPCT leg ulcer pathway.

By moving away from the previous 90-page guideline to using a pathway format, the aim was to remind practitioners that certain steps need to be taken in a logical order when managing a patient with a leg ulcer. While it seems common sense to make a diagnosis prior to starting treatment, diagnosis itself is not a usual part of nursing practice. Nurses may be used to performing initial assessments, but it requires that little extra in terms of skill and knowledge to draw conclusions when it comes to diagnosing ulcer aetiology.

The following chapters look at the development of the pathway, how it was introduced and used in practice, who was consulted and what other changes will be needed in the future to ensure its success.

The remainder of the book will provide the reader with the theory that underpins the pathway, and will allow the nurse to consider how to use this approach in his/her own work environment. The book breaks down the phases of the pathway and looks in more detail at the processes involved, such as:

- Which patients, and when, to enter into the pathway.
- Key considerations of clinical assessment, with special attention to the psychosocial dimensions related to leg ulceration.
- Clinical management, such as wound bed preparation and compression therapy, and the importance of involving the multidisciplinary team.
- Finally looking at evaluating outcomes for both the patient and a service.

It will become apparent to the reader that a cohesive partnership between primary and secondary care is a vital necessity when trying to achieve successful outcomes. In order for the pathway to be adopted into other regions, primary and secondary care trusts will need to be willing to work together for the greater benefit of the patient.

REFERENCES

Bosanquet, N., Franks, P., Moffatt, C., Connolly, M., Oldroyd, M., Brown, P., Greenhalgh, R. & McCollum, C. (1993–94) Community leg ulcer clinics: cost effectiveness. *Health Trends* **25**(4): 146–148.

Callum, M.J., Ruckley, C.V., Harper, D.R. & Dale, J.J. (1985) Chronic ulceration of the leg: extent of the problem and provision of care. *British Medical Journal* **290**: 1855–1856.

Callum, M.J., Harper, D.R., Dale, J.J. & Ruckley, C.V. (1987) Chronic ulcer of the leg: clinical history. *British Medical Journal* **294**: 1389–1391.

Carr, L., Phillips, Z. & Posnett, J. (1999) Comparative cost-effectiveness of four-layer bandaging in the treatment of venous leg ulceration. *Journal of Wound Care* **8**(5): 243–248.

Census (2001) *Wandsworth Fact Sheet: Wandsworth Borough*. Available at http://www.wandsworth.gov.uk/nr/wandsworth/asp/census/cenWandsworth.pdf

Cornwall, J.V., Dore, C.J. & Lewis, J.D. (1986) Leg ulcers: epidemiology and aetiology. *British Journal of Surgery* **73**: 693–696.

Fletcher, A., Cullum, N. & Sheldon, T.A. (1997) Systematic review of compression treatment for venous leg ulcers. *British Medical Journal* **315**: 576–580.

Marston, W. & Vowden, K. (2003) Compression Therapy: A Guide to Safe Practice. In: *EWMA Position Document: Understanding Compression Therapy*. London, Medical Education Partnership Ltd.

Moffatt, C.J., Franks, P.J., Oldroyd, M., Bosanquet, N., Brown, P., Greenhalgh, R.M. & McCollum, C.N. (1992) Community leg ulcer clinics and impact on ulcer healing. *British Medical Journal* **305**: 1389–1392.

Moffatt, C.J., Franks, P.J., Doherty, D.C., Martin, R., Blewett, R. & Ross, F. (2004a) Prevalence of leg ulceration in a London population. *Quarterly Journal of Medicine* **97**: 431–437.

Moffatt, C., Morison, M.J. & Pina, E. (2004b) Wound bed preparation for venous ulcers. In: *European Wound Management Association. Position Document: Wound Bed Preparation in Practice*. London, Medical Education Partnership Ltd.

RCN Institute (1998) *Clinical Practice Guidelines. The Management of Patients with Venous Leg Ulcers*. London, Royal College of Nursing.

Schofield, J., Flanagan, M., Fletcher, J., Rotchell, L. & Thomas, S. (2000) The provision of leg ulcer services by practice nurses. *Nursing Standard* **14**(26): 54–60.

SIGN (1998) *The Care of Patients with Chronic Leg Ulcer*. Edinburgh, Scottish Intercollegiate Guidelines Network, SIGN Publication No. 26.

A Leg Ulcer Care Pathway

2

LEARNING OBJECTIVES

Nurses involved in leg ulcer management should be able to demonstrate:

❏ An understanding of the development of the International Leg Ulcer Advisory Board's treatment pathway and its application to practice.

❏ The ability to describe the factors that influence changing practice.

❏ An understanding of the principles and process of change management used to introduce the international pathway into the Wandsworth service.

❏ An understanding of how the different phases of the Wandsworth pathway assist the patients' journey through the service.

INTRODUCTION

An integrated care pathway (ICP) has been defined as (Middleton & Roberts, 2000a, pp. 3–4):

> 'an outline or plan of anticipated clinical practice for a group of patients (client group) with a particular set of diagnosis or set of symptoms [whose aim is to] ensure evidence-based care is delivered to the patient by the right individual, at the right time'

An ICP tends to require multi-disciplinary working and a single record of care, and is particularly well suited to patients undergoing routine episodes of care such as hip replacement.

The use of care pathways for more complex chronic conditions presents a greater challenge. Patients do not necessarily fit nicely into a 'category', and care may need to vary considerably according to their individual needs and circumstances. The traditional format of integrated care pathways could therefore be seen to be too 'rigid' for this patient group. Nonetheless, there remains the need to ensure that patients with chronic leg ulceration can expect to receive evidence-based care by the right individual at the right time, and care pathways that are sufficiently adaptable provide a useful tool by which to achieve this aim.

This chapter looks at the authors' own experience of developing a leg ulcer care pathway for their area of care, and some of the challenges and achievements involved. Underpinning the pathway is recognition of the need to help the practitioner think logically and to base care on a thorough and well thought through assessment. The remainder of the book draws strongly from the pathway's framework.

THE INTERNATIONAL LEG ULCER ADVISORY BOARD'S TREATMENT PATHWAY

The production of a local leg ulcer pathway for Wandsworth PCT was aided enormously by the fact that, in 2002, the International Leg Ulcer Advisory Board developed a recommended treatment pathway (Stacey et al., 2002). This pathway has since been incorporated into the European Wound Management Association's suite of Position Documents (Marston & Vowden, 2003) (Fig. 2.1).

For the first time this pathway provides a clear consensus on the fundamental principles that should underpin a leg ulcer patient's journey. Its beauty lies in its successful combination of comprehensive depth with simple clarity. It provides a clear linear picture of what the patient journey should look like according to best available evidence, while also recognising the complexity of leg ulceration, guiding the practitioner along different paths according to the results of their assessment, and leaving room for individualised treatment options where indicated. It is particularly helpful in the area of mixed arterial and venous ulcers, providing explicit guidance on using reduced levels of compression – something that has not previously been addressed in national guidelines for leg ulcer care.

TRANSFERRING THE INTERNATIONAL LEG ULCER ADVISORY BOARD'S PATHWAY INTO PRACTICE – FIRST STEPS

Transferring an international pathway – or indeed any guideline – into local practice requires a concerted effort, and change

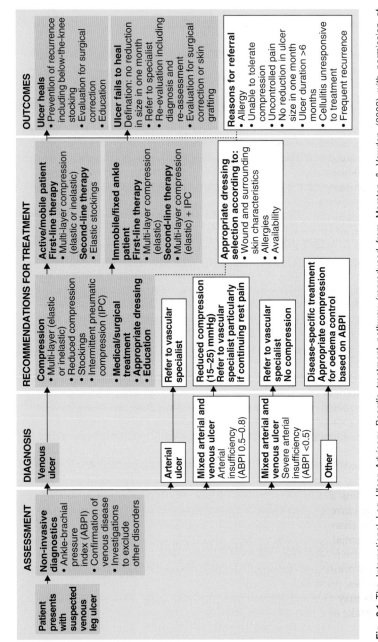

Fig. 2.1 The International Leg Ulcer Advisory Board's treatment pathway (reproduced from Marston & Vowden (2003) with permission of MEP/EWMA).

ASSESSMENT

Patient presents with suspected venous leg ulcer

Non-invasive diagnostics
• Ankle-brachial pressure index (ABPI)
• Confirmation of venous disease
• Investigations to exclude other disorders

DIAGNOSIS

Venous ulcer

Arterial ulcer

Mixed arterial and venous ulcer
Arterial insufficiency (ABPI 0.5–0.8)

Mixed arterial and venous ulcer
Severe arterial insufficiency (ABPI <0.5)

Other

RECOMMENDATIONS FOR TREATMENT

Compression
• Multi-layer (elastic or inelastic)
• Reduced compression
• Stockings
• Intermittent pneumatic compression (IPC)

• Medical/surgical treatment
• Appropriate dressing
• Education

Refer to vascular specialist

Reduced compression (15–25) mmHg)
Refer to vascular specialist particularly if continuing rest pain

Refer to vascular specialist
No compression

Disease-specific treatment
Appropriate compression for oedema control based on ABPI

Active/mobile patient
First-line therapy
• Multi-layer compression (elastic or inelastic)
Second-line therapy
• Elastic stockings

Immobile/fixed ankle patient
First-line therapy
• Multi-layer compression (elastic)
Second-line therapy
• Multi-layer compression (elastic) + IPC

Appropriate dressing selection according to:
• Wound and surrounding skin characteristics
• Allergies
• Availability

OUTCOMES

Ulcer heals
• Prevention of recurrence including below-the-knee stocking
• Evaluation for surgical correction
• Education

Ulcer fails to heal
Defination: no reduction in size in one month
• Refer to specialist
• Re-evaluation including diagnosis and re-assessment
• Evaluation for surgical correction or skin grafting

Reasons for referral
• Allergy
• Unable to tolerate compression
• Uncontrolled pain
• No reduction in ulcer size in one month
• Ulcer duration >6 months
• Cellulitis unresponsive to treatment
• Frequent recurrence

is unlikely to occur unless people with the necessary skills and knowledge take the lead in applying a multi-faceted strategy of dissemination and implementation (NHS Centre for Reviews and Dissemination, 1999). Simply sending out information rarely results in widespread uptake and changes in practice (Lomas, 1991). This can be due to a variety of reasons, but may simply be because healthcare practitioners are constantly bombarded with new information, and trying to keep abreast of change can feel like an insurmountable challenge. Healthcare organisations have a duty towards their healthcare professionals to provide routine mechanisms, structures and personnel to facilitate the uptake of change in practice. A specialist nurse or team of specialists is well placed to take on this role. They not only possess the necessary knowledge and skills, but also have a unique insight into the situation and potential barriers to change: they are a 'familiar face', and are likely to have the time and resources required.

The first step is often to simply raise awareness. In Wandsworth PCT, the leg ulcer team wrote to all district nursing teams and practice nurses, advising them of the pathway and how to access it successfully from the internet. In addition, the leg ulcer training courses were redesigned to directly reflect the pathway's recommendations. However, dissemination activities that simply raise awareness are not sufficient on their own, and must not be misinterpreted as being the same as implementation strategies that bring about change in behaviour (NHS Centre for Reviews and Dissemination, 1999).

Situational analysis

Before attempting to implement any major change, the person leading the change must ensure that he or she really understands the current situation. A situational or diagnostic analysis allows the change agent to gather information on the status quo and potential factors likely to influence the proposed change (NHS Centre for Reviews and Dissemination, 1999). These include ways of working, habits, deeply held values and beliefs, organisational issues, pressures of time and resources that healthcare professionals may face and key people who may either help or hinder the uptake of change.

Auditing a service is one means of capturing the information required, though more personal insights about team dynamics and key leaders gained through experience and observation significantly enhance the understanding and interpretation of audit results. The Wandsworth PCT's leg ulcer model of care, focusing as it does on one-to-one visits, offers an excellent opportunity for the leg ulcer team to be familiar with what happens in practice. Years of experience working on a one-to-one basis with district nursing teams and practice nurses have provided a unique insight into current standards of and variations in practice, practical challenges faced by the teams, common misunderstandings and particular areas of theory/practice gaps.

A formal audit was also conducted to confirm, formalise and quantify the leg ulcer team's perception of the current situation. This was carried out with the help of the clinical governance department, who were able to provide expertise in how to construct the audit tool and synthesise the data. It was important not to give the impression that the audit was a 'policing' exercise by the leg ulcer team – therefore keeping the results anonymous and ensuring that it was administered by the clinical governance department was essential. Each nursing team was asked to complete one audit for every patient on their caseload who had a break on their leg that had been present for four weeks or more.

Findings

The following key themes emerged from the audit and clinical observations:

- The local guidelines required updating, were not available to practice nurses, and were no longer available to all nursing teams within the PCT due to the change of geographical boundaries. More importantly, they were rarely consulted by those teams with access to them, due to their size (a large A4 file) and their location (stored on a shelf in the office), rather than being accessible when most required – in the clinical environment.
- The Trust's leg ulcer assessment tool was rarely used by district nursing teams as it was not part of the colour-coded, patient-held record. It was almost never used by practice nurses, particularly those who used computer-based records.

- There remained a tendency to base diagnosis largely on the ABPI result. Where the ABPI was above 0.8, ulcers were often assumed to be venous, with no documented evidence of venous disease. This was alarming, particularly given the previous prevalence study's finding of a large number of unusual or complex ulcer aetiologies within the Wandsworth area (Moffatt et al., 2004).
- There was widespread variation between practitioners in terms of how quickly they referred to the leg ulcer team for help with complex or unhealing ulcers, ranging from one week to over a year.

From these findings the following conclusions were drawn in relation to how the care pathway should be integrated into practice:

- It needed to be in a format that was accessible to healthcare professionals at the point of need, i.e. when with the patient.
- It needed to reflect the local patient profile, with clear guidance on assessing and managing multi-factorial or complex ulceration.
- It needed to set out clear and standardised referral pathways, reflecting local resources and emphasising the importance of including the multi-disciplinary team in diagnosis and care.
- It needed to set out definite but realistic time frames for diagnosis, referral and evaluation of care.
- It needed to be incorporated into the district nursing colour-coded, patient-held record, and to be available in a format that practice nurses could keep as a computer-held record.
- It needed to guide the practitioner through a logical process of diagnosis, dispelling any myths that diagnosis could be based on ABPI alone or that ulcers could be treated without seeking a firm diagnosis.

DEVELOPMENT OF A LOCAL PATHWAY IN WANDSWORTH

The local leg ulcer care pathway is based directly in the International Leg Ulcer Advisory Board's treatment pathway, but was adapted to meet the findings of the situational analysis. Specifically, it included more detail, particularly on multi-factorial ulcers, with distinct time frames for referral and evaluation.

Summary card

Opinion was sought from district and practice nurses on the pre-ferred format in which to present the condensed pathway. Options included a web-based document that would be instantly accessible to all practitioners and easy to update. However, at the time the Trust's IT systems were unable to support this format, and – more importantly – it did not overcome the problem of the pathway needing to be accessible in the patient's own home or the clinic room.

It was therefore decided to condense the pathway onto a laminated A5 card that would fit into the front of each district nurse's work diary. For practice nurses, the card was printed in an A4 format to be displayed on the wall. A bandaging guide, dressings guide, hosiery guide, TIME assessment tool (Falanga, 2004) and Doppler ABPI calculation guide were included on the back of the card, as well as contact details for the leg ulcer team (Fig. 2.2).

Patient record

In addition to the laminated summary card, a fuller version of the pathway was reproduced for incorporation into the patient record. This comprised a leg ulcer assessment tool and semi-pre-printed care plan printed on the district nursing colour-coded, patient-held documentation and in a format capable of being scanned in as a computer record by practice nurses (Fig. 2.3).

The semi-pre-printed care plan is designed to ensure all patients receive a plan of care that is in accordance with best practice, as well as allowing sufficient room for individualised care. As is essential to any care pathway documentation, it is laid out sequen-tially, and includes clear time frames and check-points for evalu-ation of progress along the patient journey (Middleton & Roberts, 2000b). It is also designed to save the practitioner time – something some practitioners may disagree with since it may take longer to complete than simply writing 'freehand' on a blank care plan. However, any increase in time required is likely to be temporary, and it is important to remember that:

- It takes time to become familiar with any new system (Hotchkiss, 2000).

- Some staff whose previous standard of documentation was inadequate may be forced to write more, but any properly designed documentation will involve no more writing for staff whose documentation standards were already satisfactory (Hotchkiss, 2000).
- Accurately documented assessment and care planning are likely to result in faster, more accurate diagnosis, timely referral and – in the long run – faster time to healing.

The pathway step-by-step

The pathway is divided into four stages, each designed to guide practitioners logically and methodically through best practice in assessment, management and evaluation of care.

Phase 0

The first phase sets out clear criteria for entry of patients into the pathway. All patients presenting with a wound on the lower leg should be screened and entered if the wound:

- Has been present for 4 weeks or more. A leg ulcer is simply a wound on the lower leg that fails to heal within the expected time frame (Moffatt et al., 2004). It is a symptom of an underlying disorder that is preventing normal 'acute' healing from taking place. Unless diagnosed and treated, healing is unlikely to occur. Normal healing should occur within a 4–6-week period; since it may take the practitioner more than one appointment to complete a full assessment, a 4-week period was chosen as the time-frame in which to begin assessment.
- Is a new trauma or surgical wound and the patient has known or obvious venous or arterial disease of the affected leg. There is no point in waiting 4 weeks to see if these wounds heal, since the presence of venous or arterial disease will almost certainly delay or prevent healing. Prompt investigation and treatment will enhance the chance and speed of healing, and reduce the risk of complications, pain and ineffective care.
- Appeared spontaneously. Practitioners should be suspicious of any wound on the lower leg that appears spontaneously as it may represent any one of a number of causes, including venous or arterial disease, a skin cancer, a vasculitis, pyoderma gangrenosum, or any one of the more unusual ulcer aetiologies.

(a)

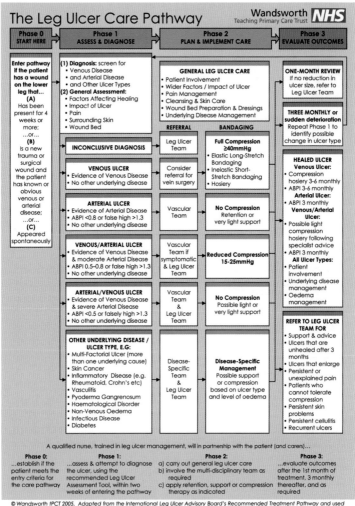

Fig. 2.2 The leg ulcer care pathway card used at Wandsworth tPCT. (a) Front, (b) back (reproduced with permission of Wandsworth Teaching PCT).

(b)

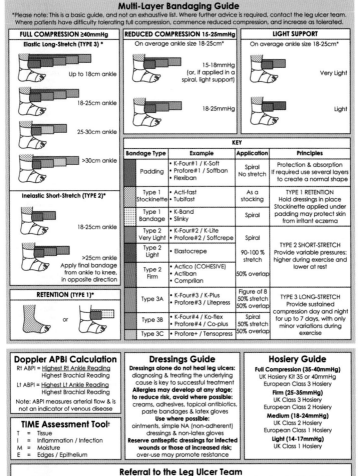

Multi-Layer Bandaging Guide
*Please note: This is a basic guide, and not an exhaustive list. Where further advice is required, contact the leg ulcer team. Where patients have difficulty tolerating full compression, commence reduced compression, and increase as tolerated.

FULL COMPRESSION ≥40mmHg	REDUCED COMPRESSION 15-25mmHg	LIGHT SUPPORT

Elastic Long-Stretch (TYPE 3) *
- Up to 18cm ankle
- 18-25cm ankle
- 25-30cm ankle
- >30cm ankle

On average ankle size 18-25cm*
- 15-18mmHg (or, if applied in a spiral, light support)
- 18-25mmHg

On average ankle size 18-25cm*
- Very Light
- Light

Inelastic Short-Stretch (TYPE 2)*
- 18-25cm ankle
- >25cm ankle
Apply final bandage from ankle to knee, in opposite direction

RETENTION (TYPE 1)*
or

KEY

Bandage Type	Example	Application	Principles
Padding	• K-Four#1 / K-Soft • Profore#1 / Soffban • Flexiban	Spiral No stretch	Protection & absorption If required use several layers to create a normal shape
Type 1 Stockinette	• Acti-fast • Tubifast	As a stocking	TYPE 1 RETENTION Hold dressings in place Stockinette applied under padding may protect skin from irritant eczema
Type 1 Bandage	• K-Band • Slinky	Spiral	
Type 2 Very Light	• K-Four#2 / K-Lite • Profore#2 / Softcrepe	Spiral	TYPE 2 SHORT-STRETCH Provide variable pressures: higher during exercise and lower at rest
Type 2 Light	• Elastocrepe	90-100 % stretch	
Type 2 Firm	• Actico (COHESIVE) • Actiban • Comprilan	50% overlap	
Type 3A	• K-Four#3 / K-Plus • Profore#3 / Litepress	Figure of 8 50% stretch 50% overlap	TYPE 3 LONG-STRETCH Provide sustained compression day and night for up to 7 days, with only minor variations during exercise
Type 3B	• K-Four#4 / Ko-flex • Profore#4 / Co-plus	Spiral 50% stretch 50% overlap	
Type 3C	• Profore+ / Tensopress	50% overlap	

Doppler APBI Calculation

Rt ABPI = Highest Rt Ankle Reading / Highest Brachial Reading

Lt ABPI = Highest Lt Ankle Reading / Highest Brachial Reading

Note: ABPI measures arterial flow & is not an indicator of venous disease

TIME Assessment Tool†

T = Tissue
I = Inflammation / Infection
M = Moisture
E = Edges / Epithelium

Dressings Guide
Dressings alone do not heal leg ulcers: diagnosing & treating the underlying cause is key to successful treatment
Allergies may develop at any stage; to reduce risk, avoid where possible: creams, adhesives, topical antibiotics, paste bandages & latex gloves
Use where possible: ointments, simple NA (non-adherent) dressings & non-latex gloves
Reserve antiseptic dressings for infected wounds or those at increased risk; over-use may promote resistance

Hosiery Guide
Full Compression (35-40mmHg)
UK Hosiery Kit 35 or 40mmHg
European Class 3 Hosiery
Firm (25-35mmHg)
UK Class 3 Hosiery
European Class 2 Hosiery
Medium (18-24mmHg)
UK Class 2 Hosiery
European Class 1 Hosiery
Light (14-17mmHg)
UK Class 1 Hosiery

Referral to the Leg Ulcer Team
For Telephone Advice, call 020 8812 4050. For an appointment, fax a Leg Ulcer Referral Form to 020 8812 4051

†From V. Falanga 'Wound bed preparation: science applied to practice.' In: Wound Bed Preparation in Practice. EWMA Position Document. London MEP Ltd, 2004, 2-5, and used with kind permission from the publishers.

Fig. 2.2 *Continued.*

LEG ULCER ASSESSMENT TOOL AND CARE PLAN

SURNAME: **Forename:**   **D.O.B:**

PHASE 0. START HERE	Date:	Sign:

_____ (name) has a wound on _____ (location) that:

☐ has been present for 4 weeks or more. Duration:

☐ is a new trauma/surgical wound, and the patient has known/obvious
   venous or arterial disease of the same leg

☐ appeared spontaneously

PHASE 1. ASSESS & DIAGNOSE Within the first 3 weeks	Date:	Sign:

STEP 1. VENOUS ASSESSMENT

A. RISK FACTORS FOR VENOUS DISEASE

Family History:	Past Medical History:	Personal Factors:
☐ Varicose veins	☐ Vein trauma*	☐ Standing/sitting occupation
☐ Venous leg ulcer	☐ High risk of DVT**	☐ Pregnancy(s)
	☐ Limited ankle function	☐ Tall
	☐ Chronic constipation	
	☐ Overweight	

* E.G. DVT, leg trauma/surgery, IV drug use, phlebitis **E.G. major surgery, long distance travel, clotting disorder, prolonged immobility

B. EVIDENCE OF VENOUS DISEASE

Venous History:	Venous Skin Changes:	Venous Pain:
R☐ L☐ DVT	R☐ L☐ Varicose veins	R☐ L☐ Tired heavy ache
R☐ L☐ Thrombophlebitis	R☐ L☐ Ankle flare	R☐ L☐ Venous rush pain
R☐ L☐ Sclerotherapy	R☐ L☐ Atrophie blanche	R☐ L☐ Neuropathic
R☐ L☐ Vein surgery	R☐ L☐ Haemosiderin staining	atrophie blanche
	R☐ L☐ Venous oedema	pain
	R☐ L☐ Varicose eczema	
	R☐ L☐ Lipodermatosclerosis	

C. CONCLUSION

R☐ L☐ Severe venous disease   R☐ L☐ Mild venous disease
R☐ L☐ No venous disease   R☐ L☐ Inconclusive diagnosis

STEP 2. PERIPHERAL ARTERIAL DISEASE (PAD) ASSESSMENT

A. RISK FACTORS FOR PAD

Family History:	Past Medical Hostory:	Personal Factors:
☐ Arterial leg ulcer	☐ Diabetes	☐ Smoker (/day)
☐ Arterial disease	☐ Hypercholesterolaemia	☐ Ex-smoker (/day)
(hypertension/stroke	☐ Hypertension	☐ Lack of exercise
/angina/MI)	☐ Angina/MI	
	☐ Cardiac bypass/angioplasty	
	☐ Stroke/TIA	

⟶

Fig. 2.3 Wandsworth tPCT leg ulcer care pathway documentation (reproduced with permission of Wandsworth Teaching PCT).

B. EVIDENCE OF PAD

Peripheral Arterial History:	**Ischaemic Tissue Changes:**
R☐ L☐ Bypass/angioplasty	R☐ L☐ Cool limb
R☐ L☐ Ischaemic related amputation	R☐ L☐ Pale limb on elevation
	R☐ L☐ Dependent rubor
	R☐ L☐ Sluggish capillary refill
Arterial Pain:	R☐ L☐ Numbness/tingling
R☐ L☐ Intermittent claudication	R☐ L☐ Hair loss
R☐ L☐ Ischaemic night pain	R☐ L☐ Trophic skin/nails
R☐ L☐ Ischaemic rest pain	R☐ L☐ Muscle wastage

C. DOPPLER ABPI (OR TOE PRESSURE)

	Right	Mono/Bi/ Tri-Phasic	Left	Mono/Bi/ Tri-Phasic
Brachial:	_____		_____	
Dorsalis pedis/Anterior tibial:	_____	_____	_____	_____
Posterior tibial/Peroneal:	_____	_____	_____	_____
ABPI:	_____		_____	
Toe:	_____		_____	
TBPI:	_____		_____	

D. CONCLUSION

R☐ L☐ Severe PAD	R☐ L☐ Mild PAD
R☐ L☐ No PAD	R☐ L☐ Inconclusive diagnosis

STEP 3. ASSESSMENT FOR OTHER POSSIBLE ULCER TYPE

A. UNDERLYING CONDITIONS WHICH MAY CAUSE OR CONTRIBUTE TO LEG ULCERATION

☐ Inflammatory disease†   ☐ Haematological disease   ☐ Non-venous oedema
☐ Vasculitis   ☐ Skin cancer   ☐ Recurrent trauma
☐ Pyoderma gangrenosum   ☐ Diabetes   ☐ Other
☐ Raynaud's disease   ☐ Infectious disease‡

†e.g. Rheumatoid arthritis, systemic lupus erythematosus, Crohn's disease, ulcerative colitis, scleroderma, etc. ‡e.g. TB, tropical infection, etc.
Further details:

B. UNUSUAL ULCER APPEARANCE/LOCATION

STEP 4. GENERAL ASSESSMENT

A. WIDER FACTORS AFFECTING HEALING

Severe pain / sleeping with legs dependent / reduced mobility / systemic steroid therapy / chemotherapy / social isolation / poor nutrition / poor general health / smoking / alcohol use / depression / ulcer present for > 6 months / ulcer > 10cm^2 / other
Details:

B. IMPACT OF ULCER ON DAILY ACTIVITIES

Details/psychosocial considerations:

$\longrightarrow$

Fig. 2.3 *Continued.*

C. PAIN

All sites and types of pain (patient's own words):

Severity, onset, frequency and duration:

Exacerbating and relieving factors and analgesic history:

D. SURROUNDING SKIN

Dry / macerated / excoriated / eczematous / other:

E. WOUND BED TIME ASSESSMENT

T = Tissue: _____% black necrotic eschar _____% slough

_____% granulation _____% overgranulation

_____% epithelialisation

I = Infection/inflammation: Clinical signs:
☐ Wound swab (if infection is suspected). Results:

M = Moisture: Level: Colour: Nature:

E = Edges: Appearance: ☐ Photo ☐ Tracing
Length and width of ulcer(s) in cm:

F. LEG MEASUREMENTS AND OEDEMA

Right Ankle _____ cm Calf_____ cm Left Ankle_____cm Calf_____cm

Nature/type of oedema:

Height to which oedema extends: calf / knee / thigh / waist

G. CONTRA-INDICATIONS TO FULL COMPRESSION

Peripheral arterial disease / cardiac or renal oedema / suspected
DVT / neuropathy / other:

H. ALLERGIES

STEP 5. DIAGNOSIS OF ULCER TYPE:

(Combine Steps 1–4 and diagnose each leg separately)

R☐ L☐ **VENOUS ULCER:** Evidence of venous disease. No other disease
involvement.

R☐ L☐ **ARTERIAL ULCER:** Evidence of arterial disease. ABPI < 0.8 or
falsely elevated > 1.3. No other disease involvement.

R☐ L☐ **MIXED VENOUS/ARTERIAL ULCER:** Evidence of venous disease
and moderate arterial disease. ABPI 0.8–0.5 or false high > 1.3.
No other disease involvement.

R☐ L☐ **MIXED ARTERIAL/VENOUS ULCER:** Evidence of venous disease
and severe arterial disease. ABPI < 0.5 or false high > 1.3.
No other disease involvement.

R☐ L☐ **OTHER ULCER TYPE:** Details:

R☐ L☐ **MULTI-FACTORIAL ULCER:** More than one underlying condition
contributing to ulceration. Details:

R☐ L☐ **INCONCLUSIVE DIAGNOSIS:** Refer to leg ulcer team.

RESULTS OF ANY INVESTIGATIONS BY LEG ULCER TEAM

⟶

Fig. 2.3 *Continued.*

PHASE 2: CARE PLAN
Valid for up to 3 months   Date: Sign:

1. PATIENT INVOLVEMENT
⇨ Provide opportunities to discuss the ulcer and its treatment, and for the patient and carers to express anxieties and ask questions.
⇨ Agree the extent to which the patient (and carers) wish to participate in care: _____

2. REFERRAL
⇨ Consult the leg ulcer care pathway for guidance on which teams to involve in care, according to ulcer type and symptoms.
   Team(s) referred to: _____

3. WIDER FACTORS/IMPACT OF THE ULCER
⇨ In partnership with the patient, and where possible, address wider factors affecting healing/impact of the ulcer on daily activities

_____

4. PAIN
⇨ Assess pain at each visit, before and after dressing changes.
⇨ Monitor analgesic use and its effect. Consider adjuvant therapies.

_____

⇨ Liaise with GP and leg ulcer team if pain remains uncontrolled.

5. CLEANSING, SKIN CARE AND DRESSINGS
⇨ Frequency of dressing changes: _____

Cleansing:
⇨ Maintain a clean technique and use universal precautions.
⇨ Wash and dry hands and apply a clean apron. Place a clean protective plastic sheet or towel under the patient's legs. Prepare a clean dressing area. Open and lay out the cleansing solutions, ointments, dressings and bandages.
⇨ Apply clean non-latex gloves (e.g. vinyl) and gently remove dressings.
⇨ EITHER Wash the leg in a clean bowl/bucket of warm tap water, lined with a clean plastic liner
   OR Soak the leg in a solution of _____
   _____(use hypo-allergenic products where possible)
   OR Irrigate with warmed normal saline.
⇨ Pat dry with clean towel/gauze swabs, taking care not to disturb the ulcer.
⇨ Change gloves.

Skin Care:
⇨ If macerated or excoriated, increase frequency of dressing changes, and apply _____barrier film.

⟶

Fig. 2.3 *Continued.*

⇨ If eczematous, commence a reducing dose of _____
_____steroid ointment.
Details:_____
_____

⇨ Apply moisturising ointment _____
using a gauze swab. Use downward strokes to prevent folliculitis. (To avoid causing allergies, use ointments in place of creams where possible).

Wound Care and Dressing:

⇨ Assess wound weekly for signs of progress using the TIME assessment tool.

⇨ Swab if clinical signs of infection are present and obtain result. If antibiotics are required, request a 14-day course.

⇨ Debridement method (if applicable): _____
_____

⇨ Wound treatment (if applicable): _____
_____

⇨ Primary dressing: _____
_____ (To reduce risk of causing allergies, use simple low-adherent dressings where possible, and avoid adhesives to the skin. To reduce risk of maceration, avoid foam dressings under compression. To reduce risk of resistance, reserve antiseptic dressings for infected wounds or those at increased risk.)

⇨ Secondary dressing(s) (if applicable) _____
_____

6. BANDAGING/HOSIERY

⇨ Select the target therapy for each leg (consult the care pathway and multi-layer bandage guide for guidance).

Right
☐ Full Elastic Long-Stretch Compression
☐ Full Inelastic Short-Stretch Compression
☐ Reduced Compression (18–25 mmHg)
☐ Reduced Compression (15–18 mmHg)
☐ Light Support
☐ Very Light Support
☐ Retention

Left
☐ Full Elastic Long-Stretch Compression
☐ Full Inelastic Short-Stretch Compression
☐ Reduced Compression (18–25 mmHg)
☐ Reduced Compression (15–18 mmHg)
☐ Light Support
☐ Very Light Support
☐ Retention

⇨ Apply the bandage or hosiery layers to achieve the target therapy (consult the multi-layer bandage guide for guidance).

⟶

Fig. 2.3 *Continued.*

⇨ Where necessary, first reshape the legs with extra layers of padding bandage, then re-measure the ankle.

⇨ Where there is risk of irritant eczema, apply a stockinette under the padding layer(s).

Right

Layer 1: _____Application:_____

Layer 2: _____Application:_____

Layer 3: _____Application:_____

Layer 4: _____Application:_____

Layer 5: _____Application:_____

Layer 6: _____Application:_____

Left

Layer 1: _____Application:_____

Layer 2: _____Application:_____

Layer 3: _____Application:_____

Layer 4: _____Application:_____

Layer 5: _____Application:_____

Layer 6: _____Application:_____

⇨ Ensure the patient is comfortable and that padding over the foot is kept safely to a minimum to facilitate applying shoes.

⇨ Re-measure the legs monthly or as required. A reduction in limb size may require a change in bandage selection.

7. ADDITIONAL DETAILS/DISEASE-SPECIFIC MANAGEMENT

PHASE 3: EVALUATE OUTCOMES After 1 month of treatment, three monthly, at sudden deterioration, and at healing

AFTER ONE MONTH OF TREATMENT:

⇨ Re-measure the ulcers. Measurements: _____

⇨ Re-assess wound bed: _____% black necrotic eschar; _____% slough; _____ % granulation; _____% overgranulation; _____% epithelialisation

⇨ If no improvement in wound bed or reduction in ulcer size, refer to the leg ulcer team. if ulcer is improving, continue care.

⇨ Action taken:_____ Date: _____ Sign: _____ ⟶

Fig. 2.3 *Continued.*

THREE MONTHLY OR AT SUDDEN DETERIORATION

⇨ If ulcer is unhealed and healing is not imminent, repeat Phase 1 to look for possible change in ulcer type. Refer to leg ulcer team for further investigation, if not previously referred.

⇨ Action taken:_____ Date: Sign:

AT HEALING

☐ **Venous ulcer**: Continue bandaging for further 4 weeks, then fit with medium to firm compression hosiery.
Monitor 3–6 monthly for hosiery review and Doppler ABPI assessment. If APBI drops, level of compression may need to be reduced.

☐ **Arterial ulcer:** Monitor 3 monthly for ulcer breakdown and Doppler ABPI measurement.

☐ **Mixed venous/arterial ulcer:** Possible light compression hosiery following specialist advice. Details: _____
Monitor 3 monthly for ulcer breakdown and Doppler ABPI measurement.

☐ **Other ulcer type/multi-factorial ulcer:** Ongoing disease-specific management and oedema management.
Details:_____

Date: Sign:

Fig. 2.3 *Continued.*

Case studies

Mrs Patel sustained a pre-tibial laceration after falling in the garden. After initial treatment in the accident and emergency department, she was referred to her practice nurse for dressings. She has some pitting oedema of both legs, and small varicose veins are visible at the top of the calf. She also complains of intermittent claudication. Unless these signs of venous and arterial disease are investigated and managed, the laceration will almost certainly ulcerate.

Mr O'Neil was discharged home to his district nursing team for dressing changes following surgery for coronary bypass grafts. The nurses notice venous skin changes affecting the leg from which the veins were harvested. Without a thorough assessment and adequate control of the underlying venous hypertension, healing is likely to be delayed.

Phase 1

Phase 1 guides the practitioner through five steps covering the fundamental aspects of leg ulcer assessment and diagnosis:

Step 1 Assessment for venous disease.
Step 2 Assessment for arterial disease.
Step 3 Assessment for other possible ulcer aetiologies.
Step 4 General assessment, e.g. of wider factors potentially delaying healing, psychosocial considerations, ulcer-related pain, surrounding skin, the wound bed, oedema, leg measurements and allergies.
Step 5 Diagnosis of the ulcer aetiology, drawing together all the information gathered.

This sequence of steps is designed to help practitioners think logically through every potential factor contributing to their patient's ulcer before concluding with a diagnosis or initiating treatment, thus facilitating better recognition of multi-factorial ulceration. It also forces practitioners to base a diagnosis of venous disease on evidence of venous disease, and not simply assume the presence of venous disease in the absence of a low Doppler ABPI reading. While it is often possible to come to a conclusion about a likely diagnosis, some ulcers can be difficult to diagnose without further specialist assessment and possible biopsy. The pathway guides the practitioner to refer these patients immediately to the leg ulcer team.

Case study

Mrs Morris was referred to her district nursing team for management of a left leg ulcer. A Doppler ABPI assessment was performed and the reading was 1.0.

In the past, the team would have assumed the ulcer was venous in origin, and commenced compression bandaging. By using the leg ulcer care pathway assessment tool, they noticed that, though there was some mild venous disease present (ankle flare), the ulcer was in an unusual location (on the calf), and very round in appearance with rolled edges. The diagnosis was inconclusive and Mrs Morris was referred to the specialist team. Further investigation confirmed the ulcer was a basal-cell carcinoma.

Phase 2

Phase 2 of the pathway sets out the fundamental aspects of leg ulcer care according to the patient's ulcer aetiology, and includes:

- Referral to the appropriate members of the multi-disciplinary team.
- General management issues, such as symptom control and management of the wound bed and surrounding skin. The documentation allows room for flexibility, while also guiding the practitioner through basic best-practice principles. Emphasis is placed on involvement of the patient in their care, according to their wishes.
- Bandage (or hosiery) selection. The documentation requires the practitioner to make a clear statement about the target therapy required, be it compression, support or retention, prior to selecting the appropriate bandage or hosiery layers required to achieve the target therapy, in accordance with the patient's ankle circumference. This safety mechanism is designed to ensure practitioners consider the aims of therapy and the individual patient's limb size, rather than issuing a 'standard' bandaging regime for all patients
- Additional disease-specific treatment. Observations in practice reveal that practitioners are poor at including interventions other than the dressing regime in the patient care plan, even when the mainstay of treatment is not the dressing regime but, for example, medication in the case of pyoderma gangrenosum.

Phase 3

The final section looks at when and how to evaluate the effectiveness of care given. The one-month evaluation is a simple test for any signs of progress by means of re-measuring the wound and re-assessing the wound bed using the TIME assessment tool (Falanga, 2004), and triggers a referral to the leg ulcer specialist team if no measurable improvement in the ulcer is observed. The three-monthly check provides a regular means of monitoring any changes to the underlying cause of the ulcer, and acts as a back up for further referral if not previously considered or arranged. The 'Healed Ulcer' section of this check (see Fig. 2.2a) sets out best practice in aftercare for the various ulcer types, to give patients the best possible chance of remaining ulcer-free.

PILOTING AND LAUNCHING THE LOCAL PATHWAY

A key component to ensuring the success of a care pathway is the early involvement and commitment of those who will use it, and the opportunity to pilot the new documentation (Hotchkiss, 2000). The pathway was written in consultation with the entire leg ulcer team, as well as with patients and other members of the multi-disciplinary team, including district nurses, practice nurses and vascular teams from the two main hospitals within the region. The assessment tool was then piloted with five district and/or practice nurses.

Once final changes were made, ten 'launch lunches' were set up at various health centres around the Trust. These included a 2-hour teaching session by the leg ulcer team on how to use the pathway and accompanying documentation. Particular emphasis was given to improving practitioners' ability to recognise and record signs of venous disease and how to use and incorporate the TIME assessment tool (Falanga, 2004) into routine practice. In addition, the pathway was presented at practice nurse forums and to the professional management committee.

UPTAKE AND IMPACT OF THE PATHWAY

Any implementation of change to professional practice requires a concerted effort if effects are to be long-lasting, and should include maintenance and re-enforcement strategies as well as plans to monitor and evaluate outcomes (NHS Centre for Reviews and Dissemination, 1999). The literature suggests that not all interventions work in every setting, and that a variety of strategies are likely to be most successful (NHS Centre for Reviews and Dissemination, 1999), including:

- **Reminders**. Reminder letters to be sent to all practitioners 3 months after the launch of the pathway.
- **Educational outreach**. The care pathway to continue to form the basis of the Trust's leg ulcer training programme.
- **Personal contact**. Referral to the leg ulcer team to be based on the care pathway, and – where referral is made without

evidence of use of the pathway – a reminder to be sent to the practitioner involved. Practitioners who remain unconfident in completing the pathway – either due to inexperience or to the complexity of the patient's ulcer – to be guided through the process by the leg ulcer team during the initial 'joint visit'.

- **Re-audit and feedback**. Results of a planned re-audit to be fed back to all district and practice nurses.

The subject of the evaluation of outcomes is dealt with in depth in Part V of this book, and will not be repeated here. Although re-audit results are not yet available, clinical observation has revealed interesting insights into the impact of the pathway. Referrals to the leg ulcer team have improved, both in terms of more appropriate time frames as well as the quality of assessment prior to referral. There appears to be a greater recognition amongst practitioners of the presence of multiple complex factors contributing to many ulcers, and the need to manage these. Most practitioners appear to have adopted the pathway documentation, are using the TIME assessment tool (Falanga, 2004) in practice and are making more informed bandage choices. As with any planned change, there remain a small number of key practitioners who have not yet adopted the pathway. This highlights the need for ongoing strategies to understand the reasons behind this, to support its uptake and to work with all practitioners to ensure equity of care for all patients.

CONCLUSION

This chapter has highlighted the importance of continuous service evaluation and development of services in response to audit findings and changes in the patient population. The pathway described in this chapter has been successfully integrated into the service and can easily be adapted to other services. Its principles encourage re-evaluation and help to ensure that patients move smoothly through the service and have ready access to specialist opinion if the diagnosis is uncertain, symptoms are uncontrolled or progress is slow.

REFERENCES

Falanga, V. (2004) Wound bed preparation: science applied to practice. In: *European Wound Management Association (EWMA) Position Document: Wound Bed Preparation in Practice*. London, MEP, pp. 2–5.

Hotchkiss, R. (2000) Maintaining momentum. In: *Integrated Care Pathways. A Practical Approach to Implementation* (S. Middleton & A. Roberts, eds). Oxford, Butterworth Heinemann, pp. 93–98.

Lomas, J. (1991) Words with action? The production, dissemination and impact of consensus recommendations. *Annual Review of Public Health* **12**: 41–65.

Marston, W. & Vowden, K. (2003) Compression therapy: a guide to safe practice. In: *European Wound Management Association (EWMA) Position Document: Understanding Compression Therapy*. London, MEP, pp. 11–16.

Middleton, S. & Roberts, A. (2000a) Introduction. In: *Integrated Care Pathways. A Practical Approach to Implementation* (S. Middleton & A. Roberts, eds). Oxford, Butterworth Heinemann, pp. 3–12.

Middleton, S. & Roberts, A. (2000b) Documentation. In: *Integrated Care Pathways. A Practical Approach to Implementation* (S. Middleton & A. Roberts, eds). Oxford, Butterworth Heinemann, pp. 46–64.

Moffatt, C.J., Franks, P.J., Doherty, D.C., Martin, R., Blewett, R. & Ross, F. (2004) Prevalence of leg ulceration in a London population. *Quarterly Journal of Medicine* **97**: 431–437.

NHS Centre for Reviews and Dissemination (1999) Getting evidence into practice. *Effective Health Care Bulletin*. University of York, NHS Centre for Reviews and Dissemination, Vol. 5, Issue 1, www.york.ac.uk/inst/crd

Stacey, M.C., Falanga, V., Marston, W., Moffatt, C., et al. (2002) The use of compression therapy in the treatment of venous leg ulcers: a recommended management pathway. *EWMA Journal* **2**(1): 9–13.

Part II
Clinical Assessment and Diagnosis

The first step in successfully managing a patient with a leg ulcer is recognising the wound as a leg ulcer. This might be quite surprising for many practitioners, but the reality is that in practice there are many incidents where wounds on the leg that have been present for many weeks or even months are not given the due concern they deserve and are (incorrectly) not treated as an ulcer. Wounds that commonly fall into this trap include pre-tibial lacerations (or other trauma wounds) and surgical incisions where veins have been harvested for coronary artery bypass graft.

This problem was one of the driving forces behind the development of the pathway – helping practitioners to identify 'when does a wound on the leg become a leg ulcer?' The literature suggests that a leg ulcer may be classed as a wound that is taking a long time to heal, anything more than 4–6 weeks. This pathway has adopted a 4-week period to allow time for busy practitioners to undertake an assessment and enter the patient into the pathway. Even with this 4-week allowance, the wound may have been present for 6–7 weeks by the time an assessment might be completed and a conclusion reached as to the problems delaying healing.

The sooner the assessment is completed and the correct treatment implemented, the greater the chance of healing the wound in a timely fashion. In light of this, some additional options for entering patients into the pathway were created to ensure that assessment and treatment was commenced more promptly in particular clinical circumstances. These options include patients with known venous or peripheral arterial occlusive disease who are at greater risk of ulcerating should they develop a leg wound. In addition, patients with spontaneous wounds having no obvious cause should also be entered into the pathway.

The next logical step in successful management is a thorough patient assessment in order to answer the questions, 'Why isn't the wound healing? What has caused this wound'? Despite the obvious nature of these questions there are many times when this does not happen in clinical practice. Practitioners often jump ahead to implementing treatment without a sound assessment to inform the treatment decisions. They are often seduced to use antibiotics or one of the many new dressings available, without realising that these items alone are unlikely to help resolve the wound because they do not address the underlying cause.

The pathway, and its accompanying assessment tool, guides the practitioner through the assessment procedure. Practitioners frequently comment on the amount of time required to complete such an assessment, but this is time well invested and will serve both the patient and practitioner well in the long run.

In the majority of cases, leg ulcers are generally related to chronic venous hypertension or peripheral arterial occlusive disease or a combination of the two. However, there are many other, albeit rarer, potential causes that practitioners need to be aware of and look for. Recognition of the multi-factorial ulcer is also growing and the potential that there could be several major contributing factors to the ulcer, which all need to be identified in order to be treated, illustrates the importance of the need for a thorough patient assessment.

Part II of this book covers the assessment process in detail. It explores both general issues related to leg ulceration and chronic wound assessment and more specific issues focusing on the different causes of leg ulceration, how they occur and how they are diagnosed.

Each chapter considers the competencies required by the person performing the assessment and contains the necessary theory to enable a healthcare professional to adequately achieve these goals. In most instances the healthcare professional most likely to be undertaking the assessment and making an initial diagnosis will be the nurse. This makes leg ulceration different to some other nursing or task-orientated duties. The responsibility of making a diagnosis may not sit lightly on some nurses' shoulders, but with an understanding of the underlying disease processes leading to ulceration and guidance from the assessment tool they will be better equipped to make appropriate decisions. When the diagnosis is inconclusive it is important they know the process for referring the patient on to a more experienced practitioner or specialist.

Assessment of Leg Ulceration

LEARNING OBJECTIVES

Nurses involved in leg ulcer management should be able to demonstrate:

❏ An appreciation of the concept of leg ulceration as a sign or symptom of another underlying problem that needs to be identified.

❏ An understanding of the main causes of leg ulceration.

❏ An awareness of the local barriers to wound healing.

❏ The ability to recognise the wider factors that can delay wound healing.

❏ The ability to collect and collate information as a part of a comprehensive patient assessment and use this information to form a diagnosis.

❏ A recognition of the patient's experience of leg ulceration and be able to use this experience to individualise treatment and care.

INTRODUCTION

Leg ulcer assessment is a highly complex skill. Underpinning the process is a knowledge of the circulatory systems of the lower limbs, an understanding of the theories as to how an ulcer develops, an awareness of the more unusual causes of leg ulceration, in conjunction with the ability to gather the necessary information to determine the cause of the ulcer and identify the wider factors that are likely to delay healing. Practitioners who lack these skills can tend to focus their attention entirely on the wound rather than the patient, not recognising there is an underlying cause that needs to be managed. Alternatively, assumptions are made about the ulcer aetiology, despite a lack of thorough clinical assessment, which often leads to misdiagnosis and long periods of ineffective and inappropriate care (Cornwall et al., 1986).

A holistic approach is absolutely essential to ensure safe and effective care, and should include a full clinical history, clinical examination of the lower limbs and wound/s, vascular assessment and any appropriate laboratory tests (Jones, 2000). More specialist investigations may be required to fully evaluate the pathology. Thus recognition of the role of the multi-disciplinary team (MDT) is critical.

Best practice

- Leg ulcer assessment and diagnosis is a complex skill. It should be undertaken by a healthcare professional trained in leg ulcer management (RCN, 1998).
- Assessment is not a one-off procedure but an ongoing one. Significant changes in the nature and aetiology of a leg ulcer can rapidly occur. General issues related to the wound bed, surrounding skin, pain and impact of the ulcer should be reviewed on a weekly basis, while a more in-depth review should occur every 3 months.

WHO DOES THE ASSESSMENT?

Historically, the majority of patients with leg ulceration in the UK have been managed almost entirely in the community, usually by district nursing teams, with limited input from GPs or hospital departments (Callum et al., 1985; Cornwall et al., 1986). Few doctors are sufficiently exposed to leg ulcer care to develop expertise or to adequately evaluate treatment options (Callum et al., 1987), so the responsibility of performing a holistic assessment to diagnose ulcer aetiology is often handed to the community nursing services.

Since the 1980s, the importance of involving the multi-disciplinary team has been acknowledged. Moreover, evidence-based leg ulcer service models have begun to reflect this change with the provision of jointly run integrated services that span the boundaries between acute and primary care (Moffatt et al., 2004).

Despite this shift, the initial assessment and diagnosis remains largely the responsibility of community and primary care nurses (Moffatt et al., 2004). These nurses should be fully qualified, with additional specific training in leg ulcer assessment and management. In most cases the results of the assessment should then prompt referral to other appropriate members of the multi-disciplinary team; this could include the GP for further medical assessment, a specialist leg ulcer team/nurse, a vascular or dermatology team, or any other specific disease management team or therapy services.

Readers are asked to refer to Chapter 12 for further information relating to the involvement of the multi-disciplinary team.

ASSESSMENT TO DETECT THE UNDERLYING CAUSE OF THE ULCER

Misdiagnosis is surely the most likely factor to lead to unnecessary delayed healing (Hoffman, 2002). It should therefore go without saying that identifying the cause of the ulcer is paramount to its successful management.

The one rule we must not forget when dealing with a leg ulcer is to remember that an underlying condition or problem is preventing the ulcer from healing. In the majority of cases the ulcer will be due to some form of vascular insufficiency, be it chronic venous hypertension, peripheral arterial occlusive disease (PAOD) or a combination of the two (Callum et al., 1985; King, 2004).

Over 40 causes of ulceration have been identified, and more often than not there is more than one contributing factor to the presence of the ulcer (Moffatt et al., 2004). Regardless of how many factors are likely to be causing the ulcer it is important to identify them all; only then can we help the patient begin to successfully manage them. Other factors are also likely to be present, perhaps not directly causing the wound but nonetheless contributing to its overall slow healing.

How did it all begin?

On first presentation, a picture needs to be built up pointing to the origins of the ulcer (Table 3.1). This information will help in deciding whether to enter the patient into the pathway and will also aid the diagnosis and treatment plan.

Many wounds may start out as the result of some form of trauma – collisions with shopping trolleys, prams and bus steps are not uncommon – and most will probably heal without special intervention. However, for patients with a past history of leg ulceration,

Table 3.1 Ulcer history (adapted from RCN, 1998).

- When and how did it occur?
- Where is it located?
- Is this the first episode of ulceration?
- Time taken to heal for previous ulcers
- Time free from ulcers
- Past treatments (successful/unsuccessful)

PAOD and/or signs of chronic venous hypertension it is probably better to assume the worst and start treating the wound as though it were an ulcer.

Many wounds appear quite spontaneously or for no obvious reason. Therefore it is wise to hold a certain amount of suspicion for these, so further assessment is beneficial in these cases.

Assessment for the principal causes of leg ulcers

Chronic venous hypertension and PAOD, or a combination of these two conditions, are frequently the primary cause of leg ulceration. Therefore the bulk of the assessment is based on screening patients for these problems, looking for both risk factors and evidence of the disease. This is achieved by exploring various aspects – the patient's family history, past medical history, personal factors, looking for tissue changes and Doppler assessment – it should then be possible to draw some conclusions in determining the presence or absence of either of these diseases. This process is described in much more detail in Chapters 4 and 5.

During the initial assessment, however, some clues, with respect to the location of the ulcer (Figs 3.1, 3.2 and Table 3.2) and its appearance (size, depth and tissue type), may point to a potential likely cause if the patient is unsure of how it began.

Consider the possibility of rarer ulcer aetiologies and multi-factorial ulceration

Numerous medical conditions can be attributed to the development of leg ulceration; these include autoimmune and infectious diseases, haematological disorders, malignancies and other inflam-

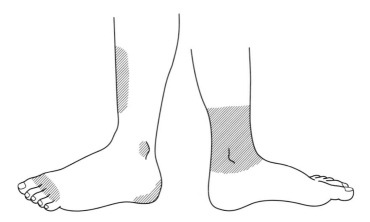

Fig. 3.1 Common sites for arterial ulceration.

Fig. 3.2 Common sites for venous ulceration.

matory conditions. Diabetes is also likely to pose problems for many patients with wounds, though it is rarely the cause of a leg ulcer except in the case of necrobiosis lipoidica; but, of course, diabetes is a major cause of foot ulceration (King, 2004).

One of the initial phases of leg ulcer assessment will be to screen the patient for any of these potential causes, which will largely be a process of elimination. However, some diseases will be more difficult to discount or identify and further investigation and referral may be required. Chapter 7 takes a much closer look at other ulcer aetiologies.

If the diagnostic process is proving inconclusive then further routine laboratory investigations may help to highlight any previously undetected significant problems, such as anaemia or polycythaemia, an inflammatory condition (be it an infection or autoimmune disorder), diabetes or a nutritional deficiency. Table 3.3 gives a list of the recommended tests (Hess & Trent, 2004).

Remember that it is always possible for more than one aetiology to be present. Just because one has been identified does not mean the search for others should be abandoned.

Table 3.2 Basic clinical descriptors of leg ulcers (adapted from Dowsett, 2005).

	Venous	Arterial	Other
Site	Gaiter region	Foot, malleoli, area of pressure	Unspecific. Be wary if ulcer is in an unusual location and developed spontaneously
Shape	Can be quite large, irregularly shaped	Can be round, with a punched-out appearance	Varied. Observe for clusters of small ulcers or ones that begin as blistering, and ulcers that rapidly increase in size
Depth	Generally shallow	Can be deep with exposed underlying structures, e.g. tendons	Variable. May be over-granulated
Edges	Tend to be flat or gently sloping	May be cliff-like	Observe for rolled or raised edges or discoloured (purple) wound margins
Tissue type	May be sloughy (pre-treatment), otherwise red granulation present	Probable devitalised tissue (slough and/or necrosis); pale granulation, if present	Variable. Observe for wounds that: bleed easily; appear to scab over and break down recurrently; look very healthy but fail to show signs of healing

Table 3.3 Laboratory tests.

- Erythrocyte sedimentation rate
- Liver function test
- Glucose
- Iron levels
- Total lymphocyte count
- U/E/Cr – electrolytes
- Lipoprotein levels
- Urinalysis

Case study

Dorothy, a 62-year-old lady, presented to her GP with a 3-week history of a painful wound on her right medial malleolus. Dorothy does not know how it started, but said she may have bumped it. She was prescribed a course of flucloxacillin and referred to the practice nurse for dressings. The practice nurse completed a leg ulcer assessment and found several possible causes for the wound. Dorothy has a medical history of:

- Systemic lupus erythematosus (SLE), for which she attends a rheumatology consultant on an outpatient basis; her disease is controlled with corticosteroids and methotrexate.
- Osteoporosis due to her long-term steroid use.
- Deep vein thrombosis in both legs (both occurred 15–20 years ago).
- Diabetes mellitus.
- Hypertension.

In terms of the wound and the surrounding skin:

- The wound is right over the bony prominence.
- It is 3 cm^2 in size and completely covered by dry sloughy tissue.
- There is localised inflammation.
- The surrounding skin is dry, and looks thin, but intact.
- The wound produces very little fluid.
- There is some localised oedema just below the ankle.
- There is some ankle flare, and atrophie blanche in the gaiter region.
- Her feet are warm to touch but quite pale in appearance.

Continued

Dorothy describes the pain as intense at times. It is generally worse at night and feels better when she is walking. She presently takes paracetamol three times a day for the pain, and is reluctant to take more or try anything stronger. Her ankle brachial pressure index was measured: right ABPI is 0.6 and left ABPI is 0.76.

This lady has a complex medical history and many factors could have caused the ulcer, or at least now be contributing to its inability to heal:

- Autoimmune disease (SLE)
- Arterial disease
- Venous disease
- Diabetes
- Medications for her SLE
- Her severe pain

The practice nurse takes the decision to liaise with the GP to arrange referral to a vascular team and Dorothy's rheumatologist for further assessment and guidance.

ASSESSMENT FOR LOCAL WOUND BARRIERS TO HEALING

In addition to the underlying pathology or pathologies preventing normal healing, it is also possible that barriers, local to the wound bed, can also impact on a wound's healing potential. Unlike acute wounds, chronic wounds such as leg ulcers fail to follow the normal pattern of repair. Instead of a balanced and ordered cellular and chemical process, disorder and imbalance prevail leading to delayed wound healing.

The main barriers to healing include:

- The presence of slough and/or necrosis
- Bacterial imbalance
- Moisture imbalance
- Cellular dysfunction
- Biochemical imbalance

A structured wound assessment tool (TIME) has been devised by the International Wound Bed Preparation Advisory Board (Falanga, 2004) to enable easy assessment of these potential barriers.

TIME stands for:

T = Tissue
I = Inflammation or infection
M = Moisture imbalance
E = Edge of wound

The TIME assessment tool should be used on initial assessment and at regular intervals thereafter.

Readers are encouraged to refer to Chapter 8 for further detail on wound bed assessment.

ASSESSMENT FOR WIDER FACTORS THAT DELAY HEALING

While accurate diagnosis of ulcer aetiology is the key to effective leg ulcer management, it is also incredibly important to identify other intrinsic or extrinsic factors (Fig. 3.3) that may be contributing to delayed healing (Jones, 2000).

The impact of some these factors on wound healing are discussed below, while others are covered in more depth in the relevant chapters.

Ulcer size and duration

Research investigating healing indicators found that the size of the wound and the length of time it had been present had a significant impact on its potential to heal (Franks et al., 1995). Ulcers greater than $5\,cm^2$ or those present for more than a year are less likely to heal than those ulcers that are smaller or present for a shorter period (Phillips et al., 2000).

While this concept is perhaps not particularly surprising it does highlight the importance of ensuring that the right treatment is started within the right time frame.

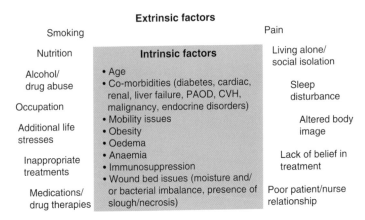

Fig. 3.3 Extrinsic and intrinsic factors that can delay wound healing (adapted from Morison & Moffatt, 1994).

Mobility

Reduced mobility can, in effect, contribute to ulceration by means of weight gain, calf muscle wastage and ineffective calf muscle pump, essentially resulting in pseudovenous disease. In turn, the presence of an ulcer can also lead to reduced mobility as a means of protecting the patient from pain, so the patient falls into a vicious circle. Therefore it is important to encourage (and help, if necessary) a patient to carry on walking in a normal fashion.

Walking normally means heel to toe, and to do this a person requires good ankle function. Assessing a patient's ankle function is just as important as their ability to mobilise generally, as the implications for delayed wound healing are equally significant. A patient may be unable to mobilise but they may have very good ankle function, and vice versa. Beware of patients who suddenly develop a fixed ankle once bandaging has been applied; remind them the bandages will not be stiff like a cast and they should be able to move their ankle relatively normally.

The reasons for a person not mobilising are many and potentially difficult, if not impossible, to resolve. Physical problems such as previous injuries or medical conditions can certainly impact on the ability to mobilise, but so too can emotional, cognitive or mental issues. Patients may need more motivation to walk, they may not feel safe when walking or there may be a lack of understanding about the benefits of walking. For some patients their mobility may be very good, but due to various factors, such as their work or a busy social life, their mobility becomes an issue because they are spending much of their day either standing or sitting with their legs dependent.

It is important to get a baseline picture of a patient's ability to mobilise as this information will be useful to help both the practitioner and patient consider:

- Is referral to a physiotherapist or occupational therapist likely to be beneficial?
- Are exercise or walking programmes appropriate?
- Is leg elevation going to be a more successful means of reversing chronic venous hypertension?
- What bandages are likely to be more suitable?
- What is the likely possibility of healing?

Smoking

Not only is smoking a major risk factor for the development of PAOD, but it has several adverse effects on wound healing. The detrimental effect of smoking on wounds has long been suspected, though this has yet to be studied in more detail. Nevertheless there is sufficient evidence that demonstrates the negative impact of smoking. Whiteford's (2003) literature review found that the three most toxic components of cigarette smoke – nicotine, carbon monoxide and hydrogen cyanide – all contribute to tissue hypoxia brought about by vasoconstriction, reduced levels of oxygen carried by haemoglobin and decreased oxidative metabolism. These components seriously impair the physiological and chemical processes that should occur naturally during wound healing.

Oedema

It is thought that oedema delays wound healing due to its effect on the microcirculatory system in preventing adequate perfusion and exchange of nutrients in the affected area. Cells are starved of oxygen and nutrients and levels of metabolic waste products become toxic (Hoffman, 1998).

There are many possible causes of oedema (Table 3.4) and the cause needs to be identified in order to manage it appropriately. Things to look for and ask include (Linnit, 2005):

- How long has the oedema been present?
- Does it affect one leg or both?
- Does it affect the feet, the ankles; does it go up to the knees, thighs or buttocks?
- Does the swelling go down at night? Does it get worse by the end of the day, or is it always the same?
- Does the patient sleep in a bed?
- Is it pitting or fibrosed?
- Are skin changes present?
- Is there a history of cardiac, renal or liver failure?

Malnutrition

The presence of a wound places great demands on the body's energy needs, therefore it is important to consider a person's total kilocalorie intake. However, it is also important to obtain these kilocalories from a diet rich in variety. Deficiencies in protein, vitamin C and zinc all contribute to poor wound strength, while deficiencies in fats, carbohydrates and vitamin A lead to impaired immunocompetence and an increased risk of wound infections.

Table 3.4 Recognising oedema.

Venous oedema may affect one or both legs with the swelling occurring mostly below the knee. It tends to resolve overnight when the legs have been elevated.

Arterial disease may contribute to oedema because the patient has to sleep with their legs dependent in order to relieve the night pain experienced.

Lymphoedema may affect one or both limbs; it can extend much further up the leg into the buttocks and groin. It may begin as a pitting oedema but over time becomes more fibrosed. It does not resolve with leg elevation.

Pitting oedema that affects both legs and does not resolve with leg elevation may be due to major organ failure or protein deficiency and needs to be investigated by a doctor.

The prevalence of malnutrition, particularly in the elderly population, is likely to be severely underestimated by practitioners. Stratton et al. (2004) studied the prevalence of malnutrition in an adult population using the Malnutrition Universal Screening Tool (MUST), and found a malnutrition risk in 30% of patients in the community (outpatients) and anywhere between 19 and 60% for inpatients.

There are some simple means of assessing a patient's nutritional intake (quantity and quality) and identifying whether there are problems or potential problems that could result in the patient being malnourished. The first step is obviously to enquire about a patient's dietary history (McIlwaine, 2003):

- Do they consider their appetite to be good, or has it changed?
- On an average day what would their meals consist of?
- Do they do their own shopping and cooking?
- Do they have any personal, cultural or religious beliefs that may have an effect on their diet?

If there are doubts about a patient a diet diary might help to identify where and how that patient could boost some variety or extra calories into their normal pattern of eating and drinking.

Weight and body mass index are also useful objective indicators for identifying either under- or over-nourished people, though as a one-off measurement it will not help to identify patients who are gradually losing or gaining weight. Nevertheless, patients are probably able to say if their clothes or rings are getting looser, or if their dentures are no longer fitting so well (Williams, 2002).

Although many nutritional assessment tools are available, consideration has to be given to who will be using them and where and to whom they are to be applied. MUST was developed for use in the community and is referred to in the Nutritional Support in Adults guideline (NICE, 2006). It is supported by numerous organisations, including the British Dietetic Association, the British Association for Parental and Enteral Nutrition, The Royal College of Nursing and Physicians and the Registered Nursing Homes Association (Harris & Haboubi, 2005). MUST is easy to use and well validated (Stratton et al., 2004); it comprises five steps, taking into account the patient's BMI, any unplanned weight loss in the past 3–6 months and any recent acute illness that has or will prevent any nutritional intake for 5 days or more. Each factor is scored and the points tallied to give a total that relates to the risk of under-nutrition – ranging from low, medium to high – guidance is also given on how to respond to each level of risk.

Other factors likely to affect nutritional intake are:

- Problems with buying, storing or preparing food – poverty, immobility or poor dexterity.
- Problems with swallowing due to neurological or neuromuscular disease.
- Poor appetite due to concurrent disease, medication or depression.
- Malabsorption problems relating to gastrointestinal disease, surgery, diarrhoea or vomiting.

Being over-nourished poses a different set of problems in regards to wound healing. In particular relation to leg ulceration, obesity can contribute to oedema by increasing the effects of venous hypertension, and restricts mobility (Jones, 2000; Hoffman, 2002).

Adequate hydration is just as important as food intake. Patients can lose large volumes of fluid in addition to protein via their wounds (Hoffman, 2002).

Once again, quality is as important as quantity. Excessive amounts of alcohol will generally have detrimental effects on the patient's general health or management of other health-related problems.

Medication/drug therapies

It is important to consider a patient's current list of medications as some have the potential to adversely affect the wound healing process. Drugs most likely to have an effect include corticosteroids, non-steroidal anti-inflammatory drugs (NSAIDs), cytotoxic drugs and tumour necrosis factor-alpha (TNF-α) inhibitors (Kindlen & Morison, 1997; Firth, 2005). Patients most likely to be taking such medication are those with autoimmune diseases (e.g. rheumatoid arthritis, systemic lupus erythematosus), malignancies or pulmonary disease.

NSAIDs have less adverse effects than corticosteroids. Corticosteroids disrupt the wound healing process during both the inflammatory and proliferative phases and delay wound closure. The risks of wound breakdown are high due to the effects of vaso-constriction and an altered immune response. The reduced levels of blood, oxygen and nutrients to the wound lead to a delay in healing and an increased risk of infection (Firth, 2005).

Cytotoxic drugs (e.g. methotrexate) are often considered cause for concern in terms of increased risk of infection and their poten-tial to interfere with the inflammatory phase of wound healing. Additional side-effects of these medications (nausea, vomiting and other gastrointestinal disturbances) can also impact on wound healing by affecting patients' nutritional intake (Firth, 2005).

Pain

Knowing and understanding a patient's level and type of pain is a vital element of leg ulcer assessment on two particular counts. One, it will help the practitioner in making a diagnosis; and, two, even moderate levels of continuous uncontrolled pain can signifi-cantly impact on a person's normal day-to-day activities – their work, rest, relationships and mental state – which, in turn, can potentially delay leg ulcer healing.

It would be highly irresponsible to assume that just because a patient does not verbalise pain they do not experience it. As carers we must encourage our patients to express their pain, and this may mean helping them to find the words to describe what they are experiencing. If we do not understand from the beginning the severity, the type and the triggers and relievers of pain how can the right treatments be chosen and the effectiveness of treatments measured?

The importance of pain assessment and management options is such that Chapter 9 covers this topic in much more detail.

Psychosocial factors

A direct link between delayed healing and psychosocial factors, such as living alone, social isolation, altered body image, poor relationship with carers and lack of belief in treatment, has yet to be clearly identified. However, from personal clinical experience these factors have frequently demonstrated their effects on both the healing potential of a wound and the patient's overall experi-ence of having a leg ulcer. Due to the impact and complexities of these factors they are covered in greater depth in Part III of this book.

Many patients deal with numerous difficult issues or health-related problems in their day-to-day lives, sometimes on top of their ulceration, in other cases despite it. The following case study is typical in regard to how the intricate nature of both physical and psychosocial problems combine to create a complex management situation. Moira's case study (summarised in Fig. 3.4) demonstrates the need for thorough assessment, for without knowing all the contributing factors it would be impossible to know who to involve, what treatments to use and what would be some realistic goals to aim for.

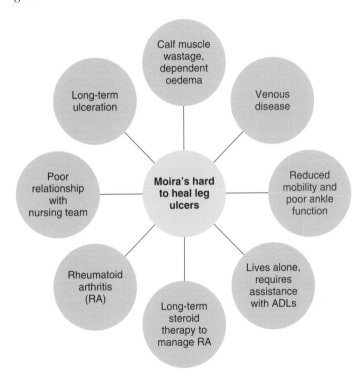

Fig. 3.4 Moira's complex leg ulceration problem.

Case study

Moira is a 64-year-old woman who lives alone in a large house. She has never married and has no children. Her only living relative is her younger brother who lives abroad. He occasionally stays with Moira when he is visiting the country once or twice a year. This lady previously worked as an editor but had to give up her work almost 10 years ago on the grounds of ill health. She has rheumatoid disease and this has been progressively worsening, resulting in increasing pain and reducing her physical abilities.

Moira strives to remain as independent as possible, though she has resorted to having a carer come in daily to help prepare some meals and do some cleaning chores. She still manages to mobilise short distances (i.e. within the house), get herself into and out of bed, dress and wash herself, albeit in a very modified manner and with the use of various aids; she is otherwise chair-bound.

She has bilateral lower leg ulceration, which has been present for over 4 years; the ulcers are largely thought to be due to a combination of both rheumatoid disease and poor venous function. Her ankle function is severely restricted and this along with her rheumatoid disease has resulted in foot deformities, which further reduces her mobility.

Moira is attended to by her district nurses, but she and her nurses do not always get along – this is often dealt with by sending agency nurses to attend to her care, which leads to a lack of consistency and, in turn, further prolongs the treatment required.

SUMMARY

- Explain the purpose of assessment to the patient.
- Assess the patient's general state of health and current status of other diseases present, including non-invasive vascular assessment.
- Determine the ulcer's aetiology; this is the most important goal.
- Use the TIME assessment tool to determine the need for wound bed preparation.
- Consider wider factors that will delay ulcer healing.
- Always remember to take into account the patient's understanding of the wound and recommended treatments.

CONCLUSION

Assessment is not just something that happens at the beginning, but is ongoing throughout any treatment. Identifying the ulcer aetiology is one of the major elements in leg ulcer assessment; however, exploring the wider issues that contribute to poor healing and that may affect treatment strategies is equally important. Having an in-depth understanding of your patient will help to find the most appropriate and successful treatments.

REFERENCES

Callum, M.J., Ruckely, C.V., Harper, D.R. & Dale, J.J. (1985) Chronic ulceration of the leg: extent of the problem and provision of care. *British Medical Journal* **290**: 1855–1856.

Callum, M.J., Harper, D.R., Dale, J.J. & Ruckely, C.V. (1987) Chronic ulcer of the leg: clinical history. *British Medical Journal* **294**: 1389–1391.

Cornwall, J.V., Dore, C.J. & Lewis, D. (1986) Leg ulcers: epidemiology and aetiology. *British Journal of Surgery* **73**: 693–696.

Dowsett, C. (2005) Diagnosing, treating and delivering care for people with venous leg ulcers. *Nursing Times Wound Care Supplement* **100**(22).

Falanga, V. (2004) Wound bed preparation: science applied to practice. In: *European Wound Management Association (EWMA). Position Document: Wound Bed Preparation in Practice.* London, MEP, pp. 2–5.

Firth, J. (2005) Tissue viability in rheumatoid arthritis. *Journal of Tissue Viability* **15**(3): 12–18.

Franks, P.J., Bosanquet, N., Connolly, M., Lorded, M.I., et al. (1995) Venous ulcer healing: effect of socioeconomic factors in London. *Journal of Epidemiology and Community Health* **49**(4): 385–388.

Harris, D. & Haboubi, N. (2005) Malnutrition screening in the elderly population. *Journal of the Royal Society of Medicine* **98**: 411–414.

Hess, C.T. & Trent, J.T. (2004) Incorporating laboratory values in chronic wound management. *Advances in Skin & Wound Care* **17**(7): 378–386.

Hoffman, D. (1998) Oedema and the management of venous ulcers. *Journal of Wound Care* **7**(7): 345–348.

Hoffman, D. (2002) Care of chronic wounds. *British Journal of Dermatology* **6**(2): 18–20.

Jones, J. (2000) Holistic assessment. *British Journal of Nursing* **9**(16): 1040–1052.

King, B. (2004) Is this leg ulcer venous? Unusual aetiologies of lower leg ulcers. *Journal of Wound Care* **13**(9): 394–396.

Kindlen, S. & Morison, M. (1997) The physiology of wound healing. In: *A Colour Guide to the Nursing Management of Chronic Wounds*, 2nd edn. (M. Morison, C. Moffatt, J. Bridel-Nixon, S. Bale, eds). London, Mosby, pp. 1–26.

Linnit, N. (2005) Lymphoedema: recognition, assessment and management. *Wound Care* **March**, S20–26.

McIiwaine C. (2003) Importance of holistic nutritional assessment in wound healing. *Journal of Wound Care* **12**(8): 285–288.

Moffatt, C.J., Franks, P.J., Doherty, D.C., Martin, R., Blewett, R. & Ross, F. (2004) Prevalence of leg ulceration in a London population. *Quarterly Journal of Medicine* **97**: 431–437.

Morison, M.J. & Moffatt, C.J. (1994) *A Colour Guide to the Assessment and Management of Leg Ulcers*, 2nd edn. London, Mosby.

NICE (2006) *Nutritional Support in Adults: Oral Nutritional Support, Enteral Tube Feeding and Parenteral Nutrition.* Developed by the National Collaborating Centre for Acute Care. London, National Institute for Health and Clinical Excellence. Available at http://www.nice.org.uk/CG032

Phillips, T.J., Machado, F., Trout, R., Porter, J., Olin, J., Falanga, V. & The Venous Ulcer Study Group (2000) Prognostic indicators in venous ulcers. *Journal of the American Academy of Dermatology* **43**: 627–630.

RCN Institute (1998) *Clinical Practice Guidelines. The Management of Patients with Venous Leg Ulcers.* London, Royal College of Nursing.

Stratton, R.J., Hackston, A., Longmore, D., Dixon, R., Price, S., Stroud, M., King, C. & Elia, M. (2004) Malnutrition in hospital outpatients and inpatients: prevalence, concurrent validity and ease of use of the 'malnutrition universal screening tool' (MUST) for adults. *British Journal of Nutrition* **92**(5): 799–808.

Williams, L. (2002) Assessing patients nutritional needs in the wound healing process. *Journal of Wound Care* **11**: 225–228.

Whiteford, L. (2003) Nicotine, CO and HCN: the detrimental effects of smoking on wound healing. *British Journal of Community Nursing, Wound Care* **December**, 8(12): S22–S26.

Venous Disease

LEARNING OBJECTIVES

Nurses involved in leg ulcer management should be able to demonstrate:

❏ An understanding of normal venous function.
❏ An understanding of venous disease (chronic venous hypertension) and its role in leg ulceration.
❏ The ability to identify those patients at increased risk of venous disease.
❏ The ability to identify the clinical signs and symptoms of venous disease.
❏ An understanding of the role of diagnostic tests for venous disease.
❏ An understanding of the priorities of venous disease management.

INTRODUCTION

Venous disorders of the leg are thought to affect up to one-third of the adult UK population (Franks et al., 1992; Evans et al., 1999). Varicose veins are possibly the most common manifestation, occurring in 10–25% of adults in the UK (Franks et al., 1992; Callam, 1994), usually due to valve incompetence often in combination with some loss of the calf muscle pump. The resulting rise in venous pressure is known as 'chronic venous hypertension' or 'chronic venous insufficiency'.

While only 1–3% of those affected do go on to ulcerate, venous disease is thought to be the largest single contributory factor to leg ulceration in the Western world. Studies in the 1980s and 1990s found evidence of venous disease in 57–80% of ulcerated legs (Cornwall et al., 1986; Callam et al., 1987; Breddin et al., 1992). Although many of these ulcers were found to be uncomplicated venous in origin, practitioners involved in leg ulcer care have – sometimes dangerously – tended to regard the majority of ulcers as 'venous', due to lack of attention to a comprehensive venous assessment (Cornwall et al., 1986) or failure to take into account other contributory aetiologies (Ruckley et al., 1982).

Over recent years there has been increased recognition of the multi-factorial nature of many leg ulcers, with fewer being attributed to venous disease alone. Studies undertaken in Sweden showed that one-third of patients suffered with complex aetiology, although venous disease was present in the majority and the dominating causative factor in 54% of cases (Nelzen et al., 1991). In the UK, the Wandsworth prevalence study found that only 43% of ulcers identified were uncomplicated venous in origin, while 35% were complex multi-factorial (Moffatt et al., 2004).

This shift may be partly due to increased awareness of non-venous aetiologies amongst healthcare professionals. However, it is also likely to be linked to an actual reduction in the prevalence of uncomplicated venous ulceration. Significant advances have been made in treatment options for venous ulceration, and nurses involved in leg ulcer care have become increasingly skilled in recognising and managing the signs and symptoms of venous disease (Blair et al., 1988; Task Force on Chronic Venous Disorders of the Leg, 1999; Cullum et al., 2001; Phillips, 2001).

The Wandsworth study found that the overall prevalence of leg ulceration fell to one-third that reported in previous studies. This suggests that possibly the biggest impact in tackling the problem of leg ulceration can be made in the area of venous disease management, and that areas which adopt a research-based leg ulcer service model can achieve excellent healing rates for uncomplicated venous ulcers.

Unfortunately, it still remains common practice among some healthcare professionals to 'assume' that an ulcer is 'venous', based on a Doppler ABPI reading of more than 0.8. Not only is this erroneous, it is also dangerous, often leading to misdiagnosis, incorrect management, delayed healing and, occasionally, loss of limb or death. This chapter guides the practitioner systematically through the process of screening patients for the presence of venous disease. Practitioners are reminded, however, that a diagnosis of venous disease does not necessarily equate to a diagnosis of venous ulceration. Although the presence of venous disease will certainly contribute to the ulcer aetiology, it may not be the only contributory factor, and other possible ulcer causes must also be thoroughly investigated.

Best practice

- Venous disease remains the largest single cause of leg ulceration, although recent research suggests this may be changing with increased numbers of leg ulcer patients presenting with complex multi-factorial aetiology. Areas that adopt a research-based leg ulcer service can significantly reduce the prevalence of venous ulceration (Moffatt et al., 2004).
- All patients who present with a leg ulcer should be screened for the presence of venous disease. A diagnosis of venous ulceration must not be based on a normal Doppler ankle brachial pressure index reading, but on clinical evidence of venous disease and/or evidence from vein scans. This involves an assessment of risk factors as well as signs and symptoms of venous disease. Where a diagnosis is inconclusive or surgery may be beneficial, non-invasive tests, such as photoplethysmography and colour Duplex scans, should be performed.
- Graduated multi-layer, high compression, long- or short-stretch bandage systems are the first-line of treatment for uncomplicated venous ulcers (Royal College of Nursing, 1998).

COMPETENCE IN VENOUS ASSESSMENT

If patients are to receive an accurate diagnosis and management of their leg ulcer based on the underlying aetiology, it is essential that all practitioners involved in their care are able to demonstrate competence in recognising and managing the signs and symptoms of venous disease.

Case study

Mrs Jackson developed a leg ulcer on her left medial malleolus. The district nurses measured her Doppler ABPI and the reading was 1.0. They assumed the ulcer was venous, and for 4 months treated Mrs Jackson with compression bandaging. During this time the ulcer deteriorated and became increasingly painful. The GP adjusted her analgesia, but did not investigate the ulcer any further. The pain became so bad that Mrs Jackson's family took her to A&E. From there she was admitted to a care of the elderly unit. The hospital staff was informed that she had a venous ulcer. No further investigations were carried out into the cause of the ulcer. After a week in hospital she was discharged home on morphine. Eventually, when the ulcer was nearly circumferential and lesions had begun to appear on the other leg, she was referred to a leg ulcer specialist, who immediately recognised that the ulcers were not venous. A biopsy confirmed pyoderma gangrenosum, and she was admitted to hospital for intravenous steroid therapy.

Had the correct diagnosis been made at the start, access to the correct treatment would not have been delayed, and much of Mrs Jackson's pain and suffering would have been avoided.

NORMAL VENOUS FUNCTION

What is venous disease, and how can practitioners best help patients understand it? Patients often get told they have bad 'circulation' – a confusing term, since the circulatory system includes not only the veins, but also the arteries, capillaries, lymphatics and the heart itself (Fig. 4.1). Is this sometimes because practitioners themselves do not fully understand the condition? It should hardly be surprising that patients are sometimes reluctant to wear compression or elevate their legs, when logic dictates that tight garments will only aggravate 'bad circulation'.

Avoid the terms 'circulation' and 'bad circulation', as these can be ambiguous. Instead, be specific about which section of the circulatory system is diseased.

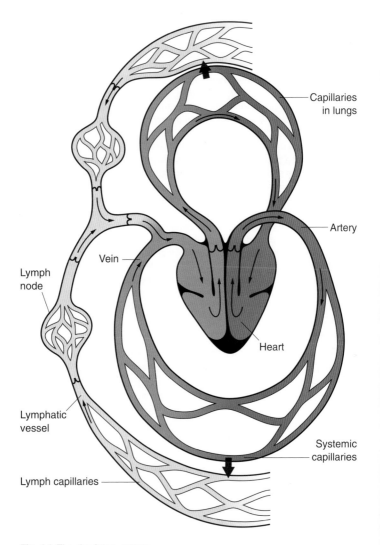

Fig. 4.1 The circulatory system.

A good understanding of the function, structure and mechanism of action of the venous system of the lower leg, as well as an awareness of the normal range of venous blood pressures, are essential prerequisites to gaining skills in recognising and managing venous disease.

Function

The venous system of the legs transports deoxygenated blood and waste products away from the capillary network in the tissues, back towards the heart, ready for re-oxygenation in the lungs and filtration in the kidneys. Not only must it be capable of carrying blood upwards, against gravity, but it also has to withstand strong gravitational forces exerted by the column of blood leading to the heart. Approximately 60% of the body's total blood volume is located in the veins at any given moment.

Structure

The veins in the leg are classified into three main categories: the deep vein, the superficial veins and the perforator veins (Fig. 4.2).

Each leg contains a deep vein lying deep within the muscles that runs the entire length of the leg. In the calf it is known as the 'anterior tibial vein', in the knee as the 'popliteal vein', and in the thigh as the 'femoral vein' – but essentially these are all sections of the same deep vein. In the groin, it joins the common iliac vein, leading to the vena cava, and eventually the heart.

The superficial veins, by contrast, are more numerous and lie outside the muscle just below the skin. They comprise the long and short saphenous veins and their tributaries. The short saphenous vein runs from the lateral malleolus (outer ankle region) and empties into the deep vein at the knee. The long saphenous vein originates in the medial malleolus (inner ankle region), and empties into the deep vein in the thigh.

The perforator veins are so-called because they pass through the muscle, transporting blood from the superficial system into the deep vein. They are located at frequent intervals along the length of the leg and are particularly abundant in the ankle region.

One-way valves are located within each perforator vein, and at various intervals along the deep and superficial veins. Their

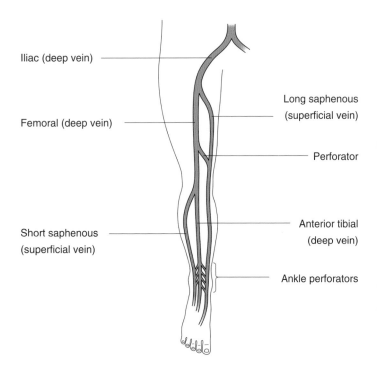

Fig. 4.2 The venous system of the leg.

function is to prevent any backwards reflux of blood towards the capillaries, only allowing blood to flow towards the heart.

Mechanism of action

So how do veins succeed in forcing blood upwards, against gravity, towards the heart? Although they are able to dilate or contract to some extent in response to the body's requirements, this is certainly not sufficient to achieve venous return. For this, they need the aid of a pumping mechanism.

The heart pump

The assumption is sometimes made that the heart pumps blood right through the arteries, the capillaries and finally the veins.

However, any noticeable difference between systolic and diastolic pressure is quickly lost in the arterioles and capillaries, where blood pressure falls to around 5–15 mmHg due to increasing resistance. The heart does exert a mild 'pull' on the veins due to the pressure gradient between the right atrium (where the pressure is around 0 mmHg) and the venous system. While this is sufficient to produce some flow when a person is horizontal, it is insufficient in aiding venous return when upright.

The respiratory pump
The respiratory pump also plays a limited part in venous return. During inspiration of air, the diaphragm pushes against the abdomen, causing pressure to rise in the intra-abdominal veins. Meanwhile, pressure within the thorax (and hence also the intra-thoracic veins and right atrium) falls, with the result that blood is drawn from the abdominal cavity into the thorax. The deeper the inspiration, the greater the venous return. However, while it is helpful to teach patients deep breathing exercises, the respiratory pump on its own is by no means sufficient to produce adequate venous return when standing or sitting.

The calf muscle and foot pumps
By far the most important factors facilitating venous return from the leg are the calf and foot muscle pumps. The foot pump (contraction of the plantar muscles during movement) squeezes and empties the veins of the foot. Likewise, during exercise, the calf muscle contracts, compressing the deep vein and forcing blood to be displaced (Fig. 4.3). The one-way valves prevent blood from refluxing, forcing it to flow only upwards, against gravity. As the muscles relax once more, the deep vein expands causing the pressure within to drop below that of the superficial veins. The resulting pressure gradient draws blood from the superficial veins into the deep vein, via the perforators. As exercise continues, muscle contraction squeezes the re-filled deep vein, forcing blood towards the heart, and so the cycle continues.

The effectiveness of the calf muscle and foot pumps depends on healthy one-way valves and good ankle function. Valve incompetence and limited ankle movement are major contributors to the development of chronic venous hypertension. Moreover, since the

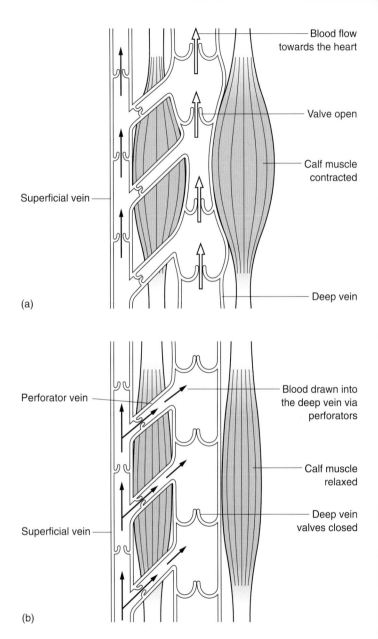

Fig. 4.3 Normal venous function showing intact valves. (a) Calf muscle contracted, (b) calf muscle relaxed.

calf and foot muscle pumps are largely inactive during sleep, a near-horizontal position is essential to achieve adequate venous return at night. Individuals who sleep in a chair or with their legs dependent are likely, over time, to develop chronic venous hypertension and dependent oedema.

Blood pressure in the veins and capillaries

As already mentioned, blood pressure in the capillary network is around 5–15 mmHg. Capillaries are delicate vessels – their walls are just one cell thick – and they are therefore unable to withstand higher pressures.

The superficial veins, though thicker walled than capillaries, are not designed to withstand prolonged high pressures, and are not generally required to do so in healthy individuals. The deep vein is able to withstand relatively high pressures during muscle contraction since it is well supported by the surrounding muscle. However, as with the superficial and perforator veins, sustained high pressure can cause the valves to become incompetent. Blood pressure within veins fluctuates according to an individual's position and level of activity. When standing, venous pressure is equal to the weight of the column of blood from the foot to the right side of the heart, and is around 80–100 mmHg (Partsch, 2003). This falls to just 10–20 mmHg when the calf muscle and foot pumps empty the veins during exercise (Fig. 4.4). Similarly, venous blood pressure is significantly reduced when an individual lies horizontally.

VENOUS DISEASE (CHRONIC VENOUS HYPERTENSION)

Venous disease occurs when the calf or foot muscle pumps are unable to effectively empty the veins, resulting, literally, in a chronic venous hypertension. Often it is a failure of the calf muscle pump due to valve incompetence (Coleridge-Smith, 1999), allowing blood to 'reflux' – to flow backwards towards the capillaries as well as forwards towards the heart. This may be due to a congenital defect of the valves, damage from a previous trauma, DVT, or prolonged back-pressure on the valves (for example, during pregnancy, pelvic tumours, obesity, or a prolonged standing occupation) (Morison & Moffatt, 1994).

Valve incompetence that occurs in the deep vein results in increased pressure on both the valve below and the

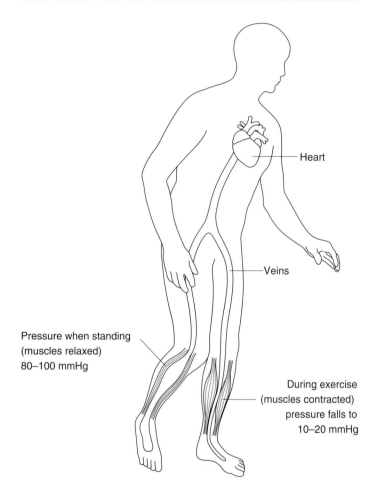

Heart

Veins

Pressure when standing
(muscles relaxed)
80–100 mmHg

During exercise
(muscles contracted)
pressure falls to
10–20 mmHg

Fig. 4.4 Venous pressures when standing and during exercise.

corresponding perforator vein valve(s). Consequently, these valves may also become incompetent, causing the superficial veins to varicose and the disease to progress (Fig. 4.5). The same 'domino effect' can occur whether the primary incompetence occurs in the perforator or superficial veins (see Fig. 4.5).

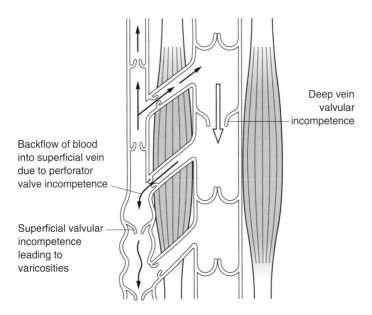

Fig. 4.5 Deep, superficial and perforator valve incompetence.

The situation is exacerbated in patients with calf muscle wastage, for example due to poor ankle mobility, long-term bandaging, arthritis and/or ulcer pain. Here the problem might be less to do with primary valve incompetence, and more to do with an inability to effectively reduce venous hypertension through exercise.

Damage to the capillary network

Chronic venous hypertension causes the pressure within the capillaries to rise above normal limits. Capillary walls are thin – generally comprising just one layer of endothelial cells supported by a basement membrane, but lacking any smooth muscle or supportive elastic tissue – and are not designed to withstand high pressures. They are also very porous. The pores are normally too small to allow larger molecules and blood cells to pass into the surrounding tissue. A rise in capillary pressure causes them to swell, stretching their delicate walls, so increasing the size of the pores and forcing blood products to leak out into the surrounding tissue.

Damage to the surrounding tissue

The exact series of events from initial chronic venous hypertension to capillary damage and tissue breakdown are not fully understood. A number of theories exist as to how exactly this happens, including the fibrin cuff theory (Browse & Burnand, 1982; Herrick et al., 1992), the white cell trapping theory (Coleridge-Smith et al., 1988), the mechanical theory (Chant, 1990) and the 'trap' growth factor theory (Higley et al., 1995). In reality, it is probably a combination of these working together that results in ulceration. These theories are summed up in Table 4.1, and their possible effect on the skin shown in Fig. 4.6.

Table 4.1 Summary of theories of venous ulceration (reproduced from Morison & Moffatt, 1994).

The fibrin cuff theory

Layers of fibrin are laid down as cuffs around the capillary wall causing a diffusion barrier to oxygen and nutrients, leading to trophic skin changes (Browse & Burnand, 1982). Herrick et al. (1992) noted that fibrin cuffs were more complex in nature and actively assembled by adjacent connective tissue in response to venous hypertension.

White cell trapping theory

Accumulation and activation of white cells in the microcirculation of patients with venous hypertension. Production of toxic metabolites leads to tissue breakdown (Coleridge-Smith et al., 1988).

Mechanical theory

Ulceration results from mechanical stress on the patient's limb. High pressure in the capillary bed leads to oedema, which in turn raises tissue pressure resulting in stretching of the skin. Ulceration is thought to arise from tissue ischaemia (Chant, 1990).

The 'trap' growth factor theory

Leakage of fibrinogen and protein-bound growth factors. The growth factors are trapped in the fibrin cuff preventing their normal use in epidermal tissue repair (Higley et al., 1995).

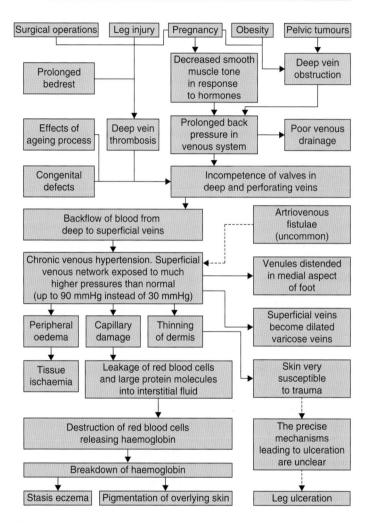

Fig. 4.6 Complications arising from venous hypertension (reproduced from Morison & Moffat, 1994).

RECOGNISING THOSE AT RISK OF VENOUS DISEASE

Risk factors are those things that predispose a person to an increased likelihood of developing a disease.

Knowing whether a patient is likely to have venous disease is useful since the signs and symptoms may be very subtle during the early stages. Practitioners also have a duty of care towards 'at-risk' patients in the form of health promotion.

Risk factors for venous disease should be assessed by looking at the patient's family history, medical history and personal factors.

Family history

- **Family history of venous disease**. There is some evidence that venous disease may be hereditary. Ask the patient if any close relatives have suffered with varicose veins, swollen legs or venous leg ulcers.

Medical history

- **Previous trauma**. Leg injury, including fractures, soft tissue injuries and burns, intravenous drug use and phlebitis, can permanently damage the veins.
- **Deep vein thrombosis (DVT)**. Many leg ulcer patients have venous disease secondary to a known or 'silent' DVT. Look for evidence that the patient may have been at increased risk and possibly suffered a silent DVT. Risk factors for DVT include a history of major surgery (particularly abdominal or orthopaedic surgery), prolonged immobility (including wearing a plaster cast), pregnancy, the oral contraceptive pill, clotting disorders and long distance travel. It is important to be aware that the effects of a DVT may only become manifest decades after the event.
- **Fixed or limited ankle function**. The calf muscle relies on good ankle function to pump blood through the veins towards the heart. Patients can lose their ankle mobility due to arthritis, injury or pain. There is also some evidence that patients with venous ulceration progressively lose their ankle function due to changes in the subcutaneous tissues. Long-term use of compression is associated with the progressive loss of calf muscle, although the reason for this remains obscure.

- **Chronic constipation**. Chronic constipation, for example due to a low fibre diet, is thought to increase the amount of pressure the veins have to withstand (Lee et al., 1999) and can lead to valve failure.
- **Obesity**. Excess body weight may exert increased pressure on the valves and is frequently associated with reduced mobility (Lee et al., 1999).

Personal factors

- **Pregnancy**. There appears to be a strong link between pregnancy and the development of varicose veins (Lee at al., 1999), possibly due to an increased risk of DVT, and/or to increased abdominal pressure. It is unclear as to whether pregnancy causes venous disease, or simply exacerbates it. Hormonal changes may also affect the muscle layer within the veins, making them vulnerable to becoming varicosed.
- **Occupations requiring prolonged standing or sitting**. These appear to increase the risk of developing venous disease, presumably due to the prolonged periods of pressure on the veins (Lee et al., 1999).
- **Being tall**. This increases the height of the column of pressure from the legs to the heart, and may increase the risk of venous disease (Lee at al., 1999).
- **Being female**. Historically, studies have tended to find that women are more commonly affected than men (Franks et al., 1992). The results of the Edinburgh Vein Study suggest that this may be changing, with chronic venous insufficiency and mild varicose veins being more common in men, though possibly more severe in women (Evans et al., 1998; Evans et al., 1999). These authors have suggested the reasons for this shift are changes in lifestyle, working practices and the environment, and the tendency for women to have fewer children. It may also be that pregnant women are becoming more aware of the risk of developing venous disease during pregnancy, and are taking preventative measures, such as wearing compression hosiery.
- **Age**. Venous disease is a common condition throughout the adult population, though prevalence does appear to increase with age (Franks et al., 1992; Callam, 1999; Evans et al., 1999).

- **Social class**. Though venous ulceration has often been thought of as a condition that affects the lower social classes, the Edinburgh Vein Study found no evidence to suggest that the prevalence of venous disease was related to any particular social class (Evans et al., 1999).

RECOGNISING CLINICAL EVIDENCE OF VENOUS DISEASE

Practitioners who manage leg ulcer patients need to develop excellent clinical skills in identifying the signs and symptoms of venous disease. This involves a thorough investigation of any venous history, venous skin changes and venous pain.

Venous history

A history of DVT, thrombophlebitis, vein surgery or sclerotherapy indicates that the veins are, to a greater or lesser extent, damaged.

Venous skin changes

Venous skin changes almost always occur in the gaiter region – between the ankle and mid calf. Occasionally, they can extend onto the foot or up to the knee. It is important to note that not all patients with venous disease present with all – or even most – of the characteristic skin changes. However, identification of just one or two signs is usually sufficient to form a diagnosis of venous disease. If in doubt, referral should be made to a specialist for further investigation.

The first step is to look for swollen blood vessels, followed by signs of leakage of blood products into the skin.

Varicose veins (Fig. 4.7)

These appear to be the most common manifestation of venous disease (Franks et al., 1992). For patients who have had a DVT that extends into the iliac veins or those with congenital venous conditions such as Klippel–Trenaunay syndrome, varicose veins may extend into the thigh or abdomen. Ask the patient to stand up – this will cause any varicose veins to fill, and be easier to spot. Check for varicose veins in the thigh and groin, as well as below the knee.

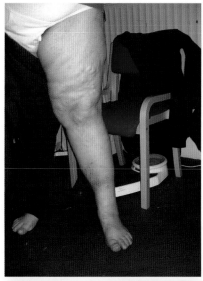

Fig. 4.7 Varicose veins.

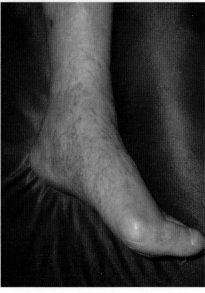

Fig. 4.8 Ankle flare and atrophie blanche.

Ankle flare (Fig. 4.8)

This is seen as tiny varicose veins on the inner aspect of the foot and ankle, and is generally due to perforator vein incompetence.

Atrophie blanche (see Fig. 4.8)

In this condition, white 'lacy' areas of avascular tissue, interspersed by visibly engorged capillaries, are seen as tiny red 'dots' just below the surface of the skin. Patches may be small or extensive, may arise on skin that has never ulcerated or at the site of previous ulceration. Some patches may be almost completely avascular, with little sign of capillaries, while others may exhibit mainly engorged capillary heads with only small areas of white scarring. It can be harder to detect on darker skin, but white areas of scarring are usually visible.

The exact pathological processes involved in the formation of atrophie blanche are not understood, but it is thought that venous hypertension leads to thrombosis and obliteration of capillaries within the skin (Vowden, 1998). The resulting localised hypoxic areas can remain static for months or years, or may progress through to ulceration. There is some evidence that atrophie blanche may be linked to a fibrinolytic disorder and that drugs that inhibit platelet thrombosis or stimulate fibrinolytic activity can be beneficial (Vowden, 1998), and some specialists advocate the use of pentoxifylline.

Patients often describe excruciating shooting or stabbing neuropathic pain. This is probably due to a combination of localised ischaemia and inflammation of the capillary walls. Although compression is necessary to reverse the venous hypertension and prevent the lesions from progressing to further ulceration, the associated pain can make the introduction of full compression intolerable.

Pain associated with atrophie blanche responds much better to low-dose, tricyclic antidepressants (e.g. amitriptyline) or anticonvulsants (e.g. gabapentin), than it does to paracetamol, codeine or opiates. NSAIDs can also be effective. Start by introducing adequate analgesia, then slowly introduce reduced compression, building it up to full compression over several weeks as tolerated. Most patients find they can reduce or stop their analgesia once the venous hypertension is adequately controlled.

Although atrophie blanche is seen most commonly in association with venous hypertension, it can also occur in a number of other dermatological conditions such as vasculitis. If pain remains uncontrolled or if other signs of venous disease are absent, referral to a leg ulcer specialist or dermatologist is necessary.

Haemosiderin staining (Fig. 4.9)
This appears as a red/brown discoloration of the skin, caused by leakage and subsequent breakdown of red blood cells from the capillary network into the skin. It may present as small localised patches, or extend over most of the gaiter region. Haemosiderin staining is usually seen as a deep-brown discoloration on darker skin.

Lipodermatosclerosis (Fig. 4.10)
The term 'lipodermatosclerosis' describes the characteristic hardening (fibrosis) of the subcutaneous fatty layer of the skin that is often seen in venous disease. It is thought to be due to leakage and the laying down of fibrin from the capillary network, fat necrosis, chronic inflammation and scarring (Browse & Burnand, 1982). It presents as a hard, woody layer just below the surface of the skin. It can be quite localised, such as around an ulcer, but often begins in the ankle region and, over months and years, gradually extends up to the mid calf area. This process can give rise to an inverted champagne bottle-shaped leg, where any soft swelling only accumulates in the calf, distorting the leg shape since the skin around the ankle is too 'tight' to stretch.

Lipodermatosclerosis can present in either an acute or chronic state (Vowden, 1998). In the acute phase the condition presents as an acute, painful inflammation, often mistaken for cellulitis, resulting in inappropriate treatment with antibiotics. However, unlike cellulitis, its borders are unlikely to change quickly and the patient will not present with pyrexia. Often the upper border over the shin will present as a characteristic inverted 'V' shape. Unless treated with compression, the leg is likely to become increasingly inflamed, and the skin may begin to break down. As in the case of atrophie blanche, the pain is likely to render full compression

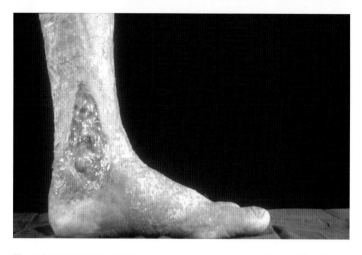

Fig. 4.9 Haemosiderin staining and classic venous ulcer on the medial malleolus.

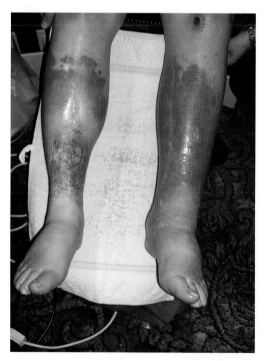

Fig. 4.10 Lipoder-matosclerosis giving rise to an 'inverted cham-pagne bottle'-shaped right leg, with pitting oedema exacer-bated by acute cardiac failure.

intolerable at first, and compression must be introduced gradually in combination with adequate analgesia. Very occasionally, a patient may need to be admitted to hospital for high leg elevation and morphine before the inflammation resolves sufficiently for compression to be tolerated. Generally, acute lipodermatosclerosis progresses to a chronic state.

Chronic lipodermatosclerosis may or may not begin with an acute episode. It tends to present as a discoloured area of leathery skin that is too tight to 'pinch up'. The colour can range from a pale to relatively dark brown. It may be harder to detect on darker skin, but a change in depth of colour can usually be seen when the whole leg is examined.

Varicose eczema (Fig. 4.11)

This is caused by irritation from blood products that have leaked into the skin. It may present as either a wet or dry eczema, can be localised to just around the ulcer, or may involve the whole gaiter region. Occasionally, the severity of the eczema, combined

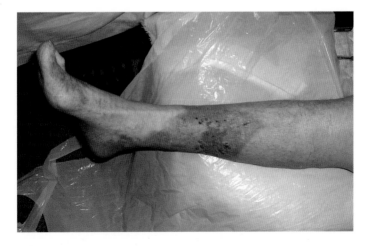

Fig. 4.11 Varicose eczema.

with scratching, can result in a much more widespread manifestation. It can be quite difficult to differentiate varicose eczema from contact dermatitis and irritant eczema – both of which are commonly associated with leg ulceration and may even be found in combination with varicose eczema. However, if there is other evidence of venous disease, and the patient has not been exposed to potential allergens or external irritants, then varicose eczema should be suspected.

Venous oedema

Here, the oedema tends to be pitting and to resolve, at least partially, at night if the patient goes to bed. It should not be confused with cardiac or renal oedema, both of which are also pitting, since treatment for these conditions will vary (Hoffman, 1998). Check for a past history, and other symptoms, of renal or cardiac oedema, such as shortness of breath; if in doubt refer the patient to their GP for review. If only one leg is affected it is unlikely to be cardiac or renal in origin, but is suggestive of venous disease of that limb. If it extends above the knee into the thigh then it is unlikely to be purely venous in origin.

Venous calcification (Fig. 4.12)

Very occasionally, patients with venous disease develop calcium stones within the skin. Over time these can make their way up to the surface, resulting in skin breakdown, and eventually the stone lifts. They are white or yellow and can initially be mistaken for slough, but are rock hard.

Venous ulcers (see Fig. 4.9)

Typically, these occur in the medial or lateral gaiter region. Ulcers higher up on the calf are unlikely to be purely venous in origin, though venous disease may be present. Venous ulcers rarely occur on the foot; when they do, it is usually due to tracking of infection, maceration from an ulcer higher up or over an area of atrophie blanche, or following the line of the lymphatics across the top of the foot due to chronic lymphangiitis (Fig. 4.13). They tend to be shallow with ragged edges.

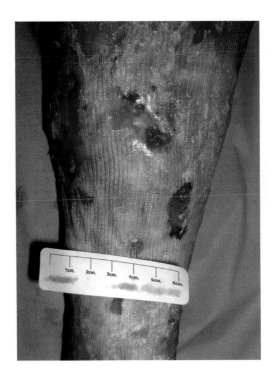

Fig. 4.12 Venous calcification.

Venous pain

The patient's description of their pain may provide valuable clues as to the presence of venous disease. Pain in venous ulceration is a complex phenomenon and is covered in detail in Chapter 9.

Clues that pain may be venous in origin include:

- A tired dull ache that is worse towards the end of the day and when standing, due to venous congestion.
- A sharp neuropathic pain associated with atrophie blanche or acute lipodermatosclerosis.

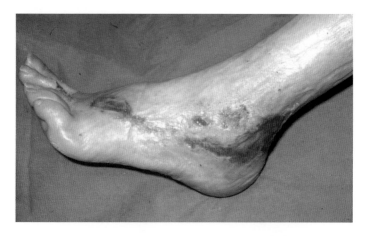

Fig. 4.13 Venous ulceration tracking onto the foot due to chronic lymphangiitis.

- A 'venous rush' pain when first getting out of bed in the morning caused by sudden venous reflux and relieved with exercise.

DIAGNOSTIC TESTS FOR VENOUS DISEASE

In most cases it is possible to diagnose the presence of venous disease without the use of a scan or other diagnostic equipment. Indeed, there is usually little or no access to scanning equipment in the community, and practitioners must rely almost entirely on their clinical assessment skills and ability to recognise the signs and symptoms of venous disease.

Sometimes venous disease is suspected but signs and symptoms are subtle, inconclusive or could be indicative of another disorder. For example, atrophie blanche can be associated with vasculitis, pitting oedema may suggest cardiac failure, and eczema may be due to contact sensitivity. In such situations diagnostic tests are invaluable. Referral for further investigation should also be encouraged, particularly if the patient is willing to consider possible vein surgery with a view to reducing the risk of recurrence.

Doppler ultrasound

Doppler ABPI measures blood flow in the arteries and is not an indicator of venous disease. Although recognition of venous disease is primarily through observation of its clinical signs and symptoms, it can be confirmed by non-invasive investigations such as hand-held Doppler assessment of venous reflux and Duplex ultrasound scanning.

While Doppler ABPI measurement cannot be used to assess for the presence of venous disease, it is possible to carry out a basic test for deep venous reflux using the same portable Doppler machine. Ask the patient to stand and face away from you. Place some ultrasound gel behind the back of their knee and locate the arterial pulse. Shift the probe slightly to one side, over the vein, and gently squeeze the patient's calf. A 'rush' of blood should be heard if the probe is correctly placed over the vein. Let go of the patient's calf and listen for a second 'rush', which indicates deep venous reflux. A similar procedure can be used to locate superficial vein incompetence in the groin. Note, however, that this is a basic test and will not detect all potential areas of vein incompetence.

Photophlethysmography

In addition to portable Doppler ultrasound, photophlethysmography can provide useful information in the community setting. While not as detailed or reliable as a Duplex scan, it can at least provide instant and relatively low-cost information regarding the presence, severity and, to some extent, location of venous disease. Unlike Doppler ABPI, it is not considered an essential tool in leg ulcer assessment at present. However, it is an important tool for use in the community, particularly amongst specialist nurses, as it is portable and can provide rapid assessment of venous function as well as information on whether venous insufficiency is within the deep or superficial system.

A number of plethysmography techniques and machines are available. Photoplethysmography uses infra-red light to detect the effectiveness of the calf muscle pump on capillary emptying and refill times during and after exercise. The test takes place with the patient seated with their feet placed flat on the floor. Note that the floor should not be unduly hot or cold as this could affect the reading. A sensor is placed on the gaiter region, and records capillary emptying while the patient undertakes ten dorsiflexions. The patient then rests for 45 seconds, during which time the machine senses and calculates capillary refill time. A refill time of less than 20 seconds indicates venous reflux. The test is then repeated several times with a blood pressure cuff applied at differing intervals along the leg, acting as a tourniquet to 'obliterate' the adjacent veins. This allows the practitioner to determine whether the incompetence is located in the deep or superficial system.

Colour Duplex

Patients referred to a scanning department for vein studies will generally undergo a Duplex (colour Doppler) scan. This non-invasive test is used to locate and map the presence of any venous incompetence, usually prior to vein surgery. Waiting lists are sometimes long. A number of the studies encourage early scanning while an ulcer is present, and some centres perform varicose vein surgery when the ulcer is open. Others prefer to wait until after healing to reduce the risk of infection. Occasionally, it can prove impossible to heal the ulcer until surgery is performed due to the severity of venous disease, and close liaison is needed between the primary care team and vascular team to ensure patients are not left waiting indefinitely for surgery.

SUMMARY

- The majority of patients with leg ulceration have some degree of venous disease.
- All patients with leg ulceration should be screened for clinical signs and symptoms of venous disease, and, where appropriate, referred to a vascular team for further investigation and possible surgery.
- The presence of venous disease suggests that the ulcer is likely to be venous in origin. However, many patients experience complex multi-factorial ulcers, where two or more disorders contribute to ulceration. Assessment should include screening for other possible ulcer aetiologies.
- Venous disease is generally managed in the first instance with compression therapy, exercise and leg elevation. Where necessary, referral to the multi-disciplinary team should be made to address wider factors affecting healing.
- Venous ulcers that fail to progress within 1 month of commencing treatment, or fail to heal after 3 months of treatment, should be referred to a specialist team for further investigation.
- Patients with venous disease should be encouraged to wear compression hosiery and consider vein surgery to reduce the risk of ulceration or re-ulceration.

REFERENCES

Blair, S.D., Wright, D.D.I., Backhouse, C.M., Riddle, E. & McCollum, C.N. (1988) Sustained compression and healing of chronic venous ulcers. *British Medical Journal* **297**: 1159–1161.

Breddin, H.K., Browse, N.L., Coleridge-Smith, P.D., Cornu-Thenard, A., Dormandy, J.A., Franzeck, U.K., et al. (1992) Consensus paper on venous leg ulcers. *Phlebology* **7**: 48–58.

Browse, N.L. & Burnand, K.G. (1982) The cause of venous ulceration. *Lancet* ii: 243–245.

Callam, M.J. (1994) Epidemiology of varicose veins. *British Journal of Surgery* **81**: 167–173.

Callam, M.J. (1999) Leg ulcer and chronic venous insufficiency in the community. In: *Venous Disease. Epidemiology, Management and Delivery of Care* (C.V. Ruckley, F.G.R. Fowkes & A.W. Bradbury, eds). London, Springer-Verlag, pp. 15–25.

Callam, M.J., Harper, D.R., Dale, J.J. & Ruckely, C.V. (1987) Chronic ulcer of the leg: clinical history. *British Medical Journal* **294**: 1389–1391.

Chant, A.D.P. (1990) Tissue pressure, posture and venous ulceration. *Lancet* **336**: 1050–1051.

Coleridge-Smith, P.D. (1999) How does a leg ulcerate? In: *Venous Disease. Epidemiology, Management and Delivery of Care* (C.V. Ruckley, F.G.R. Fowkes & A.W. Bradbury, eds). London, Springer-Verlag, pp. 51–70.

Coleridge-Smith, P., Thomas, P., Scurr, J.M. & Dormandy, J.A. (1988) Causes of venous ulceration: a new hypothesis. *British Medical Journal* **296**: 1726–1727.

Cornwall, J., Dore, C.J. & Lewis, J.D. (1986) Leg ulcers: epidemiology and aetiology. *British Journal of Surgery* **73**: 693–696.

Cullum, N., Nelson, E.A., Fletcher, A.W. & Sheldon, T.A. (2001) Compression for venous ulcers. *Cochrane Database Systematic Reviews* Issue 2, www.cochrane.org/reviews/en/ab000265.html

Evans, C.J., Allan, P.L., Lee, A.J., Bradbury, A.W., Ruckley, C.V. & Fowkes, F.G. (1998) Prevalence of venous reflux in the general population on duplex scanning: the Edinburgh Vein Study. *Journal of Vascular Surgery* **28**(5): 767–776.

Evans, C.J., Fowkes, F.G.R., Ruckely, C.V. & Lee, A.J. (1999) Prevalence of varicose veins and chronic venous insufficiency in men and women in the general population: Edinburgh Vein Study. *Journal of Epidemiology and Community Health* **53**: 149–153.

Franks, P.C., David, D.I., Moffatt, C.J., Stirling, J., Fletcher, A.E., Bulpitt, C.J. & McCollum, C.N. (1992) Prevalence of venous disease: a community study in West London. *European Journal of Surgery* **158**: 143–147.

Herrick, S.E., Sloan, P., McGurk, M., Freak, L., McCollum, C.N. & Ferguson, M.W.J. (1992) Sequential changes in histological pattern and extracellular matrix deposition during the healing of chronic venous ulcers. *American Journal of Pathology* **14**(5): 1085–1095.

Higley, H.R., Ksander, G.A., Gerhardt, C.O. & Falanga, V. (1995) Extravasation of macromolecules and possible trapping of transferring growth factor in ulceration. *British Journal of Dermatology* **132**: 79–85.

Hoffman, D. (1998) Oedema and the management of venous ulcers. *Journal of Wound Care* **7**(7): 345–348.

Lee, A.J., Evans, C.J., Ruckley, C.V. & Fowkes, F.G.R. (1999) Does lifestyle really affect venous disease? In: *Venous Disease. Epidemiology, Management and Delivery of Care* (C.V. Ruckley, F.G.R. Fowkes & A.W. Bradbury, eds). London, Springer-Verlag, pp. 32–41.

Moffatt, C.J., Franks, P.J., Doherty, D.C., Martin, R., Blewett, R. & Ross, F. (2004) Prevalence of leg ulceration in a London population. *Quarterly Journal of Medicine* **97**: 431–437.

Morison, M. & Moffatt, C. (1994) Leg ulcers. In: *A Colour Guide to the Nursing Management of Chronic Wounds*, 2nd edn (M. Morison, C. Moffatt, J. Bridel-Nixon & S. Bale, eds). London, Mosby, pp. 177–220.

Nelzen, O., Bergquist, D. & Lindhagen, A. (1991) Leg ulcer etiology – a cross sectional population study. *Journal of Vascular Surgery* **14**: 557–564.

Partsch, H. (2003) Understanding the pathophysiological effects of compression. In: *Understanding Compression Therapy, European Wound Management Association Position Document.* London, MEP, pp. 2–4.

Phillips, T. (2001) Current approaches to venous ulcers and compression. *Dermatologic Surgery* **27**: 611–621.

Royal College of Nursing (1998) *Clinical Practice Guidelines. The Management of Patients with Venous Leg Ulcers.* University of York and University of Manchester, RCN Institute.

Ruckley, C.V., Dale, J.J., Callum, M.J. & Harper, D.R. (1982) Causes of chronic leg ulcer. *Lancet* **ii**: 615–616.

Task Force on Chronic Venous Disorders of the Leg (1999) The management of chronic venous disorders of the leg: an evidence based report of an international task force. *Phlebology* **14**(Suppl.1): 52–65.

Vowden, K. (1998) Lipodermatosclerosis and atrophie blanche. *Journal of Wound Care* **7**(9): 441–443.

Arterial Disease

LEARNING OBJECTIVES

Nurses involved in leg ulcer management should be able to demonstrate:

❏ An understanding of normal arterial function.
❏ An understanding of peripheral arterial occlusive disease (PAOD) and its role in leg ulceration.
❏ The ability to identify those patients at increased risk of peripheral arterial occlusive disease.
❏ The ability to identify the clinical signs and symptoms of peripheral arterial occlusive disease.
❏ An understanding of the role and findings of diagnostic tests for peripheral arterial occlusive disease.

INTRODUCTION

Prevalence studies consistently suggest that arterial disease is the second single most common cause of leg ulceration in the Western world. The Lothian & Forth Valley study (Callam et al., 1987) found evidence of arterial disease in 21% of patients identified: with 10% of leg ulcers being due purely to arterial disease, and a further 10–15% being of mixed arterial and venous origin. Cornwall et al.'s (1986) epidemiology and aetiology study revealed similar findings, with 9% of patients with a leg ulcer due exclusively to an ischaemic element and 22% having both an ischaemic and venous cause. Adam et al. (2003) identified 100 ulcerated limbs out of 689 (14.5%) that were due to mixed arterial and venous disease, and only 2% to arterial disease. Results from the Wandsworth study (Moffatt et al., 2004) indicate that 15% of ulcers were due to a combination of venous and arterial disease, 1% were related to arterial disease with diabetes and 4% were due purely to arterial disease.

The notable factor about the prevalence of arterial disease is that, while the overall percentage rates may seem to be low in comparison to venous disease, the number of people affected increases significantly in line with advancing age. Therefore in light of a growing elderly population it is likely that prevalence levels will escalate further. Fowkes (1997) found that peripheral arterial occlusive disease affects around 30% of older people amongst the general population.

The main concerns relate to the failure to adequately screen for the presence of arterial disease in patients presenting with leg ulceration, not only the likely scenario of ineffective care, but alarmingly the potential to cause harm to the patient (see the case study below). High levels of compression therapy are dangerous when applied to limbs with severe arterial insufficiency. Moreover, patients with peripheral arterial disease who are not offered referral for vascular assessment and intervention are less likely to heal, and may experience progression of the disease resulting in amputation or even death.

Case study

Mr Jones had a mixed venous/arterial leg ulcer. He was on the waiting list for vascular intervention. Meanwhile, he was being treated successfully with a reduced level of compression therapy using a short-stretch bandage regime applied by his practice nurse.

When the practice nurse was unexpectedly taken ill, his care was transferred temporarily to the district nursing team. The team, faced with the usual time pressures, failed to perform a leg ulcer assessment or seek further information from his medical records and, instead, made assumptions about his ulcer aetiology based on the fact that he was being treated with compression therapy. Assuming he had an uncomplicated venous ulcer, his treatment was changed to an elastic high-compression system preferred by the team, which resulted in excruciating night pain and wound breakdown. He was admitted to hospital for emergency vascular intervention, and lost confidence in the ability of the district nursing team to treat him safely.

Best practice

- Patients who present with leg ulceration should be carefully screened for the presence of peripheral arterial occlusive disease (PAOD) (Callam et al., 1987).
- Doppler assessment for ABPI measurement is considered mandatory in leg ulcer assessment; palpitation of pedal pulses alone is unreliable (Vowden & Vowden, 2002).
- Nurses should be able to recognise the risk factors for PAOD. They have a responsibility to help ensure that patients with PAOD (and other forms of cardiovascular disease) receive appropriate intervention and education, with the aim of reducing cardiovascular mortality and morbidity, preventing disease progression and improving the benefit of long-term revascularisation procedures (Tierney et al., 2000; Aronow, 2005).

UNDERSTANDING NORMAL ARTERIAL FUNCTION

In order to assess for the presence of PAOD, the practitioner needs to understand both normal arterial function and arterial disease.

Function of the arteries

The arteries perform two key functions. First, they act as a network of tubes transporting oxygenated blood from the left ventricle of the heart to the tissues. Second, the muscular tone and elastic nature of the arteries enables them to sustain an adequate blood pressure and therefore blood flow during diastole. These will be described in further detail below. Other functions relate largely to the regulatory role of the endothelium, which is now recognised as playing a significant role in cardiovascular haemostasis (Jones, 2001).

Structure of the arteries

Fig. 5.1 shows the main arteries of the leg.

Mechanism of the arteries

So how do the arteries maintain an adequately high blood pressure to allow transport of sufficient blood to each of the body's organs?

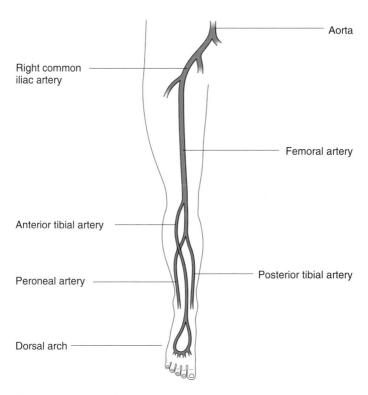

Fig. 5.1 Main arteries of the leg.

To answer this question, we must consider more closely the blood pressure within the arteries.

Pressures within the arteries

As can be seen in Fig. 5.2, the pressure generated by the heart is virtually lost by the time the blood has completed its journey back to the right atrium. This loss of pressure begins in the arterioles as they approach the capillaries. A thickening of the smooth muscle layer acts as a sphincter controlling the flow of blood into the capillary. The capillaries, being made of only one or two layers of endothelium, would be unable to withstand such high pressures

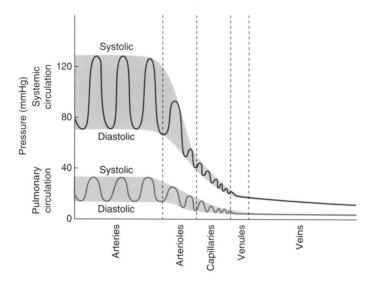

Fig. 5.2 Changing pressures within the circulatory system (reproduced from Widmaier et al. *Vander, Sherman, Luciano's Human Physiology: The Mechanisms of Body Functions, Ninth Edition* (2004) with permission of The McGraw-Hill Companies).

straight from the arterioles, thus a drop in pressure at this stage is critical.

The two key characteristics of arteries that maintain blood pressure relate to the levels of elastic fibres and smooth muscle tissue present. Certain arteries in the body can be described as being elastic (conducting) or muscular (distributing) arteries (Jones, 2001).

Arteries such as the aorta, pulmonary, common carotid and iliac arteries are highly elastic, allowing them to stretch and fill considerably during systole, much like a balloon. Thus roughly only one-third of the volume of blood that leaves the heart passes out of the arteries into the arterioles during systole. The remaining two-thirds is temporarily stored in the now expanded arteries. As ventricular contraction ends and diastole begins, the arteries recoil, much like a balloon beginning to deflate, thus pushing blood forward into the arterioles, and arterial pressure begins to fall. It is only allowed to fall a little, however, as the next ventricular contraction rapidly occurs and the cycle of systole and diastole begins again.

The more muscular arteries, such as the axillary, brachial, intercostal, femoral and popliteal, adjust their diameter (by contraction or relaxation of the muscle tissues) in response to sympathetic stimulation, thereby increasing or decreasing the resistance of blood flow. This allows the control of blood pressure by fluctuating the pressures in different arteries according to the needs of the body at any given time. For example, during exercise, when greater levels of blood and oxygen are needed by the skeletal muscles, the arteries supplying the arms and legs will dilate and arteries supplying the gastrointestinal system will constrict (Jones, 2001).

The role of the endothelium
The endothelium also plays a significant role in the maintenance of arterial pressure. It achieves this by producing and releasing factors (such as nitric oxide) which a relaxing effect on the smooth muscle of the artery resulting in vasodilation, and endothelins which have a constrictive effect (Jones, 2001).

It is this healthy functioning of the arterial network – the ability to alter the resistance of blood flow, the highly elastic walls and normal endothelial function – that enables a sufficient flow of blood to reach the body's organs.

UNDERSTANDING PERIPHERAL ARTERIAL OCCLUSIVE DISEASE AND ITS PART IN ARTERIAL ULCERATION
Arterial occlusive disease is a failure of the arteries to deliver sufficient blood to a particular part of the body resulting in tissue ischaemia (oxygen starvation); ultimately, it can lead to cellular death. If this occurs in the legs it is known as 'peripheral arterial occlusive disease' (PAOD), which, if present for a prolonged period, will lead to poorly nourished skin. Such skin is vulnerable to trauma and infection and is unable, or at least limited in its abilities, to repair itself due to poor oxygen and nutrient supply (Fig. 5.3). Aside from major trauma (severing of the blood vessels) and frostbite, there are several possible reasons why PAOD occurs.

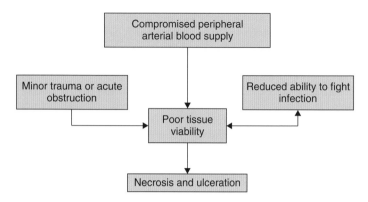

Fig. 5.3 Development of arterial ulceration (adapted from Morison & Moffatt, 1994).

Atherosclerosis

The most common cause of arterial disease is atherosclerosis, which involves the formation of fatty deposits (plaques) in the intima wall of the arteries. This gives rise to a number of complications, including the narrowing of the lumen (stenosis), the loss of arterial compliance (hardening of the artery) and endothelial dysfunction. These complications significantly reduce the pressure and therefore the volume of blood reaching the organs distal to the disease.

Atherosclerosis can affect any muscular artery in the body, and is responsible for a number of medical conditions, depending on which arteries are affected (Table 5.1). It is a major cause of death in westernised societies, primarily leading to heart disease and stroke.

While the initial stages of atherosclerosis (formation of fatty streaks) may begin in childhood, it is only in adulthood (30+ years) that atheromatous plaques really develop. Only when the lumen is occluded by 75% will symptoms be experienced (Shah, 1997). The risk factors linked with the development of atherosclerosis are well documented (Table 5.2). They can be grouped into modifiable and non-modifiable factors, although it may be argued that some factors classified as modifiable in fact have genetic links (Lusis,

Table 5.1 Effects of atherosclerosis (adapted from Ockenden, 2001).

Area of atherosclerosis	Resulting conditions
Heart	Coronary artery disease
	Angina
	Myocardial infarction
Brain	Stroke
	Trans-ischaemic attack
Kidneys	Renal failure
	Hypertension
Lower limbs	Peripheral arterial disease
	Acute/critical limb ischaemia
Thorax and abdomen	Aortic aneurysm
	Aortic dissection
Gut	Mesenteric artery disease
	Intestinal angina

Table 5.2 Risk factors for atherosclerosis (adapted from Cooke, 2001).

Modifiable risk factors	Non-modifiable risk factors	Other suspected risk factors
Cigarette smoking	Family history	Obesity
Hypertension	Advancing age	
Diabetes mellitus		Oestrogen deficiency (being male or female after the menopause)
Hypercholesterolaemia		
		Elevated levels of homocysteine
		Thrombogenic factors (affecting blood viscosity)
		Lack of exercise

2000), which may make modifications or control of these factors difficult. As atherosclerosis is the leading cause of PAOD, including both critical and acute limb ischaemia, the risk factors for both are similar.

Acute arterial thrombus or embolism

A thrombus, such as an unstable atheromatous plaque, can originate from an area of diseased artery, though other conditions can also result in thrombus formation, e.g. atrial fibrillation. When a thrombus embolises (becomes mobile within the bloodstream) it can become lodged in a smaller artery and cause an occlusion. Other substances (such as air and fat) can also embolise. For patients who develop this sudden occlusion and subsequent cessation of blood flow, the onset of symptoms – the five Ps: Pain, Pallor, Paraesthesia, Pulseless and Perishing cold – tends to be rapid and severe as there has been insufficient time to develop collateral vessels. This is an acute situation (acute limb ischaemia), though it can also occur in addition to chronic limb ischaemia. Urgent diagnosis and treatment is vital in the case of complete acute ischaemia, necessitating surgical revascularisation within 6 hours of its onset (Callum & Bradbury, 2000).

Inflammatory vascular disease

Buerger's disease (also known as 'thromboangiitis obliterans') is a rare progressive degenerative disease affecting the small- and medium-sized arteries and veins. The vessel wall becomes inflamed due to an occlusion that is surrounded by numerous non-specific immune cells, ultimately depriving cells distal to the occlusion of oxygen and nutrients (comparable to a thromboembolism), and consequently resulting in ischaemic symptoms such as intermittent claudication (Olin, 2000). However, compared to acute arterial embolisms the cause and patient profile affected is not the same, and remains somewhat perplexing.

Buerger's disease occurs predominately in young men; though it is becoming more apparent in woman, the male : female sex ratio still weighs heavily towards men at 7.5 : 1 (Mills & Porter, 1991). While the actual cause of Buerger's disease remains unknown, it has long been associated with tobacco use and, most commonly, heavy cigarette smoking. The increasing numbers of female smokers over the past century may support the theory of why the disease is now occurring a little more frequently in women. It is not fully understood what role smoking plays in the onset of the disease, but there are definite improvements in the condition with smoking cessation and recurrence of symptoms when smoking is resumed. Mills (2003) suggests that, based on more recent studies of patients with Buerger's disease, the condition appears to be an immunological one initiated by an, as yet, unknown antigen in the intimal layer of the vessel. Smoking cessation is the most important element in treating Buerger's disease. The distribution of Buerger's disease remains quite uneven across the world, with the highest incidence levels occurring in India, Japan, Korea, Sri Lanka and in Ashkenazi Jews (Olin, 2000). A couple of the theories for this pattern of distribution relate to the type of tobacco smoked in these regions or to a possible genetic predisposition (Mills, 2003).

RECOGNISING THOSE AT RISK OF PERIPHERAL ARTERIAL OCCLUSIVE DISEASE

The first step in screening a patient for the presence of PAOD is to look at whether they are likely to have the condition. This involves looking at the patient's:

- Family history
- Medical history
- Personal factors

It is important to note that the presence of PAOD also leads to a significant risk of other potentially more serious conditions, such as coronary artery disease and cerebrovascular disease, and more generally to an increased risk of cardiovascular disease (CVD) morbidity and mortality. The greater the extent or severity of the PAOD, the greater the risk of CVD (Golomb et al., 2001). Therefore a major benefit of identifying those at risk is being able to work with the patient in implementing measures to reduce progression of their disease.

Family history

- Record any family history of cardiovascular, cerebrovascular disease or peripheral arterial disease and leg ulceration (Goodall, 2001).

Medical history

- **Diabetes**. Find out if the patient has recently been screened for diabetes and obtain the result, or arrange for a fasting blood glucose test and urinalysis. It is well known that diabetes mellitus is associated with the premature and rapid progression of atherosclerosis (Jones, 2001) and is a major risk factor in the development of PAOD (Golomb et al., 2001).

- **Hypertension**. Record the patient's blood pressure in both arms, as well as details of any antihypertensive medication (Goodall, 2001). Hypertension accelerates the progression of atherosclerosis (Jones, 2001). It is commonly present in patients with PAOD. However, it is not acknowledged to be a significant factor in the development of PAOD alone, but is more significant in the presence of other risk factors (Golomb et al., 2001).
- **Cholesterol**. Record the results of a lipid profile measured within the last 12 months, or arrange for the test to be done and check if the patient is taking any cholesterol-lowering medication. High serum cholesterol levels lead to enhanced plaque formation (Goodall, 2001). Raised levels of low-density lipoproteins (LDL) increase the risk of atheroma. High-density lipoproteins (HDL) protect against plaque formation.
- **Other arterial disease**. Record any history of arterial disease affecting other parts of the patient's body, e.g. angina, myocardial infarction (MI), cardiac bypass/angioplasty, transient ischaemic attack (TIA), stroke or kidney disease.

Personal factors
- **Smoking**. Record the patient's smoking history (current or reformed and daily amount). Smoking is the most significant risk factor for the development of PAOD; it damages the vascular endothelium and increases the rate of progression of atherosclerosis (Goodall, 2001).
- **Exercise**. Record the patient's weekly exercise level (Goodall, 2001). Exercise is thought to increase HDL levels, thus protecting against atherosclerosis (Jones, 2001). The National Service Framework on Coronary Heart Disease (DH, 2000) recommends that adults undertake 30 minutes of moderately intense activity (such as a brisk walk) at least five times per week.
- **Stress**. Biochemical and immune response changes associated with stress may predispose patients to atherosclerosis (Herbert, 1997).
- **Age**. Increased age has been found to be a major risk factor for the development of PAOD (Golomb et al., 2001). In the Lothian & Forth Valley Study, no instances of arterial insufficiency were found in leg ulcer patients aged 40 years or under, but from the

age of 40 to the mid-90s, the number of patients affected rose steadily to 50% (Callam et al., 1987).

- **Gender**. The incidence of atherosclerosis appears to be higher in men than women under 70 years of age, but is similar in both sexes over the age of 70 (DTB, 2002).

RECOGNISING CLINICAL EVIDENCE OF PERIPHERAL ARTERIAL OCCLUSIVE DISEASE

Practitioners who manage patients with leg ulceration need to develop competence in recognising the clinical signs and symptoms of PAOD. This requires thorough assessment of the patient's peripheral arterial history and the presence of any ischaemic tissue changes or arterial pain.

Peripheral arterial history

- Record any history of arterial bypass or angioplasty in either leg, or previous lower limb amputation due to arterial disease.

Ischaemic skin changes

- Observe the legs closely for signs of an inadequate arterial supply (Fig. 5.4).
- Record whether the legs feel cold in a warm environment, and feel for a difference in temperature between the two limbs.
- Consider the colour of the limb (including the foot). If arterial disease is present, the limb may range from being very pale to a mottled blue due to a lack of oxygenated blood. Alternatively, it may have a deep red/purple hue (dependent rubor) appearance (Fig. 5.5). Dependent rubor is a result of the arteries in the foot vasodilating in an attempt to adequately oxygenate the limb, which results in pooling of arterial blood. This sometimes gives the appearance of either: (a) cellulitis, or (b) a well perfused limb. However, the limb will still feel cool. The position of the limb is also important to bear in mind. Dependent rubor occurs, as the name suggests, when the limb is in a dependent position. In a healthy perfused limb the colour should remain the same regardless of it being elevated or dependent. To assess for dependent rubor lie the patient in a supine position and gently elevate the patient's limb to above heart level (holding this position for a minute or so), then gently lower it noting

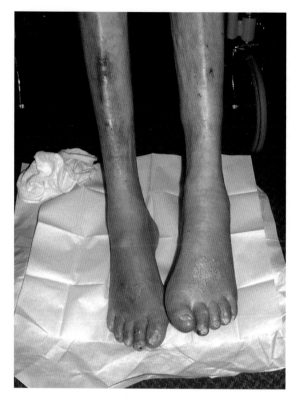

Fig. 5.4 Ischaemic limbs.

any changes in colour. If the cause for the colour change is dependent rubor, the limb becomes pale on elevation; the redness will gradually return once the limb has been lowered again.

- Check for dependent oedema. This is often a result of the patient being unable to sleep with their legs elevated (on a bed) because of ischaemic night pain. For many patients with severe night pain, the only way to get some sleep is to spend the night in a chair with their legs down.

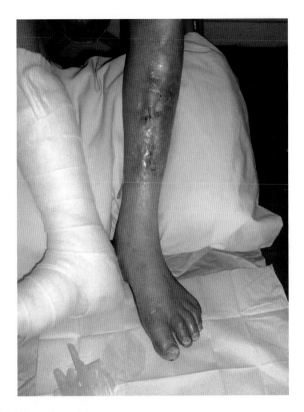

Fig. 5.5 Dependent rubor.

- Feel for pedal pulses and note any absence. **But note**: On its own, palpation of pedal pulses is insufficient to detect the presence or absence of arterial disease. The ankle brachial pressure index should be recorded in every patient.
- Note any loss of sensation (numbness/tingling).
- Look for hair loss, atrophic shiny skin, trophic changes to the nails and muscle wasting of the calf or thigh, all potentially related to arterial insufficiency.
- The site and appearance of the ulcer may give a clue as to whether PAOD is present. Ulcers due to arterial disease tend to

occur distal to the site of occlusion, and most commonly on the foot or ankle (Fig. 5.6), though they can occur anywhere on the limb. They tend to have a punched-out appearance. They may be shallow or very deep, revealing an underlying structure such as a tendon. Granulation (if present) is generally pale, and slough or black necrosis are likely to be present. Exudate levels tend to be low, except when there is concurrent infection or oedema.

Ischaemic pain

Arterial (ischaemic) pain occurs because the muscles in the leg are starved of oxygen (much like the chest pain associated with angina

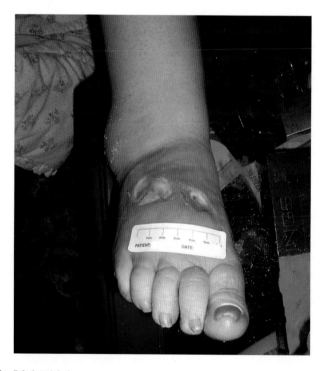

Fig. 5.6 Arterial ulcer.

or an MI). This can present itself in a number of ways depending on the severity of the ischaemia:

- Intermittent claudication is a cramp in the calves, thighs or buttocks, which occurs during exercise due to the inability of the arteries to meet the increased oxygen demands of the exercising muscle (Dumas, 1995). The pain disappears at rest when the oxygen demand is reduced, thus patients often describe only being able to walk a limited distance before having to stop to recover. Record how far your patient can walk before the onset of pain.
- Night pain occurs when the legs are elevated in bed. During sleep, the blood pressure naturally drops, and this reduced blood pressure is insufficient to maintain adequate perfusion of the legs in patients with PAOD. Patients often gain relief by hanging their leg down and out of bed, which allows the forces of gravity to facilitate arterial flow.
- Rest pain occurs even when the patient is sitting with their legs down and frequently involves the foot; it indicates a severe reduction in arterial flow below that required for normal tissue metabolism. An absolute pressure of 20–30 mmHg in the toes is often associated with rest pain (Stubbing & Chesworth, 2001).

Further details related to the assessment and management of ischaemic pain are given in Chapter 9.

UNDERSTANDING THE ROLE OF DIAGNOSTIC TESTS

The RCN (1998) recommends that all patients with a leg ulcer should have their ankle brachial pressure index (ABPI) recorded as a part of a holistic assessment. Other non-invasive and invasive tests are available, though there is probably some variation in the availability of all the possible options depending upon where the patient is seen and what is considered general practice in particular regions. The ABPI measurement, when performed according to the recommended procedure, is a useful, reliable and repeatable test requiring only a small amount of easily transportable equipment. The main costs involve the initial outlay for the equipment and staff training.

The ABPI measurement offers a simple, practical and objective means of aiding clinical judgement, and enables the identification of those patients with a compromised arterial blood supply who would benefit from further vascular assessment. Along with compression bandaging, the improved availability and incorporation of hand-held Doppler assessment into routine practice has contributed significantly to the overall improved outcomes of care for patients with leg ulcers.

Doppler ultrasound to measure the ankle brachial pressure index

The ABPI is essentially a ratio derived from comparing the blood pressure in the upper and the lower body. Using a hand-held Doppler ultrasound machine, the systolic pressure is measured in each arm (brachial) and leg (ankle) while the patient is resting. There should be little, if any, pressure variation between the limbs if peripheral arterial function is relatively normal. Significant differences, however, suggest the presence of disease. Measurement of the ABPI aids in the diagnosis of the presence and severity of arterial disease. The ABPI only measures blood flow in the arteries and is not diagnostic of venous disease. However, it is important in defining a safe level of compression for those with venous disease (Vowden & Vowden, 2001).

Measuring the ABPI

(a) Collecting the equipment needed

- Hand-held Doppler ultrasound machine with an 8-mHz probe (or 5 mHz if the limb is very oedematous).
- Headphones to detect faint pulses and to block out background noise.
- Ultrasound gel (do not use KY jelly which damages the probe).
- Manual sphygmomanometer and appropriate sized cuff (the bladder within the cuff should cover at least 80% of the size of the limb).
- Cling film or other waterproof layer to protect the ulcer and prevent cross-infection. Padding to protect the ulcer if it is painful.

- Alcohol surface wipes.
- Calculator or ABPI chart.

(b) Preparing the patient
- Explain the procedure and answer any questions.
- Ask the patient to rest as flat as is comfortable for 15–20 minutes.
- Cover the ulcer and surrounding skin with cling film. Place some padding over the ulcer if it is painful.

Time saving tips!

- Ask the patient to rest prior to their district nurse visit, or to arrive half an hour early for their practice nurse appointment and to rest quietly in the waiting room.
- Ask the patient to lie on the couch at the start of the appointment, while you complete other parts of the assessment.

(c) Measuring the brachial systolic pressure
- Ask the patient to lie flat as is comfortably possible to reduce hydrostatic pressure inaccuracies.
- Place an appropriately sized cuff around the upper arm.
- Locate the brachial pulse and apply ultrasound gel.
- Angle the probe at 45 degrees facing towards the direction of blood flow and locate the best signal.
- Inflate the cuff until the signal disappears, then slowly deflate the cuff. Record the pressure at which the signal returns.
- Repeat the procedure on the other arm.
- Record both readings.

(d) Measuring the ankle systolic pressure
- Place an appropriately sized cuff just above the ankle.
- Locate either the dorsalis pedis or anterior tibial pulse (Fig. 5.7). Apply ultrasound gel and listen to the signal.
- Record whether the signal is triphasic, biphasic or monophasic (Fig. 5.8).
- Inflate the cuff until just after the signal disappears, then deflate it slowly and record the pressure at which the signal returns.

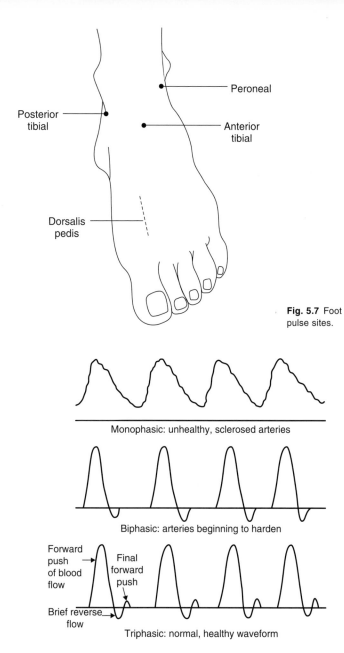

Fig. 5.7 Foot pulse sites.

Monophasic: unhealthy, sclerosed arteries

Biphasic: arteries beginning to harden

Triphasic: normal, healthy waveform

Fig. 5.8 Pulse signals.

- Repeat this procedure for the posterior tibial or peroneal pulse.
- Measure the ankle pressures in the opposite leg.
- Clean the equipment.

- To find the pulse, hold the probe near its tip, like a pen. Angle it at 45 degrees, facing towards the oncoming blood flow. Do not press, as this may close the artery. Steady your hand by resting it on the patient's limb.
- Place the cuff over the ankle with the tubing facing towards the knee, to avoid it getting in the way of the gel.

Safety and accuracy issues

- Do not attempt an ABPI assessment if there is suspected DVT, cellulitis or severe pain present.
- If the patient is unable to lie flat, elevate the legs as near to heart level as is comfortable and document the position. Note that the reading will be falsely high.
- Arterial disease can affect the upper limbs, and significant differences between brachial systolic pressures (>15 mmHg) can potentially indicate aortic arch disease. However, measuring both arms and using the highest reading significantly improves the accuracy of obtaining the nearest measurement to central systolic pressure. There are instances where only one arm can be measured and the accuracy of the test should be questioned if there are significant variations in the remaining limbs.
- The first beat may be missed if the cuff is deflated too quickly.
- An incorrect cuff size will result in inaccurate pressures. A cuff that is too short or too narrow results in overestimation of pressure, and a cuff that is too large will underestimate pressures.
- Avoid repeatedly inflating the cuff, or leaving it inflated for more than a few moments; this is uncomfortable for the patient and may alter the pressures.
- Ensure the cuff is positioned over the ankle. If it is over the calf, the result will be a 'calf brachial pressure index'.

Continued

- Remember the pressure obtained relates to the position of the cuff not the probe.
- At least two pressures should be measured from different arteries on each ankle. Pressure differences of 15mmHg or more indicate PAOD in the artery with the lower pressure. Such variations between arterial pressures should be taken into account when considering compression therapy or the need for further referral.

Calculating the ABPI

First, note down all the readings for each limb as in the example below:

	Right		Left	
Brachial	130		138	
Dorsalis pedis	130	Triphasic	70	Muffled biphasic
Posterior tibial	120	Biphasic	84	Monophasic

Next, identify the readings you will use to perform the calculation, as shown in the table below; three readings should be identified – the highest arm reading, the highest right leg reading and the highest left leg reading:

	Right		Left	
Brachial	130		**138**	
Dorsalis pedis	**130**	Triphasic	70	Muffled biphasic
Posterior tibial	120	Biphasic	**84**	Monophasic

Finally, calculate a separate ABPI for each leg, using the identified readings:

	Right		Left	
Brachial	130		**138**	
Dorsalis pedis	**130**	Triphasic	70	Muffled biphasic
Posterior tibial	120	Biphasic	**84**	Monophasic
ABPI	0.94		0.6	

ABPI = highest leg reading divided by highest arm reading.

Interpreting the ABPI
Note that this is only a guide. The ABPI must be interpreted by a qualified health professional in the context of a full clinical assessment and using all the information obtained during the Doppler assessment (i.e. how accurately the procedure was performed, the absolute pressures obtained, the variations between the pressures and the quality and type of pulse signals).

ABPI values (Vowden & Vowden, 2001; Ruff, 2003)

ABPI < 0.5: Severe peripheral arterial disease. Refer the patient to the vascular team (may need urgent referral depending upon the severity of symptoms). High compression is contraindicated. If venous disease or oedema are present, light support may be appropriate, but only following specialist guidance.

ABPI 0.5–0.9: Moderate to severe peripheral arterial disease. Refer the patient to the leg ulcer specialist and vascular team if symptomatic. If venous disease or oedema is present, reduced levels of compression therapy may be safe (following specialist guidance).

ABPI 1.0–1.3: Normal ABPI. High compression is probably safe in the absence of other contraindications.

ABPI > 1.3: May indicate a falsely high reading, especially if signals are monophasic. The ankle vessels may be noncompressible, indicating severe calcification, which is more commonly seen in people with diabetes. Falsely high readings may also be a result of incorrect positioning (i.e. legs below the level of the heart), incorrect cuff size (i.e. too small) or where there is gross oedema. Toe pressure may need to be assessed. Seek advice from a leg ulcer specialist or vascular clinic.

Doppler ultrasound for measuring toe pressures
Knowledge of toe pressures can be particularly useful in a number of circumstances, such as when:

- Falsely high readings occur due to calcification of the larger vessels (calcification rarely affects the arteries of the toe).
- Pain, or the extent of ulceration, prevents ABPI measurement.
- There is gross lower limb and/or foot oedema.

The procedure is very similar to measuring the ABPI, except for some variations in equipment and interpretation of the results.

Toe pressures can be measured using photoplethysmography, strain-gauge plethysmography and hand-held Doppler with an appropriate sized toe cuff (approximately 2.5 cm wide and 10–15 cm long).

Measuring toe pressures
(a) Preparing the equipment and patient
Prepare the equipment and the patient, and record the brachial systolic pressure in both arms exactly according to the instructions for measuring the ABPI.

(b) Measuring the toe systolic pressure using hand-held Doppler
- Place the appropriately sized cuff around the base of the great toe (the other toes can be used if the great toe is not an option).
- If possible, palpate the pulse on the distal pad area.
- Apply ultrasound gel and hold the probe towards the oncoming blood flow.
- Locate and listen to the signal (headphones usually make this much easier).
- Inflate the cuff until just after the signal disappears, then deflate it slowly and record the pressure at which the signal returns. Bear in mind that, due to the size of the cuff, inflation is much more rapid and considerable control is required to release the cuff at a slow and steady pace.
- Remove the cuff, wipe away the excess gel and clean the equipment.

Calculating the TBPI
Instead of comparing the ankle to arm pressure, the comparison is made between the toe and arm. The ratio obtained is the called

the 'toe brachial pressure index' (TBPI), and is calculated in exactly the same way as the ABPI:

TBPI = toe pressure divided by the highest brachial pressure.

	Right		Left	
Brachial	130		**138**	
Toe	**104**	Biphasic	**78**	Muffled biphasic
TBPI	0.75		0.56	

Interpreting the TBPI

Toe pressures are usually smaller than brachial pressures due to the differences in size of the arteries assessed, and so the ratios are also generally lower. It is important therefore to interpret these readings differently to ABPI measurements. Nevertheless the principles of interpretation remain the same. However, they are only a guide and must be interpreted by a qualified health professional in the context of a full clinical assessment, having followed the correct procedure and used all information obtained during the Doppler assessment.

TBPI > 0.7: Normal/satisfactory peripheral arterial supply.

TBPI < 0.65: Indicative of PAOD. Refer patient to the vascular team for further investigations (Baker & Rayman, 1999).

Pulse oximetry

The use of pulse oximetry as an additional tool for the assessment of peripheral arterial perfusion is gaining recognition and popularity. Much like Doppler assessment, it is proving to be an accurate, non-invasive tool. Regular users would argue that it is a more sensitive test than Doppler assessment (Lucke et al., 1999) and easier to use as it only requires the practitioner to place the oximeter probe on a finger and toe rather than locating arteries.

The pulse oximeter measures oxygen saturation levels of haemoglobin within tissues. Because it relies on a pulsatile blood flow, the signal will be diminished when blood flow is occluded (e.g. with a blood pressure cuff). It is on this basis that assessment of peripheral arterial perfusion can take place. This procedure is being used to good effect when deciding on the appropriate levels of compression therapy to apply when managing patients with mixed venous and arterial disease: i.e. being able to ensure that oxygen perfusion is not being compromised by high compression bandaging.

While this test offers some benefits over Doppler, there may be some problems obtaining signals from patients with extremely dystrophic toenails or if the patient is severely cyanosed or suffers from vasoconstriction.

The following is an outline of the Lanarkshire Oximetry Index (LOI) procedure (Bianchi & Stewart, 2002). As for ABPI and TBPI measurements, the correct equipment and procedure are vital to the accuracy of the test.

Measuring the LOI
(a) Preparing the equipment and patient
- As for the Doppler procedure – though the patient does not need to be lying flat.

(b) Measuring oxygen saturation
- Place the oximetry sensor on any finger and obtain a baseline reading.
- Place an appropriately sized cuff around the upper arm.
- Inflate the cuff to 60 mmHg, then continue to inflate in 10-mmHg increments approximately every 10 seconds until the pressure reaches 100 mmHg.
- Continue with 20-mmHg incremental changes until the pulse oximetry signal is lost. Record the reading at the last audible signal (e.g. if the signal disappears at 140 mmHg then the pressure recorded is 120 mmHg). If there is still a signal at 180 mmHg there is no further inflation and this reading is recorded.
- Repeat the procedure on the other arm.
- The higher reading is used to calculate the LOI.

(c) Measuring the toe pressure
- Place an appropriately sized cuff just above the ankle.
- Place the oximetry sensor on one of the first three toes.
- Begin inflating the cuff and record the reading as when measuring the finger oximetry.
- Repeat for the other leg.

Calculating the LOI

> LOI = toe pressure divided by the highest finger pressure (see example below).

	Right	Left
Brachial	120	**140**
Toe	**100**	**140**
LOI	0.71	1

Interpreting the results
Similar interpretations of the index results are applied to LOI as for ABPI measurements.

Checking the oximetry with compression in situ
- Apply an appropriate graduated compression system (bandages or hosiery).
- Place the oximetry sensor back on to one of the first three toes.
- Check the signal with the leg in the horizontal position then following elevation for 30 seconds.
- Repeat for the opposite leg if compression is applied.

Which test to use?
As with most things when there is more than one option, there are pros and cons to weigh up in each case. The problems attached to all these tests come down to what equipment and training is available in your work environment. Measurement of the ABPI

with Doppler ultrasound for assessing patients with leg ulcers is one of the key recommendations in both the RCN (1998) and SIGN guidelines (1998), and is standard practice in the Wandsworth tPCT.

Toe pressure measurement and pulse oximetry should perhaps be reserved for complex situations where there is evidence of calcified vessels (ABPI > 1.3), and/or where severe venous and arterial disease coexist. The most important elements of all these tests is that they should help in forming a diagnosis, guide or alert the practitioner to the need for referral to a vascular team for further assessment and aid management strategies.

Many other non-invasive tests can be performed, including segmental pressure measurement and exercise tests, though the 'gold standard' is colour Duplex scanning. Duplex scanning is usually performed in a vascular laboratory by a trained technician. It utilises ultrasound technology to detect blood flow, creating a colour image of the direction of flow and velocity of the blood. Areas of stenosis and occlusions can be identified and essentially mapped to help plan options for further treatment (Stubbing & Chesworth, 2001).

This may lead on to more invasive investigations such as angiography (arteriography) whereby a radio-opaque dye is injected into an artery, followed by a series of X-rays that are taken to capture the flow of the contrast media within the arteries. This procedure allows for clear assessment of the condition of the vessels; in some cases, intravascular therapy can be performed at the same time (Stubbing & Chesworth, 2001).

How often to test?

In light of the increasing risk of arterial disease in conjunction with increasing age, the importance of reassessment can not be understated. The arterial status of a patient is not static and can alter significantly enough to make previously safe treatments, such as compression therapy, no longer appropriate. This deterioration in arterial perfusion may happen over relatively short periods (Simon et al., 1994); thus 3-monthly reassessment of the ABPI, or more frequently if the clinical situation suggests it, is recommended while treatment is ongoing (RCN, 1998).

FORMING THE DIAGNOSIS

By combining the information gathered so far, it should be possible, in most cases, to determine whether or not PAOD is present and to what degree. If the outcome is unclear, the patient should be referred to a leg ulcer specialist or vascular team for further assessment.

SUMMARY

- Peripheral arterial occlusive disease (PAOD) is the second most common cause of leg ulceration.
- All patients with leg ulceration should be screened for clinical signs and symptoms of PAOD.
- Patients with PAOD should be referred on to a vascular team for further assessment and possible treatment.
- The urgency of this referral is based on the severity of the disease present – this is determined by the ABPI reading, signs present and symptoms experienced by the patient.
- Full compression therapy is contraindicated in the presence of severe arterial disease.
- If arterial disease is the only or predominate factor, the most important element in regards to treatment is to resolve the occlusion (this will usually involve angioplasty or bypass surgery): wound bed preparation and oedema control are additional important management issues.

REFERENCES

Adam, D.J., Naik, J., Hartshorne, T., Bello, M. & London, N.J.M. (2003) The diagnosis and management of 689 chronic leg ulcers in a single-visit assessment clinic. *European Journal of Vascular and Endovascular Surgery* **25**: 462–468.

Aronow, W.S. (2005) Management of peripheral arterial disease. *Cardiology in Review* **13**(2): 61–68.

Baker, N. & Rayman, G. (1999) Clinical evaluation of Doppler signals. *Diabetic Foot* **2**(1) (Suppl.): 22–25.

Bianchi, J. & Stewart, D. (2002) Pulse oximetry vascular assessment in patients with leg ulcers. *British Journal of Community Nursing* **7**(9) (Suppl.): S22–28.

Callam, M.J., Harper, D.R., Dale, J.J., et al. (1987) Arterial disease in chronic leg ulceration: an underestimated hazard? Lothian & Forth Valley Leg Ulcer Study. *British Medical Journal* **294**: 929–931.

Callum, K. & Bradbury, A. (2000) ABC of arterial and venous disease: acute limb ischaemia. *British Medical Journal* **320**: 764–767.

Cooke, J.P. (2001) Mechanisms of atherosclerosis in peripheral arterial diseases In: *Peripheral Arterial Disease Handbook* (W.R. Hiatt, A.T. Hirsch & J. Regensteiner, eds). Boca Raton, CRC Press, LLC, pp. 3–20.

Cornwall, J., Dore, C.J. & Lewis, J.D. (1986) Leg ulcers: epidemiology and aetiology. *British Journal of Surgery* **73**: 693–696.

Department of Health (DH) (2000) Reducing heart disease in the population. Chapter 1. Appendix C – Effectiveness of physical activity programmes. In: *NHS Our Healthier Nation: Modern Standards and Service Models. Coronary Heart Disease National Service Frameworks.* London, DH, pp. 41–2.

Drugs and Therapeutics Bulletin (2002) Managing peripheral arterial disease in primary care. *Drugs and Therapeutics Bulletin* **40**(1): 5–8.

Dumas, M.A. (1995) Intermittent claudication: clinical snapshot. *American Journal of Nursing* **December**: 34–35.

Fowkes, F.G.R. (1997) Epidemiology of peripheral vascular disease. *Atherosclerosis* **131**(Suppl.): S29–S31.

Golomb, B.A., Criqui, M.H. & Bundens, W.P. (2001) Peripheral arterial disease. In: *Peripheral Arterial Disease Handbook* (W.R. Hiatt, A.T. Hirsch & J. Regensteiner, eds). Boca Raton, CRC Press, LLC, pp. 57–80.

Goodall, S. (2001) Risk factor assessment for patients with peripheral arterial disease. *Professional Nurse* **17**(1): 27–30.

Herbert, L.M. (1997) *Caring for the Vascular Patient.* Edinburgh, Churchill Livingstone.

Jones, S. (2001) Anatomy & physiology of the vascular system. In: *Vascular Disease Nursing and Management* (S. Murray, ed.). London, Whurr Publishers Ltd, pp. 1–31.

Lucke, T.W., Urcelay, M., Bianchi, J., Loney, M., McEvoy, M. & Douglas, W.S. (1999) Pulse oximetry: an additional tool in the assessment of patients with leg ulcers. *British Journal of Dermatology* **141**(Suppl. 55): 65.

Lusis, A.J. (2000) Atherosclerosis. *Nature* **407**: 233–241.

Mills, J.L. (2003) Buerger's disease in the 21st century: diagnosis, clinical features, and therapy. *Seminars in Vascular Surgery* **16**(3): 179–189.

Mills, J.L. and Porter J.M. (1991) Buerger's disease (thromboangiitis obliterans). *Annals of Vascular Surgery* **5**: 570–572.

Moffatt, C.J., Franks, P.J., Doherty, D.C., Martin, R., Blewett, R. & Ross, F. (2004) Prevalence of leg ulceration in a London population. *Quarterly Journal of Medicine* **97**: 431–437.

Morison, M.J. & Moffatt, C.J. (1994) *A Colour Guide to the Assessment and Management of Leg Ulcers*, 2nd ed. London, Mosby.

Ockenden, L.J. (2001) Aetiology and pathology of vascular disease. In: *Vascular Disease Nursing and Management* (S. Murray, ed.). London, Whurr Publishers Ltd, pp. 32–68.

Olin, J.W. (2000) Thromboangiitis obliterans (Buerger's disease). *New England Journal of Medicine* **343**(12): 864–869.

RCN Institute (1998) *Clinical Practice Guidelines. The Management of Patients with Venous Leg Ulcers*. London, Royal College of Nursing.

Ruff, D. (2003) Doppler assessment: calculating an ankle brachial pressure index. *Nursing Times* **99**(42): 62–65.

Shah, P. (1997) New insights into the pathogenesis and prevention of acute coronary syndromes. *American Journal of Cardiology* **70**(12B): 17–23.

SIGN (1998) *The Care of Patients with Chronic Leg Ulcer*. Edinburgh, Scottish Intercollegiate Guidelines Network, SIGN Publication No. 26.

Simon, D.A., Freak, L., Williams, I.M., et al. (1994) Progression of arterial disease in patients with healed venous leg ulcers. *Journal of Wound Care* **3**(4): 179–180.

Stubbing, N. & Chesworth, J. (2001) Assessment of patients with vascular disease. In: *Vascular Disease Nursing and Management* (S. Murray, ed.). London, Whurr Publishers Ltd, pp. 96–136.

Tierney, S., Fennessy, F. & Bouchier Hayes, D. (2000) ABC of arterial and vascular disease: secondary prevention of peripheral vascular disease. *British Medical Journal* **320**: 1262–1265.

Vowden, K. & Vowden, P. (2001) Doppler and the ABPI: how good is our understanding? *Journal of Wound Care* **10**(6): 197–202.

Vowden, K. & Vowden, P. (2002) *Hand-Held Doppler Ultrasound: The Assessment of Lower Limb Arterial and Venous Disease*. Cardiff, Huntleigh Healthcare.

Widmaier, E.P., Raff, H. & Strang, K.T. (2004) *Vander, Sherman & Luciano's Human Physiology*, 9th edn. New York, McGraw Hill.

Diabetic Leg Ulceration

6

LEARNING OBJECTIVES
Nurses involved in leg ulcer management should be able to demonstrate:

❑ An understanding of the different types of leg ulceration that may occur in patients with diabetes.
❑ The ability to describe the factors that influence wound healing in patients with diabetes.
❑ An understanding of the assessment issues in diabetic leg ulceration.
❑ The ability to describe the clinical and psychosocial factors that influence treatment outcome.
❑ The ability to describe the different treatment issues required.
❑ An understanding of the importance of the multi-disciplinary team in providing care.
❑ The ability to describe the rare complications associated with diabetes mellitus.

INTRODUCTION
Diabetes can be one of the most devastating conditions for patients to suffer. The long-term complications are integrally linked to the length of time the patient has suffered the condition and the adequacy of their blood sugar control (Levin & O'Neal, 2001). The commonest type of ulceration in diabetes occurs on the foot, due to the effects of neuropathy. Although this book does not cover the management of diabetic foot ulceration, it will address the other forms of leg ulceration seen in these patients and discuss how neuropathy influences their management.

SKIN CHANGES IN DIABETES
Changes occur in the skin of patients with diabetes that can contribute to the development of a number of skin conditions and

forms of ulceration. Skin disorders are thought to affect about 30% of patients with diabetes (Pendsey, 2003).

The skin (the dermal layer) is measurably thicker in people with diabetes (compared to patients without) due to disturbances in collagen degradation, and it is also less elastic (Sibbald & Schachter, 1984). High blood sugar levels are thought to promote these changes (Calvet & Yoshikawa, 2001). Clinically, the skin appears thickened, waxy and tight. The patient may also have limited joint mobility. Patients with autonomic neuropathy also have reduced sweating, with the loss of its protective bactericidal effect. The stratum corneum dries, becomes brittle and fissures develop that allow the entry of bacteria. This is most often visible on the plantar surface of the foot. Sensory neuropathy leads to an insensate foot and leg, where minor trauma is not felt and ulceration may occur. Cutaneous skin problems in patients with diabetes can be grouped into three categories (Table 6.1).

A number of other skin conditions are associated with diabetes mellitus, including:

- Diabetic dermopathy 'shin spots' – atrophic brown scars usually occurring on the shin.
- Diabetic erythema – patches of reddening and purpura on the legs and feet of elderly patients with diabetes.

Table 6.1 Skin problems seen in patients with diabetes.

Skin infections (linked to poor hyperglycaemic control)	Bacterial infections (often involving more than one organism) Yeast infection, e.g. candida Fungal infections, e.g. tinea
Peripheral neuropathy	Neuropathic foot ulceration Altered sweating
Peripheral vascular disease	
Peripheral arterial occlusive disease	Trophic changes Ischaemic ulceration Gangrene (particularly affecting digits and pressure sites) Pressure ulceration (affects the heel)
Venous disease	Venous ulceration
Mixed arterial, venous and other combinations	Mixed aetiology ulceration

- Yellow-nail syndrome – yellow discoloration of the nail bed.
- Scleroderma associated with diabetes.
- Necrobiosis lipoidica (see p. 146 for details).

NAIL CONDITIONS IN DIABETES

Nail deformities are commonly associated with diabetes and can be an important contributory factor in ulceration (Figs 6.1 and 6.2). Deformities occur after trauma, fungal infection, systemic disease or because of poor nail care. Neuropathic ischaemia nearly always results in nail deformities, with a high risk of infection leading to localised gangrene of the toes. Neglect of nails due to poor health, obesity and poor vision leads to the nails becoming too long thus causing damage to the skin of the next toe. Curling of the nails can result in the nail itself becoming a pressure source, which can then lead to ulceration. Infections occurring in the nail bed are common and can spread to the foot through the lymphatics. The presence of peripheral arterial occlusive disease in this situation rapidly leads to spreading infection and distal gangrene, because the bacterial by-products cause local thrombosis of the blood supply and from this gangrene of the digits (Fig. 6.3).

FACTORS INFLUENCING HEALING

A number of factors associated with diabetes are thought to cause delayed wound healing. Peripheral arterial occlusive disease leads to reduced perfusion and low oxygen levels that result in tissue breakdown and gangrene.

Smoking is a major risk factor for peripheral vascular disease (Couch, 1986). In addition to its role in accelerating arterial disease, it is also a potent vasoconstrictor, further reducing local tissue oxygen perfusion. The oxygen is replaced by carbon monoxide to form carboxyhaemoglobin within the erythrocyte, thus reducing the amount of oxygen available to the tissues. This effect may last for up to an hour after each cigarette is smoked. Wound healing is also delayed due to abnormal platelet function and fibrinogen deposition and removal (Ford, 1990).

Many patients with diabetes are considered to be seriously immunocompromised and at risk of overwhelming sepsis. A total

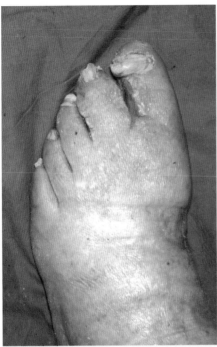

Fig. 6.1 Marked overgrowth and thickening of the nail.

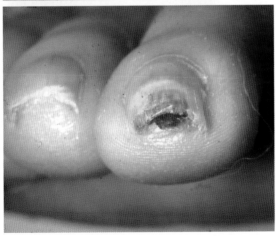

Fig. 6.2 Nail infection.

127

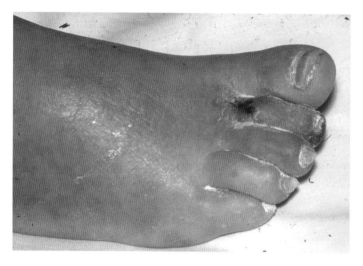

Fig. 6.3 Infection leading to thrombosis and gangrene of the toes.

lymphocyte count below 1500/ml is considered to be evidence of risk (Dickhaut et al., 1984; Armstrong et al., 1998). Reduced neutrophil activity increases the risk of opportunistic bacteria causing severe infection. The risk of infection appears to be related to levels of hyperglycaemia, with a blood glucose concentration of over 7 mmol/l being associated with delayed healing. A number of leg ulcer studies have shown that patients with diabetes with mixed aetiology ulceration have significantly reduced healing rates (Nelzén et al., 1997). Reduced serum albumin levels of less than 30 g/l due to infection, starvation, renal failure or acute stress have been shown to be linked to delayed wound healing (Sibbald & Schachter, 1984).

Nurses must be aware that the length of time the patient has suffered from diabetes and the presence of other diabetic complications, such as retinopathy and nephropathy, are important indicators that delayed wound healing may occur (The International Working Group on the Diabetic Foot, 1999).

THE IMPACT OF LEG ULCERATION IN THE PATIENT WITH DIABETES

The literature suggests that patients with diabetes face many problems when living with a leg ulcer (Aikens & Lustman, 2001). Between 58 and 80% of patients with diabetes fail to adhere to their diet or insulin prescription. Of particular importance is the psychosocial impact of the condition on the patient and their family. Of the top five predictors of long-term mortality, two are the social effects of the illness and the patients' smoking history. In 1988, Davis et al. reported that these issues were rarely addressed in treatment programmes, and sadly this is still the case. Table 6.2 outlines some of the problems reported to affect patients' psychosocial health. It is essential that assessment addresses these issues and how they influence the progress the patient will make. Access to specialist support from psychologists may be particularly useful in helping patients understand how their psychological problems impact on their condition, and will assist them in developing more effective coping strategies. These issues are discussed further in Chapter 10.

Table 6.2 Psychosocial issues affecting long-term progress in patients with diabetes.

Social factors	High divorce rate
	Being single, separated or divorced
	Being male (particularly elderly males)
	Decreased social networks
	Decreased social or family support
Psychological factors	Poor concordance with self-care regimes
	High levels of depression and anxiety
	High levels of stress
	Reduced quality of life
	Poor illness adjustment
	Poor self-esteem
	Negative attitudes to self-care
	Fear of hypoglycaemia
	Sexual dysfunction
	Eating disorders
	Alcohol abuse
	Worry about complications

ASSESSMENT ISSUES

A comprehensive assessment should be carried out using the principles described in Chapters 3, 5 and 8. It is essential that the assessment identifies the aetiology of the patient's leg ulcer as well as the compounding factors that influence treatment decisions, and whether referral for specialist opinion is required. Specific issues related to the influence of diabetes are discussed below.

Skin changes associated with ulceration in diabetes

A number of skin changes are associated with ulceration in the patient with diabetes.

General altered skin quality

- Altered skin quality – thickened, waxy, tight/rigid, dry, fissures (plantar surface of the foot must always be examined).
- Toenails – nail deformities and infections.
- Loss of hair on the lower leg.
- Interdigital maceration with erythema (usually due to chronic tinea pedis infection).

Ischaemic skin changes

- Skin colour – signs of ischaemia (red/blue on dependency and white on elevation with delayed capillary refill time).
- Reduced or absent pedal pulses associated with peripheral vascular disease.
- Trophic changes (often over areas of pressure from shoes).
- Microemboli seen on the toes (frequently associated with atrial fibrillation).

Neuropathic skin changes

- Altered sensation.
- Presence of autonomic neuropathy – red, dry skin with absence of sweating and fissures on the plantar surface of the foot.
- Prominent veins and bounding pedal pulses.
- Atrophy of the subcutaneous tissues and muscles – associated weakness.
- Prominent extensor tendons.
- Callus formation on the plantar surface of the foot.
- Presence of sub-keratotic haematoma beneath callus – highly suggestive of underlying ulceration.

- Loss of intrinsic muscles (associated with cocked up toes and hammer-toes.
- Other foot deformities – hallux valgus, prominent metatarsal heads, dropped arch, bunionette, Charcot deformity (see Figs 6.4 and 6.5).
- Infection – a small entry site may hide extensive ulceration that extends to bone. The ability to probe a wound to the bone is a strong indicator of osteomyelitis.
- Pain – the underlying cause of the pain will influence its presentation (see Chapter 9).
- Oedema – due to vasodilation caused by changes in sympathetic nerve control.

Patients with venous ulceration will also have the typical signs of venous ulceration that have been discussed in Chapter 4.

Presence of neuropathy
It is vital that nurses can effectively screen a patient for neuropathy as part of the assessment process, particularly prior to commencement of a treatment programme for leg ulceration that may involve the use of compression therapy.

Neuropathy is associated with a number of clinical conditions that may lead to ulceration, these include:

- Diabetes mellitus
- Hansen's disease (leprosy)
- Alcoholism
- Vitamin deficiencies
- Spinal lesions, such as herniated discs, tumours and spina bifida
- Malignancies
- Collagen diseases
- Pernicious anaemia
- Drug therapies
- Idiopathic (unknown cause)

The easiest way to assess sensation is using a 5.07 gauge Semmes–Wesinstein monofilament (Edmonds and Foster, 2000). This is held perpendicular to the foot and enough pressure applied until it buckles (equivalent to 10 grams of force): the test is repeated over various aspects of the foot. The patient's inability to feel the

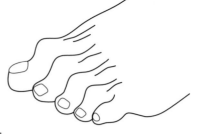

Fig. 6.4(a) Hammer-toes. Toes are held in dorsiflexion at the metatarsophalangeal joint and flexion at the interphalangeal joint.

Fig. 6.4(b) Varus deformity. The third, fourth and fifth toes shift medially. The toes appear overcrowded and may overlap each other.

Fig. 6.4(c) Hallux valgus. Deformity of the toes at the metatarsophalangeal joint. The hallus deviates laterally in relation to the first metatarsal head.

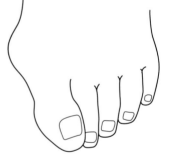

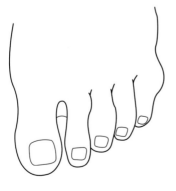

Fig. 6.4(d) Bunionette of the fifth toe. Affects the lateral part of the fifth metatarsal head. It is often associated with hallux valgus.

Fig. 6.4 Common foot deformities seen in diabetic foot neuropathy.

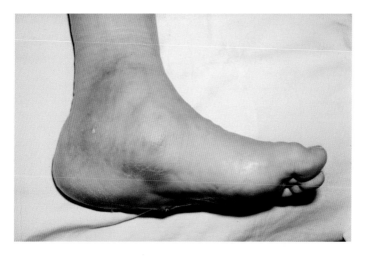

Fig. 6.5 Charcot deformity.

monofilament when it buckles is an indication that the protective sensation of the foot is lost and that severe sensory neuropathy is present (Sosenko et al., 1990). The monofilament should not be used over areas of callus as this will distort the findings. It is important to assess both limbs.

Patients with neuropathy of unknown origin should be immediately referred for a medical opinion. Patients with diabetic neuropathy should be regularly assessed and treated by the diabetic podiatrist to ensure a healthy foot is maintained. Appropriate patient education should be provided on foot care and when to seek medical advice.

Fig. 6.6 shows the sites where testing for neuropathy may occur, although there is no internationally agreed protocol. Neuropathy usually occurs bilaterally, but the severity may differ between limbs. The distribution of numbness includes the following:

- Dullness or numbness in the toes that becomes sharp at a proximal point on the leg.
- Numb feet with sensation returning in the lower leg and then becoming reduced further up the leg.
- Severe numbness extending from the toes and up the leg.

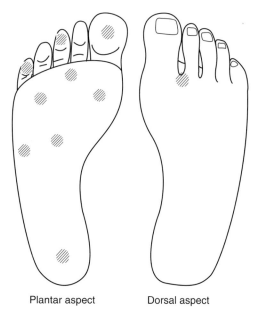

Plantar aspect   Dorsal aspect

Fig. 6.6 Sites for testing of neuropathy.

Sensory neuropathy is frequently preceded by a period of acute neuritic pain or an episode of hyperglycaemia. This period may range from a few weeks to several years. During this time the patient may complain of constant burning pain over their entire foot or leg, which is more severe at night and not relieved by changing position. Abnormal sensations such as tingling, burning and shooting pains are common. This is gradually replaced with a loss of sensation; although the two may also occur simultaneously, with some areas of the foot being numb but neuritic pain still being present. Patients report that as the numbness progresses they feel they are walking on pillows or as if their socks are rolled up beneath their feet. Many patients report their feet feel cold with overall limb weakness. This loss of protective function leads to injury to the feet and structural changes.

Development of peripheral arterial occlusive disease

Peripheral arterial occlusive disease (PAOD) occurs at an earlier age and progresses more rapidly in patients with diabetes, compared with patients without diabetes (Wilson and Kannel, 1992; Levin and O'Neal, 2001). Men and women with diabetes are affected equally. There is a difference in the distribution of disease in the patient with diabetes. Distal vessels, particularly the tibial and peroneal, are more frequently involved in patients with diabetes. In patients without diabetes, the femoral, iliac and aorta are more commonly affected.

The concept of microvascular disease in patients with diabetes has now been disproved; however, changes do occur in the micro-circulation, particularly thickening of the capillary basement membrane that influences blood flow. Other regulatory mechanisms controlling local blood flow are affected, thus influencing perfusion of the tissues. A number of risk factors for the development of peripheral vascular disease in patients with diabetes have been identified; these include:

- Genetic predisposition
- Age
- Duration of diabetes
- Smoking
- Hypertension (systolic or diastolic pressures)
- Hypercholesterolaemia
- Triglyceridaemia
- Proteinuria

Smoking, age, duration of diabetes, the disease itself and genetic factors are likely to be the most important factors.

Clinical presentation of PAOD in patients with diabetes

Many of the signs and symptoms of PAOD are similar in patients both with and without diabetes. PAOD has been discussed in Chapter 5. However, a number of important differences in the clinical presentation may occur. Intermittent claudication may occur less frequently due to the distribution of disease in the more distal vessels of the ankle and foot. Intermittent claudication depends on the development of ischaemia in the related muscle group. Despite extensive involvement of the arteries of the foot, symptoms of claudication rarely occur because of the small muscle bulk in the foot. However, pain may be experienced when walking up a hill, on a hard surface or walking fast. The sensation of pain may be obscured by the presence of concurrent neuropathy. It is very important to remember that intermittent claudication will only occur during exercise. Many patients with leg ulceration are chronically immobile due to their diabetes and other related problems such as osteoarthritis. In this situation the earliest symptoms of peripheral vascular disease may be nocturnal or rest pain and trophic tissue changes with ulceration and dry gangrene.

During the assessment process it is very important to take a careful medical history and ensure that the patient has had a recent medical assessment of their diabetes. There is a very strong association between peripheral vascular disease and coronary artery disease in diabetes (Levin & O'Neal, 2001). Patients frequently report a history of angina, myocardial infarction or other cardiovascular disorders such as transient ischaemic attacks and stroke. Arterial emboli secondary to atrial fibrillation may precede the development of severe PAOD. Assessment of the patient's arterial status can be difficult due to the calcification that occurs in the distal arteries (see Chapter 5).

> If there is any doubt about the aetiology of the ulcer, patients should be referred for expert opinion before interventions such as compression therapy are commenced.

GENERAL PRINCIPLES OF MANAGEMENT

A number of general principles apply to the care of patients with diabetes and ulceration of any kind. Nurses must address the following within their treatment plan:

- Control hyperglycaemia.
- Implement appropriate patient education.
- Teach the patient the importance of inspecting their feet daily.
- Avoid using alcohol-based products that dry the skin.
- Implement skin-care regimes that incorporate emollients to keep the skin healthy.
- Treat interdigital fungal infections promptly for a minimum of 4 weeks.

- Ensure the patient receives regular care from a podiatrist to remove callus formation and check for foot health.
- Ensure the patient's diabetes is closely monitored by the diabetic team to check for the development of other complications such as retinopathy.

USING COMPRESSION THERAPY IN DIABETES

Many textbooks state that compression therapy should not be used in the patient with diabetes. This is because of the concern that sensory neuropathy will prevent a patient detecting whether the compression is causing trauma and the risk of concurrent PAOD. However, patients with diabetes are just as likely to suffer from a venous ulcer as patients without diabetes. In this situation the treatment of choice is compression therapy. Healing may take longer but generally does occur.

In order to use compression effectively a number of issues must be addressed. A comprehensive, structured assessment that identifies the underlying aetiology is vital. If there is concern about the suitability of the patient for compression, the patient should be referred for specialist advice. The key priorities that relate to the safe use of compression in diabetes are:

- Exclusion of peripheral arterial occlusive disease.
- Assessment of peripheral neuropathy.
- Identification of vulnerable pressure sites and foot deformities.
- Identification of other factors that will influence healing, such as nephropathy.

Exclusion of PAOD

Assessment of the patient's arterial status using a clinical history and Doppler ultrasound has been discussed in Chapter 5. Recording a resting pressure index in a patient with diabetes can be difficult due to:

- Calcification of the arteries, which prevents the artery from being occluded. As a result a false, very high systolic pressure is recorded that does not give an accurate picture.
- Toe pressure measurements may be very useful in this group as calcification of the toe vessels rarely occurs.

Assessment of peripheral neuropathy and associated changes

Reduced sensation places a patient at high risk of pressure damage from inappropriately applied compression. It is important to assess the foot for:

- Areas at risk of pressure damage from compression.
- Areas of callus formation.
- Foot deformities – hammer-toes, hallux valgus, Charcot deformity, prominent metatarsal heads, dropped arch.
- Toes, interdigital infection, emboli.
- Joint function.
- Quality of the skin and signs of trauma.
- Nails, nail deformities and infection.
- Footwear.

Due to the foot deformities that frequently occur in patients with diabetes, a number of additional areas are at risk of pressure damage from compression. Fig. 6.4 highlights the typical foot deformities seen in patients with diabetic neuropathy.

Callus formation

This is rapid, particularly in patients suffering from hyperglycaemia. Common areas of callus formation are over the plantar surface of the foot, particularly where metatarsal heads are exposed. Compression bandaging traditionally extends to the base of the toes. This will mean that the compression is applied over this area, and acts as a secondary source of pressure and friction. The callus area may need to remain exposed to avoid this risk and to allow for the regular removal of callus by the diabetic podiatrist.

Sub-keratotic haematoma

Compression should not be applied without specialist advice if the patient has neuropathic foot ulceration or evidence of haemorrhage below the callus. The presence of a haematoma is highly suggestive of underlying ulceration. These patients require monitoring by the specialist leg ulcer team and will need treatment from the diabetic podiatrist.

Foot deformities

For example, hammer-toes are also areas at risk of compression damage. Other neuropathic changes include loss of the small intrinsic muscles and subcutaneous tissue in the forefoot area. High compression can result in deep pressure necrosis over the dorsum of the foot.

Pressure damage

Prominent hallux valgus (bunions), bunionettes and exposed extensor tendons are all areas at risk of compression damage. Peak pressures over these areas may be in excess of 100 mmHg, particularly over the dorsal tendon area of the foot. Pressure damage to the Achilles area can lead to sloughing and loss of the tendon with fixation of the ankle. The extensor tendon may be very prominent in these patients and will require protection. The area of the heel is rarely described as an area that is associated with compression damage. However, compression may exacerbate the risk of heel pressure ulceration in patients who are immobile and keep their limb in the same position for long periods: the loss of sensation prevents them being alerted to the need to change position. While compression bandaging should not extend over the toes, care must nevertheless be taken to ensure that compression will not exacerbate toe deformities or cause tissue damage. Crowding and overlapping of toes are common problems leading to interdigital pressure ulceration and an increased risk of infection between the toes.

Reduced mobility

Many factors influence the mobility of these patients. Reduced ankle movement is a common problem, and there are a number of reasons why this may occur. Long-term venous ulceration is associated with a progressive loss of ankle function, particularly when compression is being used. Patients who have a completely fixed ankle joint are at particular risk of delayed healing due to poor venous return. Patients with diabetes also develop reduced ankle function due to the glycosylation in the subcutaneous tissues causing stiffness and reduced function.

Footwear

It is vital to assess the patients' footwear. Patients with neuropathy are frequently found to be wearing shoes that are too tight and, therefore, their feet should be checked for signs of pressure damage (Edmonds & Foster, 2000). When compression is being considered it is important to assess how this will influence their regular footwear.

Previous history of foot ulceration

Before compression is applied, specialist advice should be sought for patients with a previous history of foot ulceration and for those wearing custom-made shoes. It is vital that the compression does not become wrinkled when the foot is placed in the shoe, as the patient with neuropathy will be unable to tell if damage is occurring.

Contraindications to compression therapy in diabetes

There are a number of clinical situations when compression should not be used in a patient with diabetes except under specialist supervision:

- Neuropathic foot ulceration over the plantar surface of the foot
- Arterial occlusive disease (ABPI < 0.8)
- Charcot deformity with ulceration

Venous ulceration may occur in a patient with concurrent neuropathic foot ulceration. In addition to the risks associated with reduced sensation, compression should not be applied over the ulcerated area as this may act as an additional pressure source and can prevent regular inspection of the foot. Similarly, a Charcot deformity with ulceration should not be treated with compression therapy. Table 6.3 outlines some of these issues and their solutions.

Although reduced compression is recommended for patients without diabetes who have a reduced ABPI of 0.6–0.8, compression should be avoided in patients with diabetes with an ABPI below 0.8 until specialist opinion has been sought.

Table 6.3 Problems associated with using compression therapy in the neuropathic foot.

Reduced sensation	Patient is unable to know if the compression is too tight and causing pressure damage.
Changes in foot structure	Potential pressure sites may become more prominent, increasing the risk of pressure damage from poorly applied compression.
Reduced ankle movement	Loss of ankle mobility reduces venous return and may lead to delayed ulcer healing.
Callus formation and neuropathic ulceration	Callus formation may be particularly rapid in the patient with poor glycaemia control. Weekly application of compression prevents regular inspection of these sites, with the risk of neuropathic ulceration developing. Adequate daily foot inspection is difficult when compression is being used.
Inadequate footwear	Current footwear (including custom-made shoes) may be unsuitable for use during compression therapy. This must be carefully evaluated to prevent damage occurring to the vulnerable at-risk neuropathic foot. Specialist podiatric advice may be required.

How to choose the correct compression

The principles of selecting a compression bandage are described in Chapter 14. Elastic or inelastic, multi-layer, high compression bandaging is the treatment of choice. When choosing a regime for a patient with diabetes the following factors may also be useful in aiding decision-making:

Elastic, multi-layer, high compression bandaging (higher resting pressure)
- Young fit patients.
- Normal ankle to brachial pressure index (ABPI) with triphasic waveforms.
- No history of cardiovascular disease.
- No previous treatment for PAOD.
- Minimal or no peripheral neuropathy.

- Varying levels of mobility, including poor mobility and those who are chair-bound.
- Control of oedema, particularly in the immobile patient.

Inelastic, multi-layer, high compression bandaging (lower resting pressure)
- ABPI > 0.8 with biphasic or triphasic waveforms.
- Good mobility – to assist the action of the bandage during walking.
- Concerns over distal perfusion at night when wearing bandaging with the foot elevated.
- Severe pain, which prevents the use of high-pressure elastic bandaging.

Self-care regimes, such as bandaging and compression garments
- Fit patients who have good eyesight and are able to undertake dressings and observe their wound for signs of progress or deterioration.
- Patients wishing to self-manage.
- Adequate hyperglycaemic control.
- Clear understanding of their condition and its treatment.
- No history of neuropathic foot ulceration.
- Ability to concord with professionally prescribed treatment.

Application of compression
The correct application of compression therapy is discussed in Chapter 14. Table 6.4 outlines additional measures that can be taken to ensure the safe use of compression in patients with diabetes.

TREATMENT OF MIXED AETIOLOGY ULCERATION
The evidence-base for the treatment of patients with mixed aetiology ulceration is poor. Few treatments have been developed and evaluated for management of this important group of patients.

Priorities of management are governed by a number of factors:

- The degree of PAOD determines the level of compression that can be safely applied.

Table 6.4 Application of compression materials in diabetes.

Limb protection	Orthopaedic wool	Pad all deformities to prevent pressure necrosis.
		Reshape the limb to protect the tibial crest, extensor tendons and forefoot.
	Foam	Apply small, soft-foam shapes to cushion deformities, or for placement in between skin folds around toe deformities.
	Dressings	Foam adhesive dressings can be used to prevent trauma and redistribute pressure.
Bandage application	Factors that can **reduce** pressure in the vulnerable limb	Large limbs have less pressure applied than small limbs (Laplace's law).
		Reduce number of layers.
		Reduce extension of the bandage.
		Reduce overlap of layers.
Correct footwear	Trainers	Larger size of trainers can accommodate compression bandaging in most cases.
	Custom-made shoes	Bandages may have to be applied from ankle to knee if neuropathic foot problems coexist. This requires **specialist** intervention to prevent oedema forming around the ankle joint.
	Adapted soft shoes/slippers	Shoes designed for the disabled can be bought from mail order catalogues.

- Control of diabetes is essential if wound healing is to occur.
- Complex medical problems such as cardiac failure are a frequent problem and often difficult to control.
- Other diabetic complications such as nephropathy may contribute to delayed healing.

- Prevention of wound complications such as infection is a major priority.

Reduced levels of compression can be used. Pressure levels should not exceed 25 mmHg unless under specialist supervision. No compression should be applied to patients with an ABPI below 0.5. Vascular referral should always be considered in those with established PAOD. Interventions such as angioplasty and reconstructive surgery, although more complex in this patient group, can improve the chances of healing due to improved perfusion.

> It is important to remember that patients with established PAOD may rapidly deteriorate. Any change in symptoms should prompt a thorough reassessment and urgent referral for a specialist opinion.

Antibiotic therapy

Antibiotics are frequently required to treat wound infections in these patients. It is essential that the correct antibiotics are prescribed and that the antibiotic sensitivities are checked. Diabetic wounds are frequently infected by a number of different organisms (polymicrobial infection) including anaerobes, and therefore a cocktail of antibiotics may be required. Advice from a microbiologist is vital in these circumstances. Hyperglycaemia is a common problem during periods of infection and can further delay healing. Osteomyelitis may be a complication of infection in such wounds. Patients who suffer repeated episodes of infection or who fail to improve with treatment should be investigated by an X-ray and magnetic resonance imaging (MRI) scan, and require specialist intervention (Edmonds & Foster, 2000; Levin & O'Neal, 2001).

Control of risk factors

The control of risk factors such as smoking can be particularly challenging in these patients as their quality of life is already significantly reduced. Patients frequently report that smoking gives them comfort, even though they have been advised of its deleterious effects. Professionals must avoid being too judgemental in their attitude and seek to try to understand how the condition is impacting on their life. A constant punitive reaction by staff may adversely affect the therapeutic relationship that is vital when nursing such complex patients.

Case study: a complex diabetic leg ulcer

Mr X is a 70-year-old gentleman who suffers with MS, type 1 diabetes and peripheral arterial disease. His MS is stable, and the diabetes well controlled. He lives alone in a council flat and, although he is wheel-chair-bound, he has good upper body mobility and manages very well independently with daily help from social services. He has never suffered with diabetic foot ulceration, and regularly attends his diabetic clinic for check-ups.

Some 3 years ago he developed an unusual ulcer over the top lateral aspect of his foot, near his ankle. Initially he was seen by his diabetic podiatrist, but the ulcer was so unusual that he was referred to the leg ulcer team. On examination, it was noted that he had some non-pitting oedema of both feet, probably due to years of dependency and immobility causing lymphoedema. His legs were very thin with calf muscle wastage. A row of superficial skin breaks were seen to track from between his first and second toe, across the top of the foot, to the lateral malleolus, following the line of lymphatic vessels and suggestive of chronic lymphangiitis. His toe pressure on the affected limb was 40 mmHg. Advice was sought from the vascular team, but angioplasty or surgery could not be offered due to the distal nature of the disease. The specialist team was very cautious about applying compression on a diabetic foot with peripheral arterial disease, and further advice was sought from the complex leg ulcer assessment clinic.

Initially, he was prescribed a 2-week course of penicillin for the lymphangiitis, followed by a 3-month prophylactic course of 250 mg phenoxymethylpenicillin (penicillin V) daily. The ulcer improved significantly and by the end of 3 months was clean and granulating. The penicillin was stopped, but the ulcer began to break down again, and the prophylactic penicillin recommenced. After another 3 months, progress had halted, and it was noted that the foot swelling had increased.

Following another in-depth assessment it was decided to commence support bandaging of his foot and leg, using an inelastic bandage and applying plenty of padding around the calf to reshape the leg. Over the course of some weeks the swelling reduced significantly and the ulcer began to improve.

Now, a year later, although complete healing has not occurred, there has been no further deterioration and his foot has been free from pain, swelling and infection.

NECROBIOSIS LIPOIDICA

Necrobiosis lipoidica is a relatively rare diabetic complication (O'Toole et al., 1999). In one-third of patients the condition appears before the development of diabetes. It is four times more common in women than men. Necrobiosis lipoidica frequently presents in young adulthood, but may occur at any time from childhood to old age. It is largely seen in Caucasians but has also been reported in Asian populations (Sawada, 1985).

The true pathogenesis of the condition is unknown. Some 85% of lesions occur on the pretibial and medial malleolar area. Lesions are usually bilateral, but asymmetrical in their presentation. Other rarer locations include the thighs, feet, arms, face, scalp and penis. The lesions appear as slowly enlarging, irregular, non-scaling plaques with a slightly elevated border and a reddish-blue periphery (Fig. 6.7).

The central part of the lesion is erythematous in the early stages of development. Later it becomes yellow or sclerotic and resembles glazed porcelain. After a time the plaque atrophies become soft and

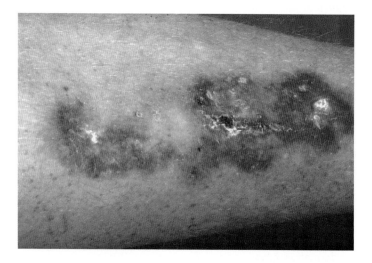

Fig. 6.7 Necrobiosis lipoidica.

brown. Telangiectasias (small dilated blood vessels) are visible on the surface. Lesions vary in size from a few millimetres to several centimetres. Single lesions may become multiple as the condition deteriorates. Some lesions ulcerate spontaneously or in response to trauma. It is thought that this is due to local destruction of cutaneous nerves by inflammation. Sensation may be absent or reduced. Secondary infection is common, leading to further tissue necrosis and delayed healing.

Assessment of the condition should be carried out using the principles discussed in Chapters 3 and 8.

Treatment priorities
The effective treatment of necrobiosis lipoidica involves:

- Appropriate wound management
- Treatment of infection
- Prevention of recurrence
- Teaching self-care regimes
- Understanding the psychosocial impact of the disorder

Hyperglycaemic control
Table 6.5 outlines some of the factors to be considered. Good hyperglycaemic control is vital for all patients with diabetes to limit the development of complications. The relationship of glycaemic control and necrobiosis has yet to be adequately examined. However, hyperglycaemia is associated with infection, a common problem for these patients.

Skin care
Emollients will help to increase the barrier function of the skin, thus reducing the portal of entry for bacteria. Practical devices such as shin pads may prevent local trauma and recurrence. Topical steroids are only useful in the early stages of the disease before atrophy occurs; steroids will further weaken the skin's resilience if the area has become atrophic. However, if the surrounding area of atrophy is affected by dermatitis a small amount of a local steroid may be useful for a very short period of 1–2 weeks until the dermatitis subsides. Daily emollients should then be applied to the affected area.

Table 6.5 Treatment priorities in necrobiosis lipoidica.

Problem	Treatment priority	Comments
Good glycaemic control	Important to reduce the risk of concurrent infection and promote wound healing	Associated link to necrobiosis lipoidica not proven. Infection associated with prolonged hyperglycaemia.
Prevention of skin trauma	Shin pads and foam dressings	Trauma is a major cause of recurrent episodes of ulceration.
Skin care regimes	Daily application of emollients	This will help to maintain skin integrity and prevent entry of bacteria.
Treatment of dermatitis	Topical steroids for 1–2 weeks	Avoid long-term use as this will further weaken the skin.
Choice of dressing	Prevention of trauma and pain are the main priorities	During periods of infection, antimicrobial dressings containing povidone iodine or silver may be required to reduce the bacterial load.
Treatment of infection	Appropriate antibiotics	Patients must seek immediate medical advice if they suspect an infection is developing.
Drug therapy	Aspirin, pentoxifylline	RCTs are lacking on these drug therapies. Drugs should only be prescribed by a specialist practitioner.
Psychological support	Seek to understand the impact of the condition on the patient	Referral for specialist psychological advice may be required.

Choice of dressings

Appropriate dressings designed to prevent skin trauma should be selected if ulceration occurs. Exudate levels are generally low, but this may increase during periods of infection; in which case, dressings designed to cope with moderate to high levels of exudate should be selected. Adequate control of exudate is vital. If exudate is left in contact with the skin the ulceration may extend rapidly due to the vulnerability of the tissues.

Antimicrobials such as povidone iodine and silver products may be useful in reducing the bacterial burden and promoting healing.

Antibiotic therapy and other therapies

Antibiotics may be required if there is evidence of clinical cellulitis (erythema, pain, oedema), for wounds can rapidly deteriorate. It is important to ensure that the organism causing infection is sensitive to the antibiotic/s given. Patients should be advised to seek immediate medical attention if they think an infection is occurring. In some cases, patients may benefit from carrying prophylactic antibiotics (penicillin) which they can begin immediately an infection develops.

Skin grafts are sometimes used for this condition, but the recurrence rate following this procedure is high. Ulceration may occur in the grafted area or surrounding area. Medical treatment is limited, although individual cases treated with aspirin and pentoxifylline have been reported with some success (Sibbald & Schachter, 1984). Both drugs influence blood flow in the microcirculation. Aspirin affects platelet aggregation and pentoxifylline alters red cell deformability. However, evidence for the routine use of these drugs is lacking, and only a specialist practitioner should prescribe such therapies.

Psychological support

Due to the young age of many of the patients with this condition it is important to assess the psychological impact and the support mechanisms they have available to them (see Chapter 10). While the recurrence rate of this condition is high, spontaneous remission frequently occurs and the patient should be given hope that improvement is possible. Effective patient education should be provided, including literature about the condition. The patient should be taught self-management strategies to aid healing and prevent recurrence. This will help the patient to feel a greater sense of involvement and control of this frustrating condition.

SUMMARY

- Diabetes mellitus causes changes in the skin and is associated with delayed healing.
- All patients with diabetes mellitus and leg ulceration should undergo a comprehensive assessment to identify the cause of the ulcer and to establish clinical and psychosocial factors that may influence decisions about treatment.
- Levels of neuropathy should be assessed in all patients with diabetes, as it is a common symptom associated with leg and foot ulceration.
- Peripheral arterial occlusive disease (PAOD) occurs at an earlier age and is more aggressive in patients with diabetes.
- Signs and symptoms of PAOD may be masked by concurrent neuropathy.
- Venous ulceration in the patient with diabetes requires compression therapy. However, it is vital to ensure the patient has an adequate arterial circulation before commencing treatment.
- Compression bandaging may require an adaptation in application technique and choice of bandage in the presence of neuropathy with foot deformities.
- Treatment priorities of mixed aetiology and ischaemic ulceration are governed by the degree of arterial disease, frequently requiring interventions such as angioplasty or reconstructive surgery to improve tissue perfusion.
- Conservative therapy should promote a healthy wound bed and control infection..
- Necrobiosis lipoidica (NL) is a relatively rare complication of diabetes that causes leg ulceration.
- Treatment includes the prevention of infection and trauma.

CONCLUSION

Patients with ulceration associated with diabetes can be some of the most challenging clinical situations that nurses deal with. Complications such as infection and arterial disease can occur at a very rapid pace and are a major factor in why the amputation rate remains depressingly high. Any significant deterioration should prompt nurses to take urgent action to involve the multi-disciplinary team in order to improve the outcome for these unfortunate patients.

REFERENCES

Aikens, J.E. & Lustman, P.J. (2001) Psychosocial and psychological aspects of diabetic foot complications. In: *The Diabetic Foot*, 6th edn (M. Levin, L.W. O' Neal, J.H. Bowker & M.A. Pfeifer, eds). St Louis, Mosby, pp. 727–736.

Armstrong, D.G., Lavery, L.A. & Bushman, T.R. (1998) Peak foot pressures influence the healing time of diabetic foot ulcers treated with total contact casts. *Journal of Rehabilitation Research and Development* **35**: 1–5.

Calvet, H.M. & Yoshikawa, T.T. (2001) Infections in diabetes. *Infectious Disease Clinics of North America* **15**: 407–421.

Couch, N.P. (1986) On the arterial consequences of smoking. *Journal of Vascular Surgery* **3**: 807.

Davis, W.K., Hess, G.E. & Hiss, R.G. (1988) Psychosocial correlates of survival in diabetes. *Diabetes Care* **7**: 538–545.

Dickhaut, S.C., Delee, J.C. & Page, C.P. (1984) Nutritional status: importance in predicting wound healing after amputations. *Journal of Bone and Joint Surgery* **66**(1): 71–75.

Edmonds, M.E. & Foster, A.V.M. (2000) *Managing the Diabetic Foot*. Oxford, Blackwell Science.

Ford, I. (1990) Activation of coagulation in diabetes mellitus in relation to the presence of vascular complications. *Diabetes Medicine* **8**: 322–329.

Levin, M. & O' Neal, L. (2001) *The Diabetic Foot*, 6th edn (M. Levin, L.W. O' Neal, J.H. Bowker & M.A. Pfeifer, eds). St Louis, Mosby.

Nelzén, O., Berqvist, D. & Lindhagen, A. (1997) Long term prognosis for patients with chronic leg ulcers: a prospective cohort study. *European Journal of Endovascular Surgery* **13**: 500–508.

O'Toole, E.A., Kennedy, U., Nolan, J.J., et al. (1999) Necrobiosis lipoidica: only a minority of patients have diabetes mellitus. *British Journal of Dermatology* **140**: 283–286.

Pendsey, S. (2003) *Diabetic Foot*. London, Martin Dunitz, Taylor & Francis Group.

Sawada, Y. (1985) Successful treatment of ulcerated necrobiosis lipoidica diabeticorum with prostaglandin E1 and skin flap transfer. A case report. *Journal of Dermatology* **12**: 449–454.

Sibbald, R.G. & Schachter, R.K. (1984) The skin and diabetes mellitus. *International Journal of Dermatology* **23**: 567–584.

Sosenko, J.M., Kato, M., Soto, R. & Bild, D.E. (1990) Comparison of quantitative sensory threshold measures for their association with foot ulceration in diabetic patients. *Diabetes Care* **13**: 1057–1061.

The International Working Group on the Diabetic Foot (1999) *International Consensus on the Diabetic Foot*. Amsterdam.

Wilson, P.W.F. & Kannel, W.B. (1992) Epidemiology of hyperglycaemia and atherosclerosis. In: *Hyperglycaemia. Diabetes and Vascular Disease* (N. Ruderman, J. Williamson & M. Brownlee, eds). New York, Oxford University Press.

Other Ulcer Aetiologies and Multi-factorial Ulceration

LEARNING OBJECTIVES

Nurses involved in leg ulcer management should be able to demonstrate:

❏ The ability to describe the different types of rare ulcer aetiologies.
❏ An understanding of how systemic diseases such as rheumatoid arthritis and scleroderma lead to ulceration.
❏ An understanding of how a comprehensive assessment will identify these types of ulcers.
❏ An understanding of the different forms of systemic and local treatment that are used.
❏ An understanding of the importance of good symptom control in promoting improved quality of life.

INTRODUCTION

There are over 40 known causes of leg ulceration reported in the literature (Falanga, 2000). Many of these are rare and related to other conditions. Patients with such conditions are usually referred directly to hospital units by their general practitioner. In 1992, Moffatt et al. reported that studies involving community ulcer services showed that patients with skin cancers and other rare aetiologies were often referred to community nurses for assessment and treatment, and this is still the case today. In these complex situations the diagnosis of the underlying aetiology is frequently incorrect and specialist medical referral can be delayed until the ulcer deteriorates or other systemic symptoms prompt referral.

It is important that nurses are aware of the systemic conditions associated with ulceration and know how to recognise the unusual features of an ulcer that requires prompt referral to a medical specialist.

A number of inflammatory conditions, such as rheumatoid arthritis, may coexist with venous or arterial disease. If these are left undetected they can, at best, prevent healing from occurring, and, at worst, lead to potentially serious complications (Falabella & Falanga, 1998). Even with appropriate intervention some of these conditions are extremely difficult to treat and are associated with prolonged periods of ulceration. While correct treatment of the underlying condition is important, appropriate wound care and control of symptoms must be equally addressed.

AUTOIMMUNE AND INFLAMMATORY DISORDERS

People with inflammatory or autoimmune disorders have an increased risk of developing leg ulceration. Examples of such disorders include rheumatoid arthritis (RA), scleroderma/systemic sclerosis, systemic lupus erythematosus (SLE), ulcerative colitis and Crohn's disease, among others. Some of these occur because of the disease process, while others occur because of the complications and treatment of the underlying disease. The presence of a systemic condition can lead to a number of different ulcer aetiologies. An example of this is seen in cases of rheumatoid arthritis when the following different ulcer types can develop:

- Vasculitic ulceration due to inflammatory changes in the blood vessels (occurs in less than 20% of ulcers) (Figs 7.1–7.3).
- Venous ulceration due to poor venous return, rapid vein refill, dependent oedema, and loss of calf muscle pump because of reduced ankle movement.
- Ischaemic ulceration due to an increased risk of peripheral arterial occlusive disease (the mechanism for this remains unclear).
- Traumatic ulceration and delayed wound healing because of fragile skin following prolonged steroid therapy.
- A combination of factors.

Roughly 5% of people with rheumatoid arthritis develop leg ulceration. About 18% of these ulcers are due to vasculitis (Pun et al., 1990).

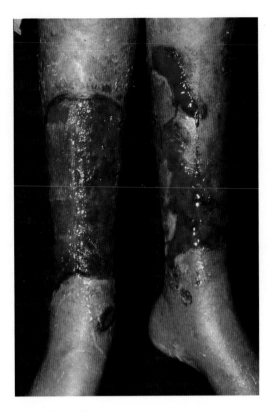

Fig. 7.1 Rheumatoid vasculitis.

Vasculitis and inflammatory ulceration

Vasculitis is an inflammation of the blood vessel wall and affects a variety of organs, including the skin. Immune complexes build up, leading to chronic inflammation and ultimately to cell death, tissue necrosis and ulceration (Sibbald, 2004). Classification of vasculitis is usually according to the size of the blood vessel affected (Cawley, 1987). Vasculitis of small- and medium-sized vessels is most commonly associated with leg ulceration. Leucocytoclastic vasculitis is the most common type that affects the skin and leads

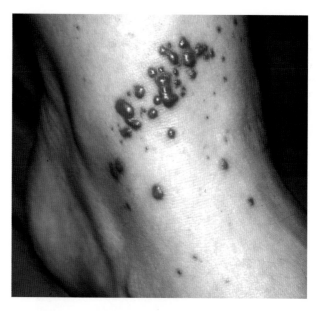

Fig. 7.2 Leucocytoclastic vasculitis.

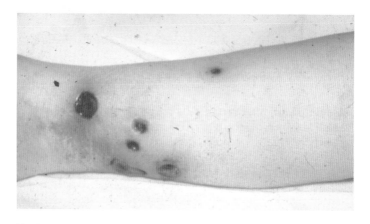

Fig. 7.3 Ulceration associated with vasculitis.

to ulceration. It tends to present initially as painful crops of purpuric lesions that appear suddenly and spontaneously (Fig. 7.2). However, the presentation may be less defined and in some cases may mimic a venous ulcer. The surrounding purpuric changes in the skin may be the most useful guide and may also be found on other parts of the body (Fig. 7.3).

Connective tissue disorders

Many inflammatory ulcers are related to collagen vascular (connective tissue) diseases and immunological conditions. These conditions include:

- Rheumatoid arthritis
- Inflammatory bowel disease
- Systemic lupus erythematosus (SLE)
- Scleroderma
- Dermatomyositis
- Polyarteritis nodosa
- Leucocytoclastic vasculitis

Other causes of inflammatory ulcers

Inflammatory ulcers are also associated with infections such as hepatitis B and C, syphilis or streptococcal infection, and with malignancy. Conditions associated with blood coagulation abnormalities, such as antiphospholipid syndrome or those in which the blood vessels are affected by excessive calcium deposition (calcinosis in scleroderma and dermatomyositis), can lead to ulceration.

IDENTIFYING THE PATIENT WITH AN INFLAMMATORY ULCER

Careful assessment, as described in Chapter 3, will provide many clues to whether the patient has an inflammatory ulcer. The following additional points may be helpful to consider:

- An underlying systemic condition may directly or indirectly cause ulceration.
- Involvement of the fingers and face with skin induration may suggest scleroderma or systemic sclerosis.

- An erythematous butterfly rash on the face and photosensitivity may indicate systemic lupus erythematosus (SLE).
- A purple–violet rash on the eyelids is distinctive of dermatomyositis.
- Hand deformities associated with rheumatoid arthritis may suggest pyoderma gangrenosum.
- Inflammatory lesions on the fingers can be important in distinguishing dermatomyositis from SLE. In dermatomyositis, purple papules or nodules occur over the finger joints, while the lesions of SLE are found between the knuckles.
- The presence of ill-defined, red streaks (livedo reticularis) indicates micro-occlusive disease, which may cause ischaemia of the skin and subsequent ulceration.
- Corticosteroid therapy may result in bulging of the posterior portion of the neck (cushingoid appearance).
- The introduction of a new drug may precede vasculitis.
- Leucocytoclastic vasculitis is associated with regular shape ulceration on the skin.
- Certain types of vasculitis, such as polyarteritis nodosa or those involving larger blood vessels, lead to areas of skin involvement and purpura that are irregular in appearance because of the chance for anastomosing vessels to modify the level of ischaemia at the skin surface.
- Ulceration is usually extremely painful and can be very rapid.

MEDICAL AND NURSING MANAGEMENT OF INFLAMMATORY ULCERS

A successful outcome is highly dependent on the ability to control the underlying disease process. While complete healing can often be achieved this is not always the case, and patients can die if the systemic effects of the condition cannot be halted.

Diagnosis is based on the patient's clinical history and results of a wound biopsy. Further tests are required to establish if other organs are affected. The treatment of vasculitis very much depends on the use of immunosuppressive or immunomodulatory agents. However, one of the first medical challenges is to exclude the possibility that a medication may have caused the vasculitis. This usually requires the removal of all medicines that are not totally necessary. Corticosteroids and immunosuppressives, such as azathioprine or ciclosporin, are used as well as the new biological agents, such anti-tumour necrosis factor (anti-TNF) drugs. Many of the treatment priorities are similar to those for the treatment of other inflammatory ulcers.

The following points should be considered when treating these patients:

- Management may be shared between the rheumatology and dermatology teams. Liaise closely with all teams involved to ensure a co-ordinated approach.
- Treatment may involve oral anti-inflammatory drugs.
- Good wound management to provide a warm moist environment.
- Appropriate exudate control to avoid maceration.
- Pain is severe and may require opiates
- If pain control is poor, the patient should be referred to a pain specialist.
- Prevention of infection (consider antimicrobials).
- Reduced levels of compression may be appropriate if oedema is a problem (Peggy & Phillips, 2002; Sibbald, 2004).
- Advanced therapies such as skin grafting may be used. These bring immediate pain relief as well as assisting wound closure once the disease process has been controlled.

PYODERMA GANGRENOSUM

It is essential that nurses recognise this condition and treat it as a medical emergency that requires immediate diagnosis and treatment by a dermatologist.

Pyoderma gangrenosum is an acute, necrotising and often excruciatingly painful ulceration that tends to occur in people with inflammatory or rheumatic disorders (e.g. ulcerative colitis, Crohn's disease, diverticulitis, RA or SLE) (Fig. 7.4). It has also been known to occur in association with diabetes mellitus and myeloma, following skin trauma or surgery, and in the absence of an associated illness but in an area of previous scarring (Margolis, 1995).

The role of pathergy

One distinctive feature of the condition is its rapid development and deterioration (pathergy) over a very short period. Biopsy

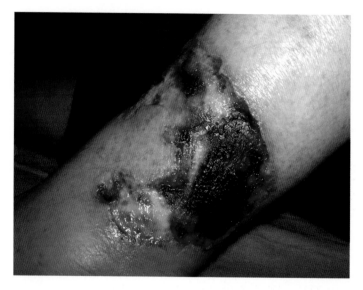

Fig. 7.4 Pyoderma gangrenosum.

or debridement both cause deterioration if performed while the disease is in its active stage.

There is no specific diagnostic test for pyoderma gangrenosum. A wound biopsy is required to aid diagnosis through the exclusion of other conditions. It is essential to rule out other causes of rapid tissue loss such critical ischaemia and infective necrotising fasciitis.

The rapid and painful deterioration associated with this condition can cause extreme anxiety, particularly until a correct diagnosis has been made and treatment instigated.

Medical and nursing management

The mainstay of therapy for pyoderma gangrenosum is systemic corticosteroids. High doses (60 mg or greater) of prednisolone are required for many weeks or months to obtain a therapeutic response. Intravenous pulse therapy with methylprednisolone is also used and patients are often hospitalised during treatment because of the danger of secondary cardiac complications. A number of other drug therapies are also used; these include (Prystowsky et al., 1989; Matis et al., 1992; de Imus et al., 2001; Gettler et al., 2003; Liu and Mackool, 2003; McGowan et al., 2004):

- Ciclosporin
- Cyclophosphamide
- Mycophenolic acid
- Azathioprine

However, due to the significant side-effects of these drugs, patients must be closely monitored by a specialist medical practitioner. Good liaison following skin trauma or surgery between the hospital and community services is required to ensure the best outcome for these patients.

> Patients should be weaned off steroid therapy slowly over a number of weeks. Nurses have a duty not just to dress the ulcer but to keep abreast of any changes made to the steroid therapy dosage, and to ensure the patient understands and takes the correct dose.

Sub-acute pyoderma gangrenosum

Not all patients with pyoderma gangrenosum deteriorate rapidly. Patients may be routinely referred to a leg ulcer service on the mistaken belief that they have a painful venous ulcer. If this condition is suspected, the following should be considered:

- Immediate referral (within 24 hours) to the leg ulcer and dermatology teams.
- If no established leg ulcer pathway is in operation, request the GP to send the patient to hospital for an urgent assessment.
- The borders of the ulcer can be marked with an indelible pen to monitor ulcer progression.
- Control of pain will usually require opiates, and should be a priority of care even before the diagnosis is confirmed.
- Use very low adherent dressings and avoid aggressive debridement or trauma at dressing removal, since disturbance can generate an even greater inflammatory response and stimulate deterioration (Sibbald, 2004).

- Prevention of infection may require the use of antimicrobials (Chakrabaty & Phillips, 2002).
- Rapid use of appropriate antibiotics if secondary infection occurs.
- If either venous disease or oedema is present, low levels of compression may be appropriate once the active inflammatory phase has subsided. Higher levels of compression may also be used if tolerated.
- When the condition is stable, debridement and skin grafting can be considered for large ulcers. If there is concern that surgery will reactivate the disease the wounds may be left to heal by secondary intention.
- Negative pressure therapy (VAC) may be used to assist debridement when the disease is stable and when large areas of ulceration are present.
- Patients should tell doctors of their condition, particularly if they are to have any other operation that may cause a further occurrence.

RHEUMATOID ARTHRITIS

RA is a chronic, progressive, inflammatory tissue disorder of unknown origin causing joint stiffness, ankylosis (fixation of a joint) and associated joint deformity. In addition, the autoimmune component of the disease can affect other systems, including the skin (Oliver & Mooney, 2002). People with RA are substantially more at risk of developing leg ulceration, and an estimated 5–10% will experience ulceration at some point in their lives (Cawley, 1987; Pun et al., 1990). About 18% of these ulcers are vasculitic (see Fig. 7.1) (Pun et al., 1990). Poor ankle mobility causing loss of the calf muscle pump and 'pseudovenous disease' is another major factor (Cawley, 1987; Moffatt et al., 2004). The general health status of many of these patients is poor. Poor nutrition due to loss of appetite, functional difficulties or fatigue are common (Ryan, 1995). These problems lead to high levels of stress and anxiety.

Recognising rheumatoid ulceration

These ulcers are often associated with high levels of rheumatoid factor and severe arthritis. However, they may also be seen in those with stable rheumatoid arthritis. The ulcers tend to have a scalloped, undulating border (Fig. 7.5). Rheumatoid ulcers should not be mistaken for pyoderma gangrenosum. They do not have the purple edges associated with pyoderma gangrenosum, nor the undermining border, and they generally do not have the necrotic or truly eschar-like ulcer base seen in pyoderma gangrenosum. Rheumatoid ulcers are often resistant to many of the treatments used for pyoderma gangrenosum. The ulcers are generally restricted to the lower extremities, whereas the ulcers of pyoderma gangrenosum may be located on other parts of the body. It is not uncommon for rheumatoid ulcers to have a component of ischaemic or venous insufficiency, which often makes the condition more difficult to diagnose. Rheumatoid ulcers are generally considered to be multifactorial in aetiology.

Medical and nursing management

The medical treatment of this condition is difficult. Many patients will already be receiving high doses of corticosteroids, and other

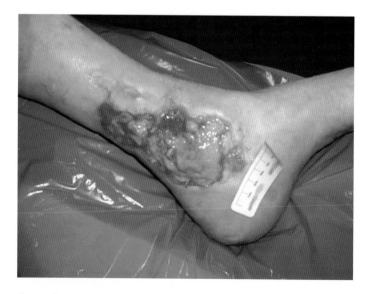

Fig. 7.5 Rheumatoid ulcer.

immunosuppressive drugs are often ineffective. Anti-TNF-alpha treatment may prove helpful in some patients. Delayed wound healing and susceptibility to infection are common problems.

Compression therapy may be of some value because of the associated venous insufficiency. However, it may cause excruciating pain in a small percentage of patients, and in these cases should not be used until the condition has stabilised and the pain reduced. Compression should always be introduced slowly (a low pressure of less than 25 mmHg) and tailored to the patient's tolerance and pain level; the level of pressure can be increased if well tolerated. The risk of tissue trauma from poor bandaging is high and limb deformities require additional padding for protection.

Great care should be taken to ensure the correct application of the bandage (see Chapter 14). A number of other factors should also be considered when managing these patients:

- The presence of rheumatoid arthritis will be contributing to poor healing, even if it is not the primary cause of the ulcer.
- If there is poor ankle mobility, venous hypertension is likely to be impeding healing. Leg elevation and ankle exercises will need to be taught and encouraged, as tolerated.
- If vasculitis is suspected, refer to the leg ulcer team for an urgent assessment.
- Liaise with the patient's rheumatologist to ensure a co-ordinated approach to care
- Monitor and control wound infection. The drugs used for RA may also reduce immunity so that fungal infections such as tinea pedis and ringworm may develop and place the patient at risk of severe bacterial infection. Osteomyelitis is a common complication and is particularly found in the toes.

SCLERODERMA

Scleroderma presents as a thickening of the skin due to the excessive accumulation of connective tissue. Scleroderma ulcers represent a spectrum of conditions manifested by skin breakdown and associated with systemic sclerosis (scleroderma). This spectrum is large: it can involve ulceration of the fingers as a result of ischaemia, as well as ulceration due to associated abnormalities in coagulation and tissue calcium deposition. Not to be forgotten is the development of ulceration purely due to indurated, tense tissues resulting from fibrosis (Fig. 7.6).

More than 90% of patients with scleroderma also have Raynaud's phenomenon. Classically, Raynaud's phenomenon presents with a triad of colour changes in the fingers and toes secondary to cold exposure or stress. Typically, there is pallor of the skin, which is followed by cyanosis, and then finally by reactive hyperaemia; the latter presents as intense redness. Some or all of the fingers and toes can be involved. A certain degree of numbness may accompany Raynaud's phenomenon. In many cases not all these symptoms are manifest.

Calcinosis is very common in the skin of patients with scleroderma and is sometimes clearly visible to the naked eye. Sometimes, angular-looking ulcers occur in the fibrotic skin of patients with systemic sclerosis and other connective tissue disorders (Essary & Wick, 2000).

Scleroderma contributes to leg ulceration in the following ways:

- Tightening and stretching of the skin, especially over bony prominences (King, 2004).

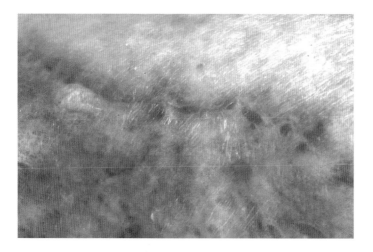

Fig. 7.6 Scleroderma.

- Poor healing due to the effect of systemic steroid or immuno-suppressive therapy.
- Secondary vasculitis.
- Severe Raynaud's phenomena of the digits that can lead to ulceration and localised gangrene in severe cases.
- Increased risk of peripheral arterial occlusive disease.

Medical and nursing management
- If scleroderma is suspected referral to a dermatologist is required for diagnosis and advice on treatment.
- Specialist wound care advice is frequently required.
- These patients have a very reduced healing potential. Areas of eschars or deep necrosis should not be debrided because the underlying vascular supply is so poor and debridement may cause gangrene leading to limb loss.
- Avoid soaking the foot in warm or hot water as this may exacerbate the Raynaud's phenomena and cause an increase in pain.
- Ensure the patient has an adequate diet. Scleroderma is associated with difficulties in swallowing due to changes in the oesophagus.
- Patients should receive education about their condition and practical ways to reduce trauma and tissue damage.

SYSTEMIC LUPUS ERYTHEMATOSUS (SLE)

SLE is a connective tissue disease causing inflammation of many of the body's organs. It tends to affect women between 20 and 40 years of age, and can cause vasculitis, venous and arterial thrombosis and Raynaud's disease (King, 2004). One study found that up to 20% of sufferers experienced vasculitic or inflammatory skin changes, and also that 5–6% of sufferers developed leg ulceration (Cawley, 1987).

As with rheumatoid arthritis, ulceration may occur because of a number of factors:

- Vasculitis or pyoderma gangrenosum.
- Peripheral gangrene due to necrotising vasculitis of the digital arteries.

- Arthritic foot changes causing poor ankle mobility, loss of calf muscle function and pressure points on the foot (Cawley, 1987).
- Delayed wound-healing, thin skin and susceptibility to infection due to long-term steroid and immunosuppressive therapy.

The principles of management are similar to those described for other inflammatory ulcers.

CUTANEOUS MICROTHROMBOTIC ULCERS

Occlusion of small dermal blood vessels (microthrombosis) leads to a number of types of ulceration. These ulcers present with severe pain, atrophie blanche, livedo reticularis and dark necrosis within the ulcer bed or at the edges. The aetiologies associated with this condition include:

- Cryofibrinogenaemia (Fig. 7.7)
- Antiphospholipid syndrome
- Coagulopathies

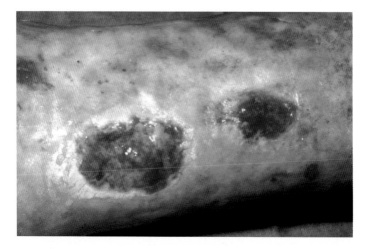

Fig. 7.7 Cryofibrinogenaemia.

- Thrombocytosis
- Idiopathic vasculitis

A high platelet count as well as other types of clotting abnormalities can lead to similar types of ulceration.

Medical and nursing management

Treatment of these types of ulcers includes anticoagulants, antiplatelet agents, high doses of pentoxifylline (800 mg three times a day) and anabolic steroids. The high-dose regimen of pentoxifylline has proven effective in patients with venous ulcers and is now being used to treat other types of ulceration. Many of these patients are under the care of haematologists and a co-ordinated approach to management is required.

Calciphylaxis is a very difficult to treat condition, in which calcium is responsible for the occlusion of blood vessels. This condition is often associated with severe renal disease and hyperparathyroidism. The ulcerations are characterised by a necrotic wound bed with eschar and areas of micro livedo. Debridement of the areas of calcified blood vessels may be required in addition to grafting. Patients should be educated about their increased risk of thrombosis, particularly during long journeys.

SKIN CANCERS

Practitioners need to be alert to malignancy occurring in ulceration, not just at the initial assessment but throughout the course of managing the ulcer (Hayes & Dodds, 2003). All patients with suspected skin cancers should be referred immediately to the dermatology team for biopsy and treatment. Skin cancer should be suspected if the ulcer:

- Is not responding to treatment (such as compression)
- Is getting larger
- Is overgranulating
- Bleeds easy
- Has rolled edges or a pearly appearance

Basal cell carcinoma (BCC, or rodent ulcer)

This appears as a small raised lesion with a pearly border (Fig. 7.8). It is relatively common, tends to grow slowly and rarely metasta-

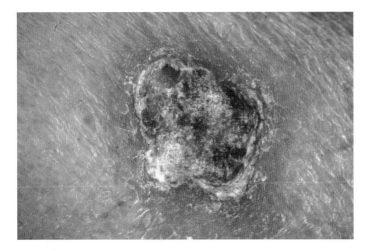

Fig. 7.8 Basal cell carcinoma.

sises. It may also appear as a scaly scab that falls off and bleeds and then re-forms but never heals. Diagnosis is through wound biopsy. BCC is generally treated by excision biopsy. Small excisions are closed with sutures, whereas slightly larger lesions may be left to heal by secondary intention. Very large rodent ulcers are very rare, but when they do occur excision is generally followed by a split skin graft.

Squamous cell carcinoma (SCC)

This is the second most common skin cancer, and can metastasise if untreated (Godsell, 2003). It usually appears as a non-healing lesion that may be crusty, scaly or indurated (Fig. 7.9). An SCC can appear on healthy skin, scar tissue or in a wound. Sun exposure is the most significant risk factor.

Marjolin's ulcer

A squamous cell carcinoma which develops in a pre-existing leg ulcer (such as a venous ulcer) is known as a 'Marjolin's ulcer' (Fig. 7.10).

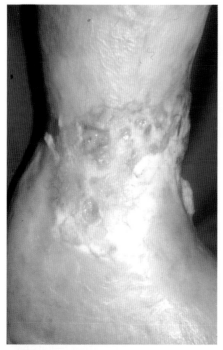

Fig. 7.9 Fungating squamous cell carcinoma.

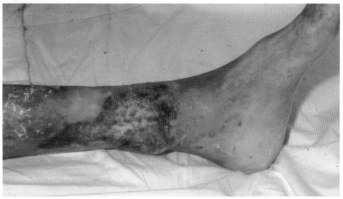

Fig. 7.10 Marjolin's ulcer.

Treatment is dependent on the spread of the cancer and the presence of metastases. While excision is the treatment of choice this may be difficult to achieve if the tumour is within an ulcerated area. Wide excision is usually followed by a skin graft. Radiotherapy is rarely used because of the effects on the wound healing process. If patients refuse active treatment, regular shaving of the extruding wound can help to prevent offensive exudate production during the palliative stage of treatment. Use of antimicrobial agents, such as povidone iodine, silver products and metronidazole gel, can help to reduce the bacterial burden from these wounds.

Malignant melanoma

This is the most serious skin cancer as it tends to metastasise very rapidly. Fig. 7.11 shows a pigmented malignant melanoma lesion. Prognosis depends on the depth of the lesion, and early detection and intervention are vital. Some lesions do not contain pigment and appear as ulcerated inflamed lesions. Melanomas on the heel and plantar surface of the foot may be wrongly diagnosed as pressure ulceration (Godsell, 2003). Treatment frequently involves a combination of excision and chemotherapy, according to the spread of the lesion.

Kaposi's sarcoma

This arises from blood vessels within the skin as multiple small purple or brownish nodules or plaques which may ulcerate (King, 2004). It often occurs on the legs or feet, where it can be mistaken for venous ulceration (Walsh, 2002). In addition, it can also occur as a result of immunosuppression secondary to AIDS.

Bowen's disease (intraepidermal carcinoma)

Generally, this carcinoma presents as a very slow-growing, pink scaly plaque (Fig. 7.12), which can be mistaken for psoriasis, discoid eczema or BCC (Walsh, 2002). It can also look like a weeping blister or an area of over-granulation. In some patients, an area of Bowen's disease can change to become an invasive squamous cell carcinoma.

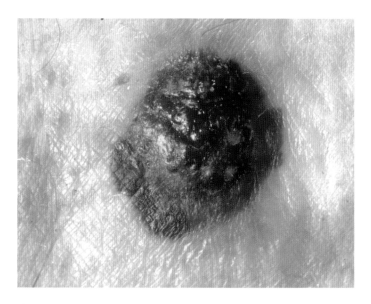

Fig. 7.11 Malignant melanoma.

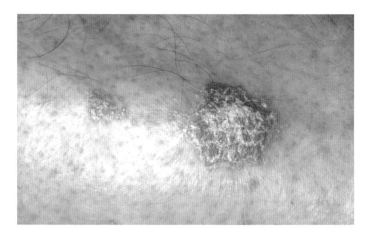

Fig. 7.12 Bowen's disease.

INFECTIVE CAUSES OF ULCERATION

With the increase in international travel it is increasingly possible that rare infective-type ulcers may be seen in those who have travelled to tropical areas. Tuberculosis is on the increase and can present as a skin ulcer (Fig. 7.13). Fig. 7.14 shows a tropical ulcer in a child living in Africa. Osteomyelitis (Fig. 7.15) may occur as a consequence of ulceration or may be the precipitating cause.

Infected insect bites that fail to heal are a common phenomenon. Infection develops deep within the dermis and healing may take many months to occur.

> If an infective ulcer is suspected it is important to liaise with a microbiologist and refer the patient for specialist treatment.

OEDEMA

Medical causes of oedema must be identified and treated systemically before treating oedema due to venous disease.

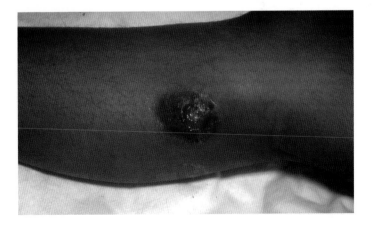

Fig. 7.13 Ulcer due to tuberculosis.

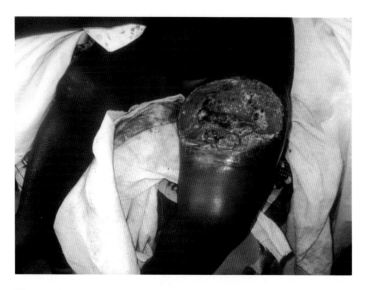

Fig. 7.14 Tropical ulcer.

Non-venous oedema

Oedema will always delay or even prevent healing (Hofman 1998). It is essential to identify the underlying cause of the oedema. Medical causes of oedema include cardiac failure, liver disease and renal failure. All patients should undergo a thorough medical examination to exclude these causes and appropriate treatment commenced (see Chapter 3 on assessment).

Venous oedema

This is a pitting oedema that tends to go down at night and develop during the course of the day. It may affect one or both lower legs. Oedema and tissue changes extending into the thigh indicate that concurrent lymphoedema has developed (phlebolymphoedema). This is particularly common in patients with post-thrombotic syndrome where extensive concurrent damage to the lymphatics has occurred.

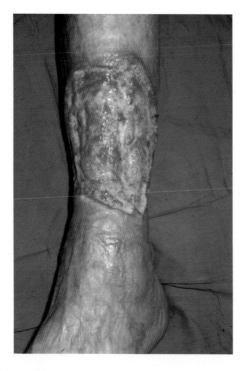

Fig. 7.15 Osteomyelitis.

Cardiac oedema

This is also a pitting oedema which, depending on its severity, may affect just the lower legs or extend into the thighs (and in decompensated heart failure may even reach the genitals and lower abdomen). Patients generally complain of breathlessness on exertion or on lying down. It affects both legs. If it is allowed to persist, it can cause erythema, blistering of the skin, lymphorrhoea and eventually ulceration. Appropriate medical intervention includes diuretic therapy; advice should be sought from the leg ulcer specialist before compression is commenced.

> Bilateral high compression should **never** be applied to patients with decompensated heart failure because this will increase the pre-load to the heart.

Renal oedema
This may present in much the same way as cardiac oedema, and can also occur in patients with uncontrolled renal failure.

Lymphoedema
This is a dense, protein-rich oedema caused by failure of the lymphatics. Unlike other oedemas, it is non-pitting and does not resolve when the patient goes to bed at night (pitting may occur during the very early stages of development). It can occur in one or both legs, and may extend into the thigh or even higher. If uncontrolled it may cause ulceration, as seen in Fig. 7.16 which shows a patient suffering with phlebolymphoedema and underlying osteomyelitis.

Other skin changes include deep skin folds and crevices, papillomatosis (cobblestone appearance), hyperkeratosis and leakage of

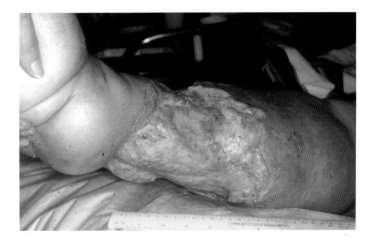

Fig. 7.16 Ulceration due to phlebolymphoedema and osteomyelitis.

lymph fluid (lymphorrhoea). A positive Stemmer's sign indicates the presence of lymphoedema. This sign is tested for by attempting to pinch up a fold of skin on the top of the foot at the base of the second toe (Board & Harlow, 2002); fibrotic skin changes associated with lymphoedema will prevent the skin from being pinched up, i.e. the positive Stemmer's sign. In Wandsworth, over one-third of patients with venous ulceration have concurrent lymphoedema (Moffatt et al., 2004). Patients with lymphoedema should be referred for specialist advice. A full exploration of the treatment of lymphoedema lies outside the scope of this book.

SICKLE CELL DISEASE

Up to 70% of people with sickle cell anaemia are likely to develop a leg ulcer (Serjeant, 2001). Ulceration often begins during the mid to late teens and is most frequent in males of Caribbean origin. The exact mechanisms are not fully understood, but it is thought to involve a combination of chronic anaemia, venous hypertension, trauma and localised microcirculatory damage, due to the affected cells clumping in the small vessels. Fig. 7.17 shows typical sickle cell ulceration.

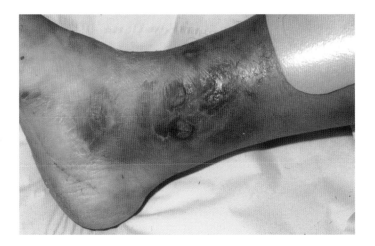

Fig. 7.17 Sickle cell ulceration.

- Sickle cell ulcers tend to be slow to heal and recurrence is common.
- Ulceration occurs most frequently in those with sickle cell disease, but it can also occur in those with sickle cell trait.
- Ulceration is rare in those with beta-thalassaemia.
- Ulcers have a similar appearance to those of atrophie blanche.
- They occur around the malleoli and tend to be painful and sloughy and are frequently misdiagnosed as a venous ulcer.

Medical and nursing management

There is, as yet, no evidence-based treatment for sickle cell ulceration. Management requires a co-ordinated approach, with the haematology team playing an important advisory role. Blood transfusion (simple 'top up' or exchange) has been successfully used in an uncontrolled manner to treat sickle cell leg ulcers. This effect may be directly due to the relief of tissue anoxia as a result of the corrected haemoglobin concentration, and also by limiting the ischaemia arising from repeated episodes of vaso-occlusion (Chernoff et al., 1954; Serjeant, 2001).

Pain may be severe, excruciating and neuropathic in origin. Simple analgesia is inadequate and opioid analgesia and neuroleptic drugs may be required. Referral to a pain specialist is frequently necessary. Additional management issues include:

- Wound debridement. Adequate pain relief during and after the procedure is essential.
- Support or compression therapy, which may aid healing.
- High leg elevation overnight, which may drastically improve the chances of healing.
- Prevention of wound.
- Systemic antibiotics reserved for acute infection with cellulitis. Treatment may need to continue for a number of weeks due to poor tissue perfusion. Consultation with a microbiologist is helpful if recurrent infections occur.
- Avoidance of standing for long periods.

Skin grafts may be very effective at reducing pain, although the recurrence rate is high. Following grafting, compression therapy must be used as soon as the patient is mobile to prevent graft rejection.

Psychological support is essential. Many of these patients are young and are therefore struggling with careers and the financial implications of this disabling condition.

Hydroxyurea is a drug used to treat sickle cell disease by increasing the level of fetal haemoglobin and reducing the effects of sickling. However, a major side-effect of this drug is the development of severe leg and foot ulceration that resolves when the drug is stopped.

SUMMARY

- Approximately one-third of leg ulcer patients suffer with complex leg ulcers from more than one cause.
- Ulcers may be due to a variety of causes. Any unusual appearance should be recorded and the patient referred for an urgent specialist medical assessment.
- The majority of leg ulcer patients in the UK are assessed and treated by community nurses – the nurse therefore has a vital role to play in referring patients on for detailed assessment. Studies show that nurses are very slow to refer on for specialist assessment.
- Successful treatment of these types of ulcers usually requires the use of systemic regimens such as corticosteroid therapy and methotrexate.
- Control of the disease is an essential component of ulcer treatment. This can be very difficult to achieve due to the complexity of the illness.
- Much can be achieved by appropriate wound care and choice of dressings that promote a healthy wound and deal with problems such as exudate control.
- Symptom control is a key priority, irrespective of whether the ulcer will heal or not.
- Communication between all members of the multi-disciplinary team is essential to optimise the potential for ulcer healing and ensure appropriate management.
- Patients with long-term conditions become experts in their condition and should be actively involved in decisions about their treatment.

CONCLUSION

This chapter considers some of the rare types of ulcers that may be seen in clinical practice. In almost all cases these patients require specialist intervention. While it is acknowledged that these patients present a real clinical challenge, there is no doubt that appropriate treatment and control of symptoms can improve the outlook for many of these distressing conditions.

REFERENCES

Board, J. & Harlow, W. (2002) Lymphoedema 2: classification, signs, symptoms and diagnosis. *British Journal of Nursing* **11**(6): 389–395.

Cawley, M.I. (1987) Vasculitis and ulceration in rheumatic diseases of the foot. *Baillière's Clinical Rheumatology* **1**(2): 315–333.

Chakrabaty, A. & Phillips, T.J. (2002) Diagnostic dilemmas: pyoderma gangrenosum. *Wounds* **14**(8): 302–307.

Chernoff, A.I., Shapleigh, J.B. & Moore, C.V. (1954) Therapy of chronic ulceration of the legs associated with sickle cell anaemia. *Journal of the American Medical Association* **155**: 1487–1491.

de Imus, G., Golomb, C., Wilkel, C., Tsoukas, M., Nowak, M. & Falanga, V. (2001) Accelerated healing of pyoderma gangrenosum treated with bioengineered skin and concomitant immunosuppression. *Journal of the American Academy of Dermatology* **44**(1): 61–66.

Essary, L.R. & Wick, M.R. (2000) Cutaneous calciphylaxis. An under-recognized clinicopathologic entity. *American Journal of Clinical Pathology* **113**(2): 280–287.

Falabella, A. & Falanga, V. (1998) Uncommon causes of ulcers. *Clinics in Plastic Surgery* **25**(3): 467–479.

Falanga, V. (2000) *Text Atlas of Wound Management*. London, Martin Dunitz.

Gettler, S., Rothe, M., Grin, C. & Grant-Kels, J. (2003) Optimal treatment of pyoderma gangrenosum. *American Journal of Clinical Dermatology* **4**(9): 597–608.

Godsell, G. (2003) Recognising the signs of skin cancer. *Nursing Times* **99**(31): (Suppl.), 44–45.

Hayes, S. & Dodds, S. (2003) The identification and diagnosis of malignant leg ulcers. *Nursing Times* **99**(31): (Suppl.), 50–52.

Hofman, D. (1998) Oedema and the management of venous ulcer. *Journal of Wound Care* **7**(7): 345–348.

King, B. (2004) Is the leg ulcer venous? Unusual aetiologies of lower leg ulcers. *Journal of Wound Care* **13**(9): 394–396.

Liu, V. & Mackool, B.T. (2003) Mycophenolate in dermatology. *Journal of Dermatological Treatment* **14**(4): 203–211.

Margolis, D.J. (1995) Management of unusual causes of ulcers of lower extremities. *Journal of Wound, Ostomy, Continence Nursing* **22**(2): 89–94.

Matis, W.L., Ellis, C.N., Griffiths, C.E. & Lazarus, G.S. (1992). Treatment of pyoderma gangrenosum with cyclosporine. *Archives of Dermatology* **128**(8): 1060–1064.

McGowan, J.Wt, Johnson, C.A. & Lynn, A. (2004) Treatment of pyoderma gangrenosum with etanercept. *Journal of Drugs in Dermatology* **3**(4): 441–444.

Moffatt, C.J., Franks, P.J., Oldroyd, M., Bosanquet, N., Brown, P., Greenhalgh, R.M. & McCollum, C.N. (1992) Community leg ulcer clinics and impact on ulcer healing. *British Medical Journal* **305**: 1389–1392.

Moffatt, C.J., Franks, P.J., Doherty, D.C., Martin, R., Blewett, R. & Ross, F. (2004) Prevalence of leg ulceration in a London population. *Quarterly Journal of Medicine* **97**(7): 431–437.

Oliver, S. & Mooney, J. (2002) Targeted therapies for patients with rheumatoid arthritis. *Professional Nurse* **17**(12): 716–720.

Peggy, L. & Phillips, T.J. (2002) Diagnostic dilemmas: systemic lupus erythematosus and antiphospholipid syndrome. *Wounds* **14**(6): 221–226.

Prystowsky, J.H., Kahn, S.N. & Lazarus, G.S. (1989) Present status of pyoderma gangrenosum. Review of 21 cases. *Archives of Dermatology* **125**(1): 57–64.

Pun, Y.L.W., Barraclough, D.R.E. & Muirdue, K.D. (1990) Leg ulcers in rheumatoid arthritis. *Medical Journal of Australia* **153**(10): 585–587.

Ryan, S. (1995) Nutrition and the rheumatoid patient. *British Journal of Nursing* **4**(3): 132–136.

Ryan, S., Reddy, A., Natsheh, D., Queen, D. & Sibbald, R.G. (2004). An epidemiological profile of pyoderma gangrenosum patients attending a wound care clinic. Presented at the *2nd World Union of Wound Healing Societies' Meeting*, Paris, 8th–13th July 2004.

Serjeant, G. (2001) *A Guide to Sickle Cell Disease. A Handbook for Diagnosis and Management*. Jamaica, Sickle Cell Trust.

Sibbald, G. (2004) Rare causes of leg ulcers, rare infections. Presented at the *2nd World Union of Wound Healing Societies' Meeting*, Paris, 8th–13th July 2004.

Walsh, R. (2002) Improving diagnosis of malignant leg ulcers in the community. *British Journal of Nursing* **11**(9): 604–613.

Assessing the Wound Bed and Surrounding Skin

8

LEARNING OBJECTIVES

Nurses involved in leg ulcer management should be able to demonstrate:

❏ An understanding of normal wound healing.
❏ An understanding of chronic wound healing.
❏ An understanding of the local barriers to wound healing and how to identify them.
❏ The ability to perform a general skin assessment.
❏ An understanding of skin conditions frequently associated with leg ulceration.

INTRODUCTION

Wound and skin assessment is a key component in effective wound management. It can provide useful information towards diagnosis, guide choices of appropriate dressings and provide the ability to monitor progress or problems in the healing process (Doughty, 2004).

Best practice

- The RCN (1998) leg ulcer guidelines recommend the use of a formal assessment tool.
- The SIGN (1998) guidelines recommend serial measurements of the leg ulcer, including a description of the wound bed.
- Accurate and regular skin and wound assessment will help guide the practitioner in diagnosis and management options, and to monitor progress and deterioration of the wound.
- The TIME framework offers a simple but comprehensive means of wound assessment, based on the principles of wound bed preparation (Falanga, 2004)

CHRONIC WOUND HEALING

As we saw in the introduction to Part II, leg ulcers fall into the category of chronic, not acute, wounds. In order to understand this further, we need to remind ourselves of what 'normal' acute wound healing looks like.

Wound healing normally follows a well-defined but complex series of cellular and biochemical interactions, affecting and affected by local and systemic factors, forming a sequence of overlapping phases. 'Normal' acute wound healing relies on a well-organised fluctuation of various cellular components to clear away debris and bacteria and promote cell growth and migration (Douglass, 2003). Chronic wounds, by contrast, fail to advance through this orderly process, with the result that healing is disrupted (Enoch & Harding, 2003).

There are numerous opportunities for the wound healing process to go wrong or get stuck when managing a leg ulcer. This can be due to not identifying one of the underlying causes, the presence of additional systemic factors, such as those we have already looked at in Chapter 3, and problems at the local wound site, which we will explore more in this chapter. Each of these components has the potential to interrupt the normal healing process, though often it will be a combination of them all. If the factors that can delay healing are identified and addressed then wound healing should be able to proceed as normal. However, it is not always possible to control all the potential elements, and this can lead to disruption of the healing process by altering the usual time frames and patterns of cellular and biochemical events (Romanelli & Mastronicola, 2002).

Chronic wounds appear to get stuck in a constant inflammatory state due to various triggers, such as the presence of excessive exudate levels, necrotic or sloughy tissue and heavy bacterial load. The ongoing inflammatory state leads to high levels of matrix metalloproteinases (MMPs), which in turn damage the extra-cellular matrix, compromising cell migration and connective tissue formation. Excess levels of MMPs create a chemical imbalance within the wound, preventing progression from the inflammatory phase due to their damaging effects on growth factors and the target cell receptors, thus resulting in cellular dysfunction and senescence (Romanelli & Mastronicola, 2002).

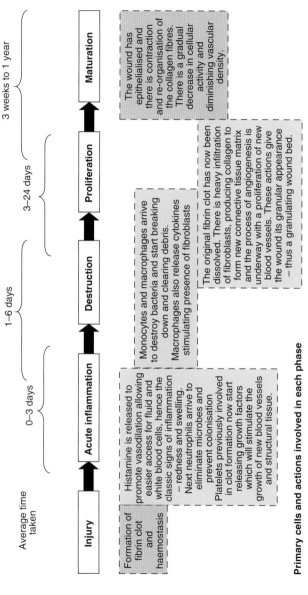

Primary cells and actions involved in each phase

Fig. 8.1 Acute wound healing.

Wound bed preparation (WBP) aims to remove or control these local wound barriers in order to promote a healthy wound bed and promote healing (Falanga, 2000; Douglass, 2003). Chapter 13 will cover the management aspect of WBP in detail; however, the principles of WBP are equally important from an assessment perspective. The European Wound Management Association (EWMA) Advisory Board on WBP (Schultz et al., 2003) has proposed a framework for assessment and management in the form of the acronym – TIME (see Fig. 8.2) – which offers a practical means of remembering and incorporating the understanding of WBP into routine practice. It involves four main observations (Falanga, 2004):

- Tissue management
- Inflammation and infection control

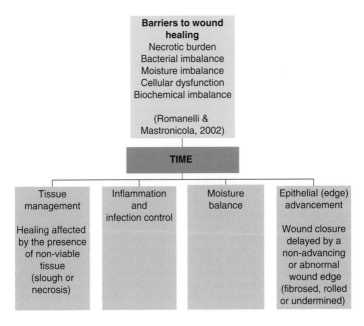

Barriers to wound healing
Necrotic burden
Bacterial imbalance
Moisture imbalance
Cellular dysfunction
Biochemical imbalance

(Romanelli & Mastronicola, 2002)

TIME

Tissue management	Inflammation and infection control	Moisture balance	Epithelial (edge) advancement
Healing affected by the presence of non-viable tissue (slough or necrosis)			Wound closure delayed by a non-advancing or abnormal wound edge (fibrosed, rolled or undermined)

Fig. 8.2 The TIME framework (adapted from Falanga, 2004).

- Moisture balance
- Epithelial (edge) advancement

USING TIME TO ASSESS THE WOUND

It is vital to perform a baseline assessment if progress is to be monitored and treatments evaluated. Thereafter, the frequency of reassessment can be performed according to the individual patient's needs. Generally speaking, weekly assessment is reasonable for a chronic wound (Doughty, 2004) unless there is notable deterioration.

It is worth remembering that the purpose of assessment and subsequent reassessments and associated documentation is to build up a picture or permanent record. This is particularly important when several practitioners share the care. But even when care is consistently provided by one person it is not always possible to remember how something appeared a week or so ago, and harder still to remember if it is any different from a month ago. Therefore it is essential that the information recorded is accurate, relevant and useful.

Something commonly seen in practice regarding wound assessment documentation is: 'Wound healing, care attended as per plan'. It is difficult to determine from this statement if any assessment has really taken place at all, and thus is essentially a meaningless comment. A structured wound assessment tool can help capture useful information and demonstrate more accurately wound progression and deterioration.

One of the simplest wound assessment tools available is the TIME assessment tool born out of the wound bed preparation framework (Watret, 2005). TIME assessment provides a quick and effective means of detecting those barriers likely to affect chronic wound healing, and also provides a simple documentation framework.

Tissue management

Necrotic or sloughy tissue (essentially dead tissue) is commonly present in chronic wounds to varying degrees. In most instances, the presence of necrosis or slough in cases of leg ulceration is usually indicative that the wound bed is hypoxic and/or the underlying cause of the wound has not yet been managed or identified – not forgetting that many leg ulcers have more than one underlying cause. The presence of slough or necrosis can be a useful reminder that the practitioner has failed to identify all the underlying conditions and that further assessment and referral needs to be undertaken. In some instances where successful management of the underlying disorder is very difficult – e.g. inoperable peripheral arterial occlusive disease, rare autoimmune conditions and sickle cell disease – ongoing tissue management or maintenance debridement (Falanga, 2004) will play a much greater role.

The problem with non-viable tissue

Necrotic tissue acts as both a focus for infection, providing a breeding ground for bacteria, and a barrier to healing. This therefore places a greater burden on cells by prolonging the inflammatory response, thus leading to cellular dysfunction and ultimately delayed wound healing. It potentially conceals dead spaces and makes accurate wound measurement difficult. The presence of necrosis may have greater systemic effects on the patient by increasing the metabolic load required by the body in an attempt to promote autolytic debridement. In addition, the appearance and odour of the wound may cause the patient significant psychological stress; many patients will believe they have gangrene (Vowden & Vowden, 2002; Falanga, 2004).

Identifying non-viable tissue

Non-viable tissue includes slough (yellow, soft fibrinous tissue) and eschar (brown/black dry leathery tissue). In addition, some very long-term leg ulcers frequently develop a fibrosed base, giving granulation a pale shiny appearance as though there is a clear film over its surface (Moffatt et al., 2004). Removal of non-viable tissue by debridement is beneficial in that it removes dead, devitalised or contaminated tissue and any foreign material, which therefore helps to reduce the number of toxins and other substances that inhibit healing (Enoch & Harding, 2003). Debridement options are covered in greater detail in Chapter 13.

Any form of debridement should only be performed following thorough assessment.

Surgical or sharp debridement should **only** be performed by an appropriately trained and qualified clinician.

Assessing the wound bed

In terms of wound bed assessment, the tissue present will give clues to its possible stage of healing and to potential problems that will delay healing. Practitioners need to assess the wound bed for the presence of necrosis, slough, granulation and epithelium: or, at the very least, record the colour/s of the wound bed, e.g. black/brown/yellow/green/white/red or pink.

Necrotic tissue is black or brown in colour, depending upon the presence of any moisture. Sloughy tissue is often referred to as 'pus' and, while this may be part of its make up, fibrin and other proteinaceous material are also present (Fig. 8.3).

Healthy granulation tissue is red or pink in colour, demonstrating an adequate vascular supply, with a raspberry skin-like appearance (Fig. 8.4). Take note of unusual granulation (i.e. exuberant or over-granulation, friable, very pale or dark granulation) as it may indicate infection or another unusual ulcer type. Epithelium has a paler appearance and may even appear white. Epithelium may develop at the wound margins or form small islands across the surface of the wound.

Using the Wandsworth tPCT assessment tool, practitioners are requested to estimate the percentage of the various tissue types identified. For example, Fig. 8.3 shows there is approximately 35% necrosis, 35% slough and 30% granulation (the total should obviously amount to 100%). Over the course of treatment, providing it is appropriate, these values should alter with decreasing amounts of slough and necrosis and greater amounts of granulation and epithelium.

Inflammation and infection control

Infection and inflammation are essentially two separate issues, and while they are often related they are not mutually exclusive. The presence of inflammation is not necessarily the result of infection and inflammation may not always present when a chronic wound such as a leg ulcer is infected.

As a part of assessing the wound and surrounding skin for signs of inflammation and infection, the patient's susceptibility to infection must also be considered. For instance, how likely are they to develop an infection and, in regards to their general state of health,

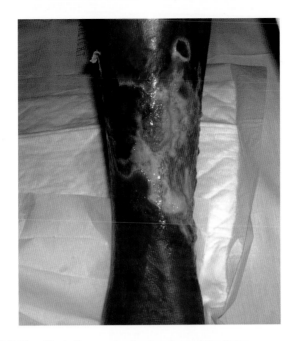

Fig. 8.3 Wound bed with necrosis, slough and granulation tissue.

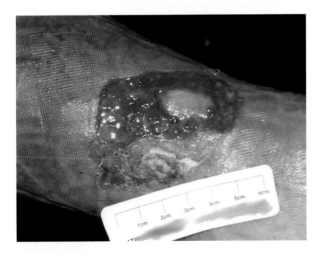

Fig. 8.4 Granulating wound with islands of epithelium.

what are the potential consequences? Factors affecting a patient's defence against infection include:

- Immunosuppression
- Medication
- Diabetes mellitus
- Alcohol or drug abuse
- Age (the very young and the very old have lowered immune responses)
- Comorbidities
- Ischaemia
- Malnourishment or obesity

Inflammation

Inflammation may occur for numerous reasons, and wound infection is certainly one such reason. However, it may also occur in relation to one of the autoimmune/inflammatory disorders discussed in Chapter 7, such as vasculitis or pyoderma gangrenosum (PG) (Sibbald et al., 2003). Inflammation that particularly presents on the lower leg in the gaiter region may indicate the early stages of chronic venous hypertension (CVH), or a particularly active phase of CVH leading to haemosiderin staining and lipodermatosclerosis. It can be a confusing clinical situation as the classic signs of inflammation or infection will be present. The limb will be red and swollen, it may feel warm to the touch and the patient may be reporting increased pain from the site. This is commonly incorrectly identified as cellulitis and treated with numerous courses of antibiotics, but to no avail (Cox, 2002). Ultimately, there are many possible causes for lower leg inflammation and a differential diagnosis must be made. See Table 8.1 for other possible causes of inflammation.

Assessing inflammation: Things to consider when assessing a patient with lower leg inflammation (Cox. 2002):

- How long has the inflammation been present? Cellulitis will have a shorter history rather than the more slowly progressive skin changes related to CVH.
- Is it spreading? Cellulitis will spread proximally (see Fig. 8.5); an indelible pen can be used to mark the affected area and

Table 8.1 Other potential causes of lower leg inflammation (Cox, 2002).

- Varicose eczema
- Contact allergy
- Acute or chronic oedema
- Deep vein thrombosis
- Compartment syndrome
- Arthritis, or other inflammatory joint conditions
- Haematoma
- Necrotising fasciitis
- Eosinophilic fasciitis
- Erythema nodosum/panniculitis
- Non-infective cellulitis

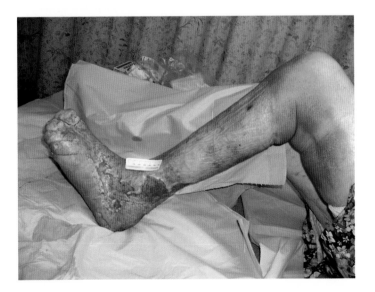

Fig. 8.5 Spreading cellulitis.

thereby monitor the inflammation over the course of a few days.
- Is the patient presenting with systemic signs of infection? For example, are they febrile, generally feeling unwell?

- Is it affecting one or both legs? Cellulitis is unlikely to affect both legs simultaneously.
- Has the patient already received antibiotic therapy? If so, what was the effect?
- Does the patient have other risk factors or medical history or signs of venous disease?
- How does the patient describe the associated pain and does anything relieve it? A cellulitis is likely to give continual pain, whereas there may be some relief when walking or resting with the legs elevated if it is related to CVH.
- Does the patient have any history of autoimmune or other inflammatory conditions?
- Are there obvious risk factors for cellulitis, such as a history of chronic lower leg oedema, toe web maceration, recent surgery (particularly vein harvesting) or blunt object injury?

The main problem with inflammation, aside from identifying its cause, is the pain and discomfort associated with it; therefore the sooner it is diagnosed the sooner the correct treatment can be implemented. Management of inflammatory conditions is covered in more depth in Chapters 7 and 13.

Infection

All chronic wounds contain bacteria, but the mere presence of bacteria does not necessarily equate to infection or delayed wound healing (Vowden & Cooper, 2006). Indeed, the presence of some bacteria are thought to enhance healing and act as a defence against more pathogenic types (Cooper, 2005). What is important is the balance that needs to be maintained between the host (the person) and the normal skin flora.

Of course, the presence of a wound can seriously alter the balance, providing bacteria with a salubrious environment in which to replicate and giving them direct access to the bloodstream. Fortunately, the protection offered by the skin is not the only hurdle bacteria encounter on their path to destruction. As already identified in the wound healing process (see Fig. 8.1), cells within the dermis and epidermis rapidly detect the presence of pathogens and an immune response is mounted to swiftly bring the situation back under control.

The process of maintaining balance, however, is far more

complex than described above, and there are several prime factors that affect or result in an imbalance (Dow et al., 1999; Enoch & Harding, 2003), including:

- The number of bacteria present
- Their type and virulence
- The strength of the host defence

In regards to host defence, numerous factors will affect the patient's susceptibility to infection and these should be identified during the initial patient assessment (see p. 190).

A bacterium's virulence relates to its ability to cause harm to its host. This will largely depend upon the bacterium's ability to detect and adapt to its changing environment and on its functional characteristics that enable it to protect itself from the host's immune system, such as the release of enzymes to allow invasion into deeper tissue and the production of toxins. Bacteria also have the ability to work synergistically to increase their virulence, by means of quorum sensing. It was originally thought that quorum sensing (sending chemical signals) only occurred between similar species; however evidence now seems to suggest that this communication can occur between different species. In addition, a new theory regarding polymicrobial communities is emerging relating to the potential for biofilms to occur. Biofilms are essentially communities formed of a variety of microbes that attach and then contain themselves within a slimy substance thus protecting them from phagocytosis, antibiotic and antimicrobial treatments (Cooper, 2005).

Different levels of bacterial balance have been categorised, ranging from contamination to colonisation to infection (see Table 8.2) (Cooper, 2005). An additional category between colonisation and infection has recently been created and is referred to as 'critical colonisation' (Kingsley, 2001). Critical colonisation has been suggested as a state where an imbalance occurs in the wound's bacterial flora and that this actually places the wound under some degree of burden, so preventing or delaying healing.

The term 'critical colonisation' does seem, in practice, to act as a useful means of trying to explain or understand those patients whose wounds might present with a couple of subtle signs of infection (for example, a dark granulating wound bed or some increase in odour or exudate), but where there is no significant

Table 8.2 Bacterial balance to imbalance (adapted from Cooper, 2005).

Contaminated	Characterised by the presence of non-replicating micro-organisms.
Colonised	As the term suggests, bacteria are setting up home and replicating, but without causing any damage to the host.
Infection	Invasion and destruction of healthy tissue by bacteria overwhelming the host defence. The classic signs of infection include advancing erythema, heat, swelling, pain, fever, odour and presence of pus.

inflammatory or systemic response and where for no other obvious reason the wound fails to show any signs of healing. However, the term has caused some controversy and no doubt will continue to do so until it can be quantified (White et al., 2005).

More recently, The European Wound Management Association (EWMA) have proposed a four-stage guide to detecting early wound infection (Vowden & Cooper, 2006). This guide endeavours to characterise this state between colonisation and infection (see Fig. 8.6) more definitively to help guide management.

The problem with bacterial burden: The problems related to bacterial imbalance are perhaps more obvious than the other barriers. A persistent, heavy bacterial presence leads to an ongoing production of inflammatory mediators, causing the wound to remain in a constantly inflamed state. This leads to fragile granulation tissue, a reduced number of fibroblasts and disorganised collagen production, the end result essentially being delayed healing and reduced tensile strength of the wound.

Indeed, the result of infection can be far more serious than delayed wound healing. Hence, careful observation of the wound for signs of bacterial imbalance and infection is crucial to prevent a more permanent disability and death. This can actually become quite difficult when dealing with a chronic wound, since it is possible that the chronically inflamed state has led to down-regulation of the immune response. Put simply, it is as though the cells have become tired of constantly acting as though infection or a foreign body has been present all along. This means the cells are unable to mount the necessary response when a true situation of increasing

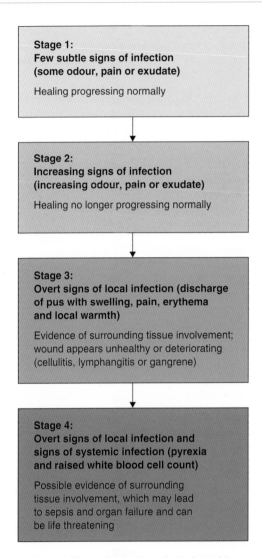

Stage 1:
Few subtle signs of infection
(some odour, pain or exudate)

Healing progressing normally

Stage 2:
Increasing signs of infection
(increasing odour, pain or exudate)

Healing no longer progressing normally

Stage 3:
Overt signs of local infection (discharge
of pus with swelling, pain, erythema
and local warmth)

Evidence of surrounding tissue involvement;
wound appears unhealthy or deteriorating
(cellulitis, lymphangitis or gangrene)

Stage 4:
Overt signs of local infection and
signs of systemic infection (pyrexia
and raised white blood cell count)

Possible evidence of surrounding
tissue involvement, which may lead
to sepsis and organ failure and can
be life threatening

Fig. 8.6 Clinical stages of increasing host reaction to bacterial presence (reproduced from Vowden & Cooper (2006) with permission of MEP/EWMA).

bacterial load develops that puts the body at risk of bacterial invasion. The classic cardinal signs of infection are therefore unlikely to be present and may lull the practitioner into a false sense of security.

Identifying infection: Diagnosis of infection is based on the presence of signs and symptoms, not a swab result. Some or all of the following clinical signs of infection may be present (Cutting & Harding, 1994):

- Cellulitis (but may be absent due to the effect of steroids, ischaemia, diabetes).
- Wound breakdown.
- Altered/unexpected pain or tenderness (may be absent in diabetes/neuropathy).
- Delayed healing.
- Discoloration (dull dusky granulation/green).
- Friable granulation tissue that bleeds easily.
- Pocketing at the base of the wound.
- Bridging of soft tissue and epithelium (fragile).
- Abnormal odour.
- Increased/seropurulent/haemopurulent exudate.
- Abscess formation.

Routine swabbing of chronic wounds is poor practice as all chronic wounds contain bacteria. Reserve bacterial sampling for where infection is suspected.

Wound swabs should be taken when infection is suspected as results will help guide antibiotic therapy. The semi-quantitative swab technique is the most practical means of assessing bacterial burden on a routine basis, and is generally considered to be adequate (Dow et al., 1999). However, its limitations must be recognised. To ensure best results practitioners should follow the technique below (Sibbald et al., 2003):

- Cleanse the wound with saline to remove surface debris and previous dressing material.
- Ideally, aspirate any pus present into a sterile syringe.
- Moisten the tip of the swab in sterile saline (or culture medium if exudate levels are low).

- Roll the swab by rotating it from the top to the bottom of the wound in a zigzag fashion, sampling the whole surface area (but avoiding areas of slough/necrosis).
- Place the swab directly into the transport medium.
- Complete the microbiology form in as much detail as possible.
- Transport the swab to the lab as soon as possible.
- Ensure results are retrieved and the appropriate action taken – recording the results in the patient's notes, liaising with the GP to ensure that appropriate treatment is prescribed. In some cases it may be helpful to also liaise directly with the microbiology team.
- Interpret the results of wound swabs with caution in view of their limitations, considering them in conjunction with the holistic assessment of the patient and the inflammatory response present.

Moisture balance

Since Winter's (1962) leading work on the benefits of moist wound healing was reported, this theory has formed a major cornerstone in wound management practice. The fact that Winter's work was based on acute wounds has not prevented this theory being applied to chronic wounds. More recently, however, questions have been raised as to whether the principle of moist wound healing is in fact transferable to chronic wounds (Parnham, 2002). There is a growing awareness that there are differences between the fluid from acute and chronic wounds and that, rather than being beneficial to healing, chronic wound fluid can be potentially damaging to the wound environment (Falanga, 2004).

Changes in the volume and nature of exudate provide valuable information about the underlying state of the wound and may give an indication of increasing bacterial load or infection (Vowden & Vowden, 2003).

The problem with excess levels of chronic wound fluid

Chronic wound exudate differs markedly from acute wound exudate in that it has a potentially adverse effect on wound healing (Schultz et al., 2003). It also has a damaging effect on the surrounding skin (Vowden & Vowden, 2003). Chronic wound fluid contains high levels of matrix metalloproteinases which damage extracellular matrix materials. It is sufficiently toxic to the extent that it reduces the proliferation of keratinocytes, fibroblasts and endothelial cells and the process of angiogenesis (Falanga, 2004).

Not only is the content of chronic wound fluid a problem, but more generally constant high levels of fluid, which are frequently associated with chronic wounds due to the ongoing nature of inflammatory or proliferative phases, are thought to have an effect on growth factors, essentially trapping them (Falanga, 2004).

Excess fluid levels not only affect the wound, but can also seriously impact on the condition of the surrounding skin, resulting in maceration and excoriation. When fluid stays in contact with healthy skin for long enough the keratinocytes begin to absorb fluid and swell. The keratinocytes will usually recover once they have the opportunity to dry out. However, if dressings are left in situ for many hours or even days longer than what their fluid handling capabilities are designed or able to do, the keratinocytes are unlikely to recover, leaving the surrounding tissues weak and more prone to trauma and further chemical attack from wound exudate (Fletcher, 2002).

Assessing exudate levels

Assessing the amount of exudate produced by a wound is a means of observing for signs of improvement or deterioration, and will help guide the practitioner to successful management strategies. Increasing levels of exudate may alert the practitioner to increasing bacterial levels, uncontrolled oedema or another underlying cause as yet unidentified. If the treatment is correct then exudate levels should respond accordingly by gradually reducing.

The following information should be recorded at each dressing change:

- **Volume**. Objectively measuring the amount of fluid produced by a wound is quite difficult. Dressings can be weighed or attempts made to collect fluid for a limited period in a drainage bag; however, the practicalities of these activities on a day-to-day basis are doubtful. Most practitioners will use words such as light, moderate or heavy, or use symbols such as +, ++ and +++, in an attempt to record the levels of exudate. The main problem with these more subjective assessments is how other carers will perceive the information and how some consistency can be ensured (Fletcher, 2002). One possible means of recording exudate levels could be to document how much of a dressing was saturated with fluid at the time of changing, or where the fluid went through to (i.e. layer 1 or 2) in the case of bandaging. There is still some element of subjectivity, but it is somewhat more informative than hazarding a guess at an amount.

- **Colour and nature**. Both give some indication of the possible stage of wound healing along with signalling potential problems (Fletcher, 2002). For instance, fluorescent green is often a classic sign of heavy pseudomonas colonisation, while a liquefied slough or necrosis may also lead to a very thick offensive exudate. Other notable colours and signs are:
  — serous (thin, clear, watery)
  — serosanguineous (pink/reddish colour, thin and watery)
  — purulent (milky or yellow, thick fluid, possibly malodorous)
  — haemorrhagic (red blood cells are the major component).
- **Odour**.

In addition to noting specific characteristics of the exudate, assessment of the surrounding skin will also help in highlighting the amounts of exudate produced and whether the current treatment is effective at controlling, or at least handling, the level of fluid produced:

- **Maceration**. This will appear as soggy, spongy white tissue frequently around the wound margins. If the exudate is not better managed at this point then the skin will continue to erode and the ulcer size increase.
- **Excoriation**. This presents as a moist inflammatory condition, often with superficial epithelial erosion (Fig. 8.7).

Epithelial (edge) advancement

Epithelial advancement essentially relates to the closing of the wound by the process of epithelialisation. In chronic wounds this process may be delayed for a number of reasons:

- The presence of devitalised tissue.
- The presence of infection.
- Too much or too little exudate.

- Fibrosed, rolled or undermined wound edges.
- Underlying problems of chemical imbalance and cellular dysfunction.

All these factors can make it difficult, near impossible, for new endothelial cells to migrate and move across the wound surface.

It is the practitioner's duty to observe for these potential factors that are likely to delay healing so they can be managed accordingly, though it will not be possible to assess the chemical picture and cellular activity in routine practice at this stage. However, the simplest means of monitoring a healing or non-healing wound will be by measuring its size and depth on a regular basis.

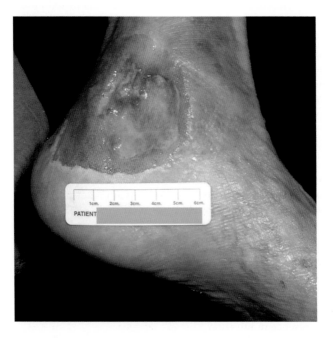

Fig. 8.7 Wound margins excoriated, with maceration visible distally.

The problem with chemical imbalance and cellular dysfunction

The usual orderly process of wound healing is basically disrupted in a chronic wound. The degradation of the extracellular matrix, constant high levels of matrix metalloproteinases (MMPs) and malfunctioning protease inhibitors leads to cells that are no longer active or able to respond (to messenger cells and growth factors) and divide.

Measuring the wound

Wound measurement provides baseline parameters against which future measurements can be compared (Flannagan, 2003). Ulcer size is a prognostic indicator for healing, larger ulcers taking longer to heal (Phillips et al., 2000).

There is no single wound measurement method readily available to the majority of practitioners that is free from limitations. The method chosen will vary with the site and type of wound, though tracing is frequently recommended in the literature (Flannagan, 2003). Estimation of wound size is not acceptable, as it lacks reliability (Bale, 1993). A combination of the following methods is likely to improve the accuracy of this critical element of wound bed assessment.

Linear measurements: This is a simple and practical approach, though limited, particularly for irregularly shaped wounds (Bale, 1993), and it does not account for wound depth.

1. Cover the wound with cling film/wrap or similar transparent protective material.
2. Use a tape measure (more appropriate for going around body contours) to measure the maximum length.
3. Take a second measurement to record maximum width (at right angles to the maximum length).
4. Document the measurements in the patient's records.

Wound tracing: Ulcer tracing is generally considered to be the method of choice (Flannagan, 2003). The technique is quick, inexpensive, requires minimal training, provides instant results and allows any surface area reduction to be calculated. The main source of error is the subjectivity involved in people's interpretation of the wound edge (Bohannon & Pfaller, 1983). It also fails to take into account wound depth.

Wound tracing charts/mapping grids can be obtained from some pharmaceutical companies, or some transparent dressings or the packaging they come in can be used in a similar fashion (though they may not have a printed grid).

1. Cover the wound with cling film if the chart does not have a backing sheet.
2. Place the chart over the ulcer and trace the wound edges using a permanent marker.
3. Dispose of the cling film/backing sheet in accordance with the local clinical waste protocol.
4. Label the tracing with the date, patient's name, hospital number and/or date of birth and location of the wound then file it in the patient's notes.

Photography: Photography is initially a more expensive option than tracing. However, with the development of digital cameras this may prove a more cost-efficient option, and certainly offers advantages in terms of communicating with other members of the multi-disciplinary team for those practitioners working in more isolated locations. Photography offers particular advantages including reliable recording of the colour and appearance of the wound tissue and surrounding skin. The accuracy will be limited if the ulcer extends around the leg, though a poor photographer technique is generally the main source of error. Patient consent is an issue and must be resolved during all stages of the assessment and management process. However, some healthcare trusts may have a policy specifically relating to the act of photographing patients, and request that a signed consent must be obtained. Patients should be made aware of the purpose of the use of photography and how that information will be used, and to whom it will be available.

1. Ideally place the limb over a plain, light background.
2. Place some form of measuring scale (i.e. disposable paper ruler) alongside the wound.

3. Use a Polaroid or digital camera (check the manufacturer's instructions for the correct focusing distance to ensure a clear picture).
4. Label the photo and place it in the patient's notes.
5. Take subsequent photos from the same distance to minimise changes of scale.

Measuring depth: This is somewhat more complex than assessing the surface area of a wound, and in reality is generally going to be a greater issue with other chronic wounds such as pressure sores and diabetic foot wounds rather than leg ulcers.

In the majority of instances the depth of leg ulcers will largely be assessed based on the tissue or other structures (e.g. tendon) visible in the wound bed.

In some cases it may be possible to fill a wound with saline (or similar isotonic fluid) using the volume dispensed as a guide to the wound depth. However, this will only be appropriate for wounds that do not extend to underlying structures and where there actually is sufficient depth to test. The patient will also need to understand the purpose of and be able to co-operate with the procedure. The position of the wound may make this process very difficult.

If undermining is suspected, a sterile measuring probe should be used to gently explore the extent and depth of the cavity or sinus.

ASSESSING THE SURROUNDING SKIN

We have already explored the importance of assessing the lower limb for those specific skin changes that indicate the presence of venous, arterial disease, diabetes and other unusual cases of ulcers in Chapters 4–7. This section will pick up further on some more general aspects of skin assessment, and then look a little closer at some particular skin problems often related to leg ulceration.

Assessing the surrounding skin involves (Lawton, 1998):

- Explaining to the patient the importance of assessing the skin condition of both legs.
- Ensuring a suitable environment in which to perform the assessment: one which is warm and where there is sufficient light and privacy.

- Looking at the whole of the lower limbs, being aware that varicosities and or oedema may extend to the abdomen, and paying particular attention to the toes, toe webbings and nails for oedema and/or fungal infection.
- Feeling the skin to assess the type and extent of oedema.
- Observing the skin condition for any signs of redness, scaling, crusting, exudate, excoriation, blistering, erosions or pustules.
- If lesions are present, noting whether the lesions are the same or whether there are notable variations.
- Considering the patient's history:
  — How long have any skin changes been present?
  — Is there any related family history?
  — Are there known allergies?
  — Has the patient had similar lesions previously, and how were they treated?
  — What medication is the patient taking? Were any new drugs commenced prior to the skin changes occurring?
- Noting sensations such as pain, soreness, itching and the presence of neuropathy.

When assessing patients with darker skin tones always bear in mind that skin changes or lesions may present differently than in those with a lighter skin. For example, skin changes that may be red or brown on light skin may appear to have a possible bluish tone or be almost black on darker skin (Manning, 2004).

Eczema

The presence of eczema alongside leg ulceration is not uncommon and may be a result of endogenous or exogenous factors. Although the causes are due to different factors, the different eczema types may be difficult to tell apart initially, and may even be confused with other inflammatory skin conditions. In addition, it is possible that both endogenous and exogenous eczema types present together. Thus, further assessment by the multi-disciplinary team may be required in order to reach an accurate differential diagnosis.

Table 8.3 presents the primary features of endogenous and exogenous eczema, while Fig. 8.8 shows a case of contact dermatitis.

Table 8.3 Eczema associated with leg ulceration.

Endogenous (varicose eczema)	Exogenous (irritant eczema, allergic eczema or contact dermatitis)
Predominantly occurs in the gaiter region	Irritant eczema is a non-immunological inflammatory reaction to a product applied to the skin. For example, many patients find the padding or wadding used under compression therapy to be quite irritating due to the fibres rubbing against already sensitive skin, rather than actually having an allergy to cotton
Appears as erythematous, scaly skin	Allergic eczema (otherwise known as 'contact dermatitis') is a result of allergens being absorbed via the skin, resulting in an immune response. The most common allergens related to leg ulcer management include: rubber/latex, topical antibiotics, lanolin, emulsifiers, preservatives, adhesives and perfumes
May be wet or dry	
Weeping skin can lead to further excoriation and secondary infection	The patient will have to have been exposed to the allergen previously in order for the body to have produced antibodies to the product, this may occur over a very short or extended period
If uncontrolled, skin may ulcerate	Where the skin has been in contact with the allergen it often becomes red, itchy, scaly and can produce exudate
Varicose eczema should improve following the application of compression therapy (Soo & Mortimer, 2004)	The response may be localised but in the case of severe reactions there may be a systemic response
	Patch testing is required to confirm the causative allergen, so patients will need to be referred to a dermatologist (Cameron, 2004)

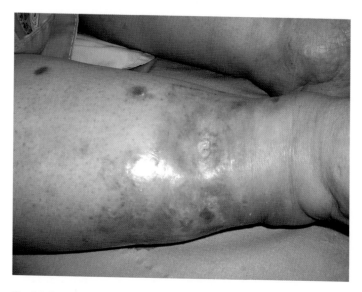

Fig. 8.8 Contact dermatitis.

Folliculitis

Inflammation of the hair follicle as a result of bacterial or fungal infection, though most commonly due to *Staphylococcus aureus*, is referred to as 'folliculitis'. It may present as pustules within or near the follicle with localised inflammation. Folliculitis can be triggered by blockage of the hair follicle (particularly by greasy emollients) and is likely to be exacerbated by infrequent skin cleansing. It may also develop as a result of a secondary infection following some other break in the skin, such as an insect bite or eczema. Depending upon the extent of the lesions, antibiotic therapy may be required; however, the best means of management is prevention. When caring for a patient with a leg ulcer, the surrounding skin often requires as much attention as the wound – washing and moisturising the skin on a regular basis. As hair follicles grow in a downwards direction, lotions/emollients should be applied using stokes from the knee to the toe so as to direct products away from the follicle (Goldstein & Goldstein, 1997; Linnitt, 2000).

Dry skin

Dry skin (xerosis) is a common problem affecting people of all ages, generally presenting on the dorsal and lateral surfaces of the arms and legs. It tends to appear as fine white scales, though the level of scaliness can significantly increase depending upon how well the stratum corneum is hydrated (Engelke et al., 1997).

The skin may become dry for a number of reasons:

- Age
- Chronic oedema
- Dehydration
- Malnutrition/mineral deficiencies
- Medications
- Smoking
- Stress
- Frequent use of soaps and other surfactants
- Sun exposure/environmental factors

The problem with dry skin is the impairment or loss of its protective capabilities against infection. It can also be uncomfortable, with patients reporting itching and stinging sensations. Many patients who undergo weekly bandaging for their leg ulcers report severe itching sensations. Skin cells are normally shed constantly when we move, wash and dress ourselves. However, this process is affected in patients who have a bandage in situ for up to a week, thus large amounts of dry skin can build up resulting in discomfort. When planning treatment, the effect of treatments on the surrounding skin as well as the wound should always be considered: weekly treatment may be inadequate for some patients. For the majority of patients, soaking the leg (for short periods) in warm water with some gentle exfoliation (to the surrounding skin) will remove excess skin scales. For patients with very dry skin, adding an emollient (non-perfumed) to the water should be considered, followed by an emollient such as white soft paraffin and liquid paraffin (50:50) to moisturise the skin prior to re-application of the bandages.

Lymphatic skin changes

Particular skin changes related to lymphoedema may present along with multi-factorial leg ulceration. The problem of high-protein chronic oedema, fibrosis of the dermis and subcutaneous tissues as well as a chronic inflammatory state can lead to severe skin changes and limb distortion. The extent of the skin changes present may range from thickening of the dermis to the more classic picture of 'elephantitis', depending upon the length of time and degree of lymphatic failure present.

Specific changes include (Keeley, 2000; Linnitt, 2000):

- **Hyperkeratosis** – presenting as a build-up of dry horny skin scales due to excessive keratin production.
- **Deep skin folds** – particularly affecting the toes and around the ankle.
- **Papillomatosis** – solid papules or nodules giving a cobblestone appearance over the skin surface.
- **Lymphangioma** – dilated lymph vessels producing a blister-like appearance on the surface of the skin, which may contain clear or blood-stained fluid.
- **Lymphorrhoea** – where there is leakage of lymph (clear) fluid.

Although the management of lymphoedema lies outside the scope of this book, the basic principles of management revolve around good skincare (as suggested for dry skin and in Chapter 13), exercise and support or compression therapy (depending upon other conditions present).

Fungal infections

Fungal infections affecting the feet, such as tinea pedis, are common, persistent and highly contagious, and the presence of a fungal infection can significantly increase the risk of inducing a cellulitic event. It usually results from poor hygiene and environmental conditions, which provide the moist warm conditions favoured by fungi. Tinea pedis is generally characterised by an itchy, dry scaly rash between the toes that may progress to a more inflamed and moist state, with the patient reporting a severe burning sensation. Skin scrapings should be sent for examination to confirm the diagnosis since tinea pedis may be mistaken for candida infections, psoriasis or discoid eczema (Smoker, 1999). For those patients particularly vulnerable to developing infection, every effort should be made to resolve this condition – it can usually be managed with topical antifungal agents such as imidazole or allylamine compounds (Cox, 2002). Systemic treatment may be required for more persistent infections.

SUMMARY

The essential factors to note about the wound include:
- Location.
- Number of wounds.
- Size and depth.
- Appearance of the tissue, e.g. necrotic, sloughy, granulated, epithelium, or colours such as black/brown/yellow/green/white/red and pink.
- Condition of the wound edges, e.g. flat, cliff-like, rolled or any discoloration.
- Presence of undermining.
- Signs of infection or inflammation.
- Nature and levels of wound exudate.
- Presence of odour.
- The condition of the surrounding skin, e.g. eczematous, macerated, excoriated or indurated.

(Collier 2003; Doughty 2004)

CONCLUSION

Assessing the wound bed and the surrounding skin are important elements of the holistic patient assessment, providing further clues to aid diagnosis and to highlight additional problems or challenges that may need to be addressed when planning and implementing care. Practitioners tend to be very good at focusing on the wound, though this is sometimes to the exclusion of everything else, but possibly not so good at recording their observations and using all the available information to make the most appropriate choices for their patients. The classic scenario being: struggling with exudate levels, but using a hydrogel because the wound is a bit sloughy; and, ultimately, not considering the cause for both the exudate and slough.

The TIME framework is a useful tool for documenting the condition of the wound and helping practitioners plan treatments. An effective means of communication is vital when the care of a patient is shared between several practitioners, especially when it comes to ensuring that more formalised reviews and referral pathways are observed in a timely manner – a brief TIME assessment will be far more useful to your colleagues than: 'Care attended to as planned'!

Always take into account the condition of the surrounding skin; remember the patient is being treated not just the wound. Consider how the skin presents at the initial assessment and whether any changes are taking place during treatment. In some circumstances, managing the surrounding skin can be equally if not more challenging than the wound itself, so always remember to seek further advice from a dermatologist should management prove to be very problematic. Chapter 13 looks in more detail at the management of the wound bed and surrounding skin.

REFERENCES

Bale, S. (1993) Wound assessment. *Surgical Nurse* **6**(1): 11–14.

Bohannon, R.W. & Pfaller, B.A. (1983) Documentation of wound surface area from tracing of wound perimeters. *Physical Therapy* **63**(10): 1622–1624.

Cameron, J. (2004) Demystifying allergic contact dermatitis and venous leg ulcers. *British Journal of Dermatology Nursing* **8**(2): 11.

Collier, M. (2003) The elements of wound assessment. *Nursing Times (Wound Care Suppl.)* **99**(13): 48–49.

Cooper, R.A. (2005) Understanding wound infection. In: *European Wound Management Association (EWMA) Position Document: Identifying Criteria for Wound Infection.* London, MEP Ltd, pp. 2–5.

Cox, N.H. (2002) Management of lower leg cellulitis. *Clinical Medicine* **2**(1): 23–27.

Cutting, K.F. & Harding K.G. (1994) Criteria for identifying wound infection. *Journal of Wound Care* **3**(4): 198–201.

Doughty, D.B. (2004) Wound assessment: tips and techniques. *Advances in Skin and Wound Care* **17**: 369–372.

Douglass, J. (2003) Wound bed preparation: a systemic approach to chronic wounds. *Wound Care* **June**: 26–34.

Dow, G., Browne, A. & Sibbald, R.G. (1999) Infection in chronic wounds: controversies in diagnosis and treatment. *Ostomy/Wound Management* **45**(8): 23–40.

Engelke, M., Jemsen, J-M., Ekanayake-Mudiyanselage, S. & Proksch, E. (1997) Effects of xerosis and ageing on epidermal proliferation and differentiation. *British Association of Dermatologists* **137**(2): 219–225.

Enoch, S. & Harding, K. (2003) Wound bed preparation: the science behind the removal of barriers to healing. *Wounds: A Compendium of Clinical Research and Practice* **15**(7): 213–229.

Falanga, V. (2000) Classifications for wound bed preparation and stimulation of chronic wounds. *Wound Repair and Regeneration* **8**(5): 347–352.

Falanga, V. (2004) Wound bed preparation: science applied to practice. In: *European Wound Management Association (EWMA) Position Document: Wound Bed Preparation in Practice*. London, MEP Ltd, pp. 2–5.

Flannagan, M. (2003) Wound measurement: can it help us monitor progression to healing? *Journal of Wound Care* **12**(5): 189–194.

Fletcher, J. (2002) Exudate theory and the clinical management of exuding wounds. *Professional Nurse* **17**(8): 475–478.

Goldstein, B.G. & Goldstein, A.O. (1997) Bacterial diseases. In: *Practical Dermatology*, 2nd edn (A.O. Goldstein & B.G. Goldstein, eds). St Louis, MO, Mosby, pp. 71–77.

Keeley, V. (2000) Clinical features of lymphoedema. In: *Lymphoedema* (R. Twycross, K. Jenns & J. Todd, eds). Oxon, Radcliffe Medical Press Ltd, pp. 44–67.

Kingsley, A. (2001) A proactive approach to wound infection. *Nursing Standard* **15**(30): 50–58.

Lawton, S. (1998) Assessing the skin. *Professional Nurse (Study Suppl.)* **13**: 14.

Linnitt, N. (2000) Skin management in lymphoedema. In: *Lymphoedema* (R. Twycross, K. Jenns & J. Todd, eds). Oxon, Radcliffe Medical Press Ltd, pp. 118–129.

Manning, J. (2004) The assessment of dark skin and dermatological disorders. *Nursing Times (Wound Care Suppl.)* **100**(22).

Moffatt, C., Morison, M.J. & Pina, E. (2004) Wound bed preparation for venous leg ulcers. In: *European Wound Management Association (EWMA) Position Document: Wound Bed Preparation in Practice*. London, MEP Ltd, pp. 12–17.

Parnham, A. (2002) Moist wound healing: does the theory apply to chronic wounds? *Journal of Wound Care* **11**(4): 143–146.

Phillips, T.J., Manado, F., Trout, R., et al. (2000) Prognostic indicators in venous ulcers. *Journal of the American Academy of Dermatology* **43**(4): 627–630.

Romanelli, M. & Mastronicola, D. (2002) The role of wound bed preparation in managing chronic pressure ulcers. *Journal of Wound Care* **11**(8): 305–310.

Royal College of Nursing (1998) *Clinical Practice Guidelines. The Management of Patients with Venous Leg Ulcers*. University of York and University of Manchester, RCN Institute.

Schultz, G.S., Sibbald, R.G., Falanga, V., Angello, E., Dowsett, C., Harding, K., Romanelli, M., Stacey, M.C., Teot, L. & Vanscheidt, W. (2003) Wound bed preparation: a systematic approach to wound management. *Wound Repair and Regeneration* **11**(2) (Suppl. 1): S1–S28.

Sibbald, R.G., Orsted, H., Schultz, G.S, Coutts, P., Keast, D, International Wound Bed Preparation Advisory Board, Canadian Chronic

Wound Advisory Board (2003) Preparing the wound bed: focus on infection and inflammation. *Ostomy/Wound Management* **49**(11): 23–51.

SIGN (1998) The care of patients with chronic leg ulcer. Edinburgh, Scottish Intercollegiate Guidelines Network, SIGN Publication No. 26.

Smoker, A. (1999) Fungal infections. *Nursing Standard* **13**(17): 13–19.

Soo, J. & Mortimer, P. (2004) Recognising and treating the symptoms of varicose eczema. *British Journal of Dermatology Nursing* **8**(4): 14–16.

Vowden, K. & Vowden, P. (2003) Understanding exudate management and the role of exudate in the healing process. *British Journal of Nursing* **8**(11) (Suppl.): 4–13.

Vowden, P. & Cooper, R.A. (2006) An integrated approach to managing wound infection. In: *European Wound Management Association (EWMA). Position Document: Management of Wound Infection*. London, MEP Ltd, pp. 2–6.

Vowden, P. and Vowden, K. (2002) *Wound Bed Preparation. World Wide Wounds*. http://www.worldwide-wounds.com/2002/april/Vowden/Wound-Bed-Prepararation.html

Watret, L. (2005) *Standardised Assessment Tools and the Management of Complex Wounds*. Huntingdon, Wound Care Society Publication.

White, R., Cutting, K. & Kingsley, A. (2005) Critical colonisation: clinical reality or myth? *Wounds UK* **1**(1): 94–95.

Winter, G. (1962) Formation of scab and the rate of epithelialisation of superficial wounds in the skin of the young domestic pig. *Nature* **193**: 293–294.

Part III
Psychosocial Dimensions of Assessment and Management

Since the 1980s, research has demonstrated the significant burden that leg ulceration places on the patient. Protracted periods of non-healing ulceration reduce the patients' ability to enjoy life and are associated with an overall reduction in their quality of life status. In some situations this leads to spiralling depression and an inability to tolerate treatment.

Pain affects up to 80% of patients with leg ulceration. Chapter 9 addresses the assessment and management of pain and provides guidance on how to use both analgesia and other methods of pain relief. The complex issues of pain management frequently require expert advice and specialist intervention from the multidisciplinary team. The primary goal of all nursing care for patients with leg ulceration must be that symptoms such as pain are successfully managed.

Chapter 10 considers the psychological consequences of leg ulceration and the strategies that can be used to identify patients at risk of depression and psychological distress. Chapter 11 extends this theme by considering the problem of concordance with therapy. This is frequently the most complex issue reported by nurses and often reflects problems in the relationship between professional and patient. One of the most damaging effects is labelling the patient as 'non-compliant' and blaming them for their failure to heal. This chapter discusses why this occurs and provides advice on how to overcome these issues and build a successful therapeutic relationship.

Assessment and Management of Pain

LEARNING OBJECTIVES

Nurses involved in leg ulcer management should be able to demonstrate:

- ❑ An understanding of the importance of pain in leg ulceration.
- ❑ The ability to describe the different forms of pain and how they present clinically.
- ❑ An understanding of the clinical, social and psychological issues that surround the experience of pain.
- ❑ An understanding of how different ulcer aetiologies lead to different pain manifestations.
- ❑ An understanding of the assessment of pain within a holistic framework.
- ❑ The ability to describe pharmacological and other methods of pain control.
- ❑ The ability to describe the appropriate wound care strategies that can reduce pain.
- ❑ An understanding of the importance of referral for specialist advice and the range of interventions available.

INTRODUCTION

Pain is a major, often unrecognised factor in leg ulceration (Hollinworth, 1995; Hofman, 1997). Many factors influence the development and experience of pain in patients with leg ulceration. The development of pain may indicate a number of possible causes including a change in the aetiology of the ulcer, as is the case in deteriorating peripheral arterial occlusive disease (PAOD). It may also indicate that an infection is developing or that a treatment is not suiting the patient. In some cases it may signal that the treatment is being poorly or inappropriately applied, such as over-tight compression bandaging. Changes in pain intensity or the level of coping with pain may indicate that the psychological status of the patient has changed and that the pain is now becoming more intrusive. What is clear from these diverse situations is that pain is a major factor in the lives of many patients with leg ulceration and that it requires careful assessment and appropriate, timely intervention.

PROFESSIONAL ATTITUDES TO PAIN IN LEG ULCERATION

Professional attitudes have frequently underestimated the pain associated with conditions such as venous ulceration while acknowledging other clinical conditions such as ischaemic ulceration to be very painful. Research has shown that over 80% of patients with venous ulceration experience pain, with many describing it as excruciating (Franks & Moffatt, 1998a). Nursing research, in particular, has explored the impact it has on the lives of patients (Charles, 1995). The experience of unremitting pain leads to feelings of helplessness and hopelessness and is a major factor that reduces overall quality of life (Krasner, 1998). Pain levels in patients with leg ulceration are significantly higher than in people without ulceration but of a similar age and sex (Moffatt, 2004a). Effective ulcer treatment leading to healing has a significant effect on eliminating ulcer pain (Franks et al., 1994). While the greatest improvement in pain does occur in those with complete ulcer healing, improvements can also be seen in those whose ulcer fails to heal but to whom appropriate care is being delivered.

THE EFFECTS OF UNCONTROLLED PAIN

Uncontrolled pain affects many other dimensions of life, including sleep deprivation (Franks & Moffatt, 1998b). A number of studies in the chronic illness literature report the important link between uncontrolled pain and the development of depression (Alison et al., 1991; Dworkin & Breitbart, 2004). The quality-of-life literature on leg ulceration indicates that the emotional state of patients is affected, with particular influence on young patients seeking to develop intimate relationships and in those who are attempting to work (Phillips et al., 1994).

NURSING MANAGEMENT OF PAIN

Pain control must be a goal of all treatment strategies irrespective of the underlying aetiology, the overall prognosis or other complex medical and psychosocial issues that surround the patient.

Despite the growing awareness of these issues, nurses often failed to adequately assess pain or provide effective management (Hollinworth, 1995), and this is still the case today. They frequently fail to prescribe analgesia prior to a painful wound procedure even though they are aware that the patient is suffering with moderate or severe pain (Choniere et al., 1990). A number of authors have concluded that nurses' knowledge of pain management is poor and that this contributes to poor practice (Kitson, 1994). Complex pain manifestations such as hyperalgesia, which will be discussed in this chapter, result in extreme pain even with minimal touch. Nurses' lack of understanding of the physiology of pain leads to a poor appreciation of pain intensity. Such patients can be dealt with harshly by nurses who perceive the patient is exaggerating their pain. Attitudes to different patients are influenced by whether the patient is considered to be difficult or emotionally draining. These attitudes lead to professional labelling of patients and the development of social defences such as 'distancing' and 'denial', which are used to protect nurses from feeling overwhelmed about inflicting pain on their patients (Moffatt, 2004a). While these can be helpful coping strategies, when used in excess they lead to poor practice.

USING THE CHRONIC PAIN LITERATURE

While there is a growing interest in understanding pain in leg ulceration, there is, as yet, little evidence to support claims of which intervention strategies are the most effective. Recommendations made in this chapter are therefore drawn from published research into chronic pain, which contains many useful approaches to reducing the suffering of patients (Jenner et al., 1991). Although some of the research was published 15 or more years ago, the findings are still as valid today. So far, the focus has been on ulcer healing as the most important outcome, but this may have been at the expense of developing treatments for symptom control.

MECHANISMS OF PAIN

Pain is a highly complex phenomenon, which extends beyond a simple description of how pain is transmitted through complex neural pathways and is interpreted in the cortex of the brain. Pain is highly individual, complex and dynamic and is influenced by physiological, psychological, emotional and social factors (Briggs & Hoffman, 1999). A comprehensive review of the physiology of pain is beyond the scope of this chapter, but further key texts are provided in the references at the end of this chapter. Patients with leg ulceration suffer with chronic pain, which is defined by being present for more than 7 weeks. Table 9.1 presents definitions of pain drawn from a recent consensus document (2004).

PAIN IN VENOUS DISEASE AND VENOUS ULCERATION

Some patients have difficulty describing their symptoms, and do not necessarily consider they are experiencing pain. Common phenomena such as burning, sharp sensations and feeling they are walking on glass are often difficult for patients to identify as pain, referring to them rather as unpleasant symptoms. However, these descriptions do not fit with their own belief or previous experience of pain.

Varying patterns of pain and discomfort are experienced by patients with venous disease. Patients report aching heavy legs, particularly in the calf region, which is often relieved when the

Table 9.1 Definitions of pain.

The publication, *Principles of Best Practice. Minimising Pain at Wound Dressing Procedures: A Consensus Document* (World Union of Wound Healing Societies, 2004), has a number of useful descriptions of the different types of pain and their manifestations:

Nociceptive pain may be defined as an appropriate physiological response to painful stimulus. It may involve acute or chronic inflammation.

. . . the prolonged inflammatory response may cause heightened sensitivity in both the wound (primary hyperalgesia) and the surrounding skin (secondary hyperalgesia).

Neuropathic pain has been defined as an inappropriate response caused by a primary lesion or dysfunction in the nervous system.

[Neuropathic pain] . . . is often associated with altered or unpleasant sensations whereby any sensory stimulus such as light touch or pressure or changes in temperature can provoke intense pain (allodynia).

Adapted from WUWHS (2004).

patient can lie or sit with their limb elevated and is worse during periods of heat. The symptoms are probably directly linked to the development of venous hypertension (high pressure in the superficial veins and microcirculation) which is relieved on high elevation. Some patients also report restless legs and irritation over varicosities, particularly at night.

Venous claudication

Venous claudication is a relatively rare phenomenon that occurs in patients who develop extremely severe venous hypertension, with the pressure in the venous microcirculation almost reaching that in the arterial microcirculation. Patients experience severe, unremitting pain that often feels bursting in nature. It can be similar in presentation to the pain experienced in compartment syndrome, where severe swelling causes constriction of the circulation with the attendant risk of anoxia and tissue death.

Atrophie blanche

This is a common manifestation in venous disease, but the true pathology of this condition is debated. Overall, histologically, patients with atrophie blanche have fewer capillaries than normal individuals. Moreover, these fewer capillaries contain micro-thrombi which make them appear dilated. It is thought the pain may be due to localised ischaemia or a vasculitic process with inflammation and blockage of the capillaries. The ulcers are frequently deep and punched out, resembling small ischaemic ulcers (Fig. 9.1). Pain levels may be very high. These areas may remain after the ulcer heals or may develop within an area of healed ulceration. Patients report long-term sensitivity and pain. The areas are particularly vulnerable to ulcer breakdown.

Venous ulcer pain

The pain of venous ulceration may include nociceptive pain due to inflammation, as well as symptoms of neuropathic pain. Patients frequently report an increase in pain during dressing procedures and on exposure to air, which slowly improves after the wound is redressed. High levels of exudate are associated with increased pain, particularly if there is adherence to the primary dressing or if there is friction of the dressing against the wound. Patients

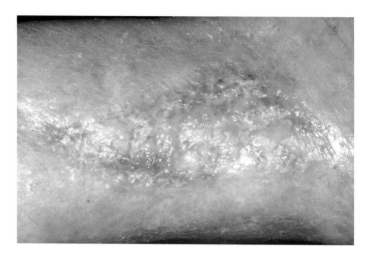

Fig. 9.1 Atrophie blanche is associated with severe pain.

report sharp, spontaneous shooting pains that are not associated with movement (ectopic discharge). Other features of neuropathic pain, such as burning, tingling or creeping sensations, are also reported.

Periods of acute cellulitis are frequently preceded by an increase in pain in the ulcer area, which can often be the most important clinical sign of a systemic infection. This occurs prior to any other changes in the wound or surrounding skin.

While the mechanisms for this remain unclear, pain usually decreases as the oedema resolves and as levels of exudate are reduced. Research has shown that the introduction of compression is associated with decreases in the levels of those serum cytokines involved in acute inflammation, and that this occurs in parallel to ulcer healing (Murphy et al., 2002). Traditional advice on exercise and leg elevation may actually increase levels of pain in a proportion of patients (Hofman, 1997). Bursting and burning pain (venous rush pain) is frequently reported when getting out of bed in the morning, probably due to the rapid refill within the damaged veins.

- Pain in venous ulceration is common.
- Pain does not indicate peripheral arterial disease (assuming a normal ABPI).
- Pain may occur when compression is first applied.
- Pain may increase over the first few weeks of treatment.
- Pain can be successfully controlled.
- Pain will decrease with ulcer healing.

PAIN IN PERIPHERAL ARTERIAL OCCLUSIVE DISEASE (PAOD) AND ISCHAEMIC ULCERATION

Varying types of pain are associated with PAOD. The presentation and severity is linked to the advancement of disease, and varies from patients with mild intermittent claudication to those with severe ischaemic pain due to critical limb ischaemia and gangrene.

Intermittent claudication

The distribution of pain is related to the area of stenosis or occlusion in the artery or arteries. Calf pain is the commonest and is related to disease affecting the femoral and popliteal arteries. Pain in the buttocks is associated with disease in the iliac vessels or the aorta. Patients frequently report that their exercise tolerance has reduced and the distance they can walk without pain is reducing. Pain that persists after exercise has stopped is not due to intermittent claudication but may be due to other causes, such as spinal nerve entrapment or arthritis. The stage of intermittent claudication is often missed in patients with ischaemic leg ulceration due to their low levels of activity. As the disease progresses they may develop pain at night, which is due to the fall in peripheral perfusion as the blood pressure drops causing neuritic pain. Relief occurs when the patient hangs their leg over the side of the bed, thus increasing distal perfusion through increased peripheral blood pressure.

Rest pain in critical limb ischaemia

Rest pain is intense, unremitting and is often only partially relieved by opiates. It generally occurs in the foot or toes, but patients may also report that it extends up the leg particularly if an ulcer is present. Pain is worse when the patient is in a supine position; so many hours are spent sitting in a chair with the limb dependent, which leads to dependency oedema.

Development of rest pain indicates that critical limb ischaemia has developed and that the blood supply is no longer able to supply the nutritional requirements of the skin. Skin breakdown, ulceration and gangrene quickly follow.

Exacerbation of pain is experienced when:

- The patient moves
- The affected area is in contact with bed-clothes
- The skin or ulcer is touched
- The area comes into contact with hot or cold objects
- The limb is elevated

While this situation is usually due to chronic atherosclerosis, an arterial embolism may cause the sudden development of these symptoms in a small proportion of patients (Fig. 9.2). The five P's

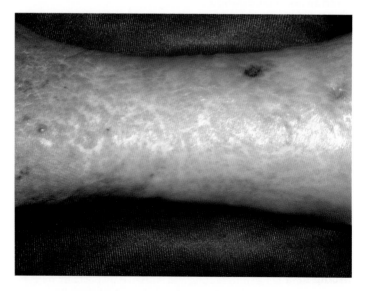

Fig. 9.2 Clinical appearance following an arterial embolism. This condition leads to severe, sudden pain.

are a useful tool for remembering the signs and symptoms associated with this condition:

- Pain
- Pallor
- Pulseless
- Paraesthesia
- Perishing

Phantom limb pain

A proportion of patients with critical ischaemia will require amputation. Phantom limb pain can be a pervasive problem and is reported in approximately two-thirds of patients (Jensen et al., 1984; Houghton et al., 1994). Research suggests that the level of phantom pain may be related to the degree of pain the patient experiences preoperatively, although not all studies concur with this opinion. In many centres preoperative epidural therapy is given to reduce the risk of limb pain (Nikolajsen et al., 1997). Phantom pain is generally intermittent and most often described as a shooting, pricking or boring pain.

A number of factors have been shown to aggravate the pain (Houghton et al., 1994):

- Emotional distress
- Stump touch or pressure
- Prosthetic wear
- Weather changes
- Mental attention on the limb

Pain relief occurs with (Pohjolainen, 1991):

- Massage of the stump
- Distraction
- Rest
- Cold or heat
- Stump movement

Stump pain

Stump pain occurs in around 21% of patients, and some believe that stump and phantom pain are related (Jensen et al., 1984).

Patients may also experience other non-painful sensations related to their lost limb.

PAIN IN MIXED ARTERIAL AND VENOUS ULCERATION

Nurses are frequently perplexed when dealing with mixed aetiology ulceration (venous and arterial ulceration combined). The associated pain is usually related to the reduced blood supply and compounded by the symptoms of venous ulceration. Tolerance of low levels of compression is variable, so pain levels are an important guide in deciding how much compression is appropriate for each individual patient (see Chapter 14).

DIABETIC NEUROPATHY

Nurses frequently associate diabetic foot neuropathy with an insensate foot, however many patients suffer severe symmetrical neuritic pain that is worse at night (Edmonds & Foster, 2000). It is burning in nature and frequently accompanied by paraesthesia and discomfort when in contact with clothing or shoes. This can be so severe that patients are unable to tolerate wearing shoes and normal clothing. The pain leads to sleep problems, including restless legs and cramps. Some patients also report deep aching pain and spontaneous shooting sensations. Although the pain is often precipitated by poor diabetic control, it is also reported after stabilising diabetic control.

Differentiating the cause of pain at night in diabetic patients can be difficult. Diabetic neuropathy and arterial occlusive disease both cause pain and sleep disturbance. The most useful differentiation is that ischaemic pain is relieved by hanging the leg over the side of the bed, while walking tends to make the pain worse. In contrast, walking often relieves neuropathic pain. A proportion of patients suffers with severe ischaemia and neuropathy. The symptoms of ischaemia can be severely masked by the neuropathy and patients may not report pain even in the presence of gangrene.

INFLAMMATORY CONDITIONS

Many inflammatory conditions causing leg ulceration, such as rheumatoid arthritis, pyoderma gangrenosum and other forms of vasculitis, are associated with extreme pain in and around the ulcer site (Jayson, 1999). Pain intensity can be severe and opiates are required to alleviate this.

SICKLE CELL ULCERATION
This is extremely painful. The deep, punched-out ulcers produce pain that is similar in character to the pain associated with atrophie blanche, with neuropathic symptoms such as burning and shooting sensations (Embury, 1996).

INFECTION
Osteomyelitis is a rare but important complication of ulceration. The symptoms of osteomyelitis are often difficult to detect clinically. Some patients complain of an underlying joint pain that is gnawing or aching in character, and of pain when they move the joint (McLain & Weinstein, 1999).

PSYCHOSOCIAL DIMENSIONS OF PAIN
It is now well recognised that pain is a complex, multi-factorial phenomenon and that psychological and social issues play a major role (Wall & Melzack, 1999; Williams, 2004). The leg ulcer literature has shown that many patients suffer from social isolation and low levels of social support, both of which may worsen the pain experience (Keeling et al., 1996; Franks & Moffatt, 1998a). While support from family can have positive effects, in some relationships the patient's pain behaviour may be reinforced by family reactions, preventing effective adaption and leading to a situation called 'learned helplessness' (Garafolo, 2000). The beliefs of the patient and their family may also influence the pain experience (Low, 1984).

Patients vary significantly in their ability to cope. Research into chronic illness has shown that pain intensity does not correlate with functional disability (Wall & Melzack, 1999). Effective coping requires the mobilisation of flexible coping strategies that allow the patient to make adjustments to their situation (Turner et al., 2000). One particularly negative coping style is catastrophising, in which patients focus on and exaggerate only the negative effects of life (Turner et al., 2000). Underlying personality traits such as optimism and pessimism also affect the experience of pain (Geisser, 2004).

Very little research has been undertaken to examine the cultural and ethnic diversity associated with leg ulceration. It is important for nurses to understand how cultural beliefs and attitudes may affect the pain experience and how the different groups access traditional health services.

ASSESSMENT AND CONTINUOUS EVALUATION OF PAIN

Practitioners need to develop a therapeutic relationship that enables them to listen carefully and empathically to the patient and family. It is important to remember that not all patients talk about their pain. Particular attention should be paid to care and observation in those with cognitive impairment, language difficulties or the frail elderly (Walker et al., 1990). Assessment of pain should be undertaken at each leg ulcer treatment and be carried out by a skilled practitioner. A careful description of the pain experience provides a great deal of information for the practitioner.

The layered approach to pain developed by the World Union of Wound Healing Societies (2004) has been adapted in this chapter for the assessment and management of leg ulcer pain (Fig. 9.3). It is

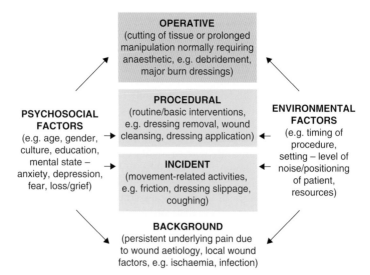

Fig. 9.3 The layered approach to leg ulcer pain (reproduced from the World Union of Wound Healing Societies (2004) with permission).

a useful tool to help practitioners assess the different components of pain the patient may be experiencing. Patients frequently have additional sources of pain, such as that from osteoarthritis and rheumatoid arthritis, that significantly influence their experience.

Pain should be believed and respected.

Background pain
Felt at rest and significantly influenced by the underlying aetiology of the ulcer, background pain is often present almost continuously in the following patient groups:

- Rest pain in critical limb ischaemia
- Acute inflammatory conditions
- Rheumatoid arthritis (rheumatoid vasculitis)
- Pyoderma gangrenosum
- Haematological conditions such as sickle cell disease

Other influencing factors that may lead to continuous background pain include:

- Infection in the ulcer
- Poor control of oedema
- Acute dermatological skin conditions
- Tight or poorly applied compression

Other background pain from conditions such as arthritis and cancer may significantly influence the overall pain experience.

Incident (breakthrough) pain
This occurs during activities of daily living, such as walking and standing, or slippage of the dressing on the wound.

Procedural pain
Procedural pain occurs during the routine treatment of the patient's leg ulcer. One of the most painful aspects is dressing removal, but routine cleansing or exposure of the wound may also lead to high levels of pain. Rough handling of the wound may exacerbate pain and fear. Anticipatory anxiety over dressing procedures

may develop, worsening the overall experience for the patient (Andrasik, 1994).

Operative pain

This is associated with particular procedures, such as debridement, that require significant cutting of dead material at the interface with live sensitive tissue in the wound. The pain associated with this type of procedure is very severe. Debridement should only be undertaken with either a local or general anaesthetic. The pain following debridement may last for hours once the anaesthetic has worn off. Patients may require additional analgesia during the next few days (Briggs & Nelson, 2001).

Coping with pain

It is very important to assess how the patient is coping with their pain (Arathuzik, 1991). The algorithm in Fig. 9.4 outlines questions that should be asked during an assessment and how these should be linked to pain management strategies. Although this algorithm was developed by Walker et al. (1990) for the nursing management of elderly patients with pain, it is useful for patients with leg ulceration.

Using pain assessment tools

The World Union of Wound Healing Societies (2004) consensus paper on the assessment of wound pain reviews the different methods for assessing pain. They make a number of useful recommendations:

- Pain assessment should be routine and systematic.
- The choice of pain assessment tool will depend on the individual needs of the patient (no one tool is suitable for all patients).
- The same assessment tool should be continued on an individual patient.
- Visual scales using faces are useful, as are visual analogue scales where a patient is asked to point to the position on a line that best represents their level of pain.
- Numerical and verbal scales are useful.

- Pain diaries allow for a detailed account of the pain experienced during a particular period, and can identify triggers and the effect of pain management strategies.

MANAGEMENT OF PAIN
Using analgesia to control background, incident and procedural pain

Background and incident pain associated with leg ulceration should be controlled by the appropriate use of analgesics from different classes of drugs. The World Health Organization has developed a three step-ladder approach ('The analgesic ladder') for the control of cancer pain (WHO, 1996). This approach can be used to control background pain in leg ulceration. If simple analgesics (e.g. non-steroidal anti-inflammatory drugs (NSAIDs), paracetamol) do not control pain, weak opioids such as codeine should be introduced or combined with simple analgesics. Stronger opiates such as morphine may be required if pain relief is not achieved. Opiates are required for controlling the pain associated with critical limb ischaemia. However, they may also be needed for patients with ulceration due to other aetiologies, including venous ulceration.

> The underlying aetiology of the ulcer should not be used to determine whether opiates are required to control pain.

Doctors are often reluctant to prescribe opiates because they fear patients will develop addiction. However, there is little evidence that this occurs if they are being used appropriately as an analgesic (Twycross, 1999).

Care must be taken to ensure the correct dose of analgesia is prescribed, and that this is under constant review. Twycross in discussing the use of opioids states (Twycross, 1999, p. 434):

'the right dose is the dose which relieves the pain.'

The dosage of morphine may range from 30 mg daily to 1200 mg daily or more. The effective use of morphine should render the patient free from pain for a period of 4 hours, but without unacceptable side-effects such as nausea and constipation.

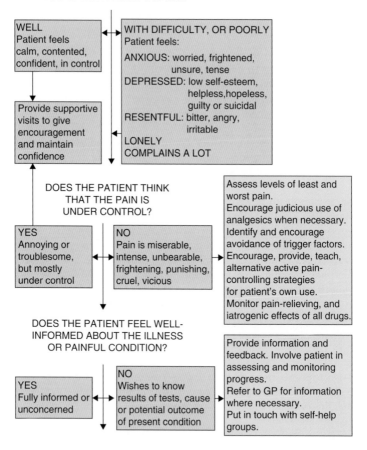

Fig. 9.4 Assessment of how a patient is coping and appropriate intervention strategies (reproduced from Walker et al. (1990) with permission of Blackwell Publishing).

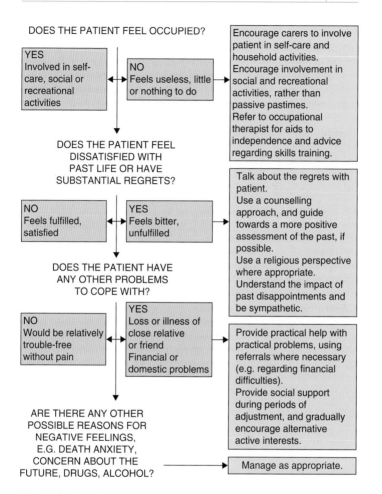

DOES THE PATIENT FEEL OCCUPIED?

YES
Involved in self-care, social or recreational activities

NO
Feels useless, little or nothing to do

Encourage carers to involve patient in self-care and household activities.
Encourage involvement in social and recreational activities, rather than passive pastimes.
Refer to occupational therapist for aids to independence and advice regarding skills training.

DOES THE PATIENT FEEL DISSATISFIED WITH PAST LIFE OR HAVE SUBSTANTIAL REGRETS?

NO
Feels fulfilled, satisfied

YES
Feels bitter, unfulfilled

Talk about the regrets with patient.
Use a counselling approach, and guide towards a more positive assessment of the past, if possible.
Use a religious perspective where appropriate.
Understand the impact of past disappointments and be sympathetic.

DOES THE PATIENT HAVE ANY OTHER PROBLEMS TO COPE WITH?

NO
Would be relatively trouble-free without pain

YES
Loss or illness of close relative or friend
Financial or domestic problems

Provide practical help with practical problems, using referrals where necessary (e.g. regarding financial difficulties).
Provide social support during periods of adjustment, and gradually encourage alternative active interests.

ARE THERE ANY OTHER POSSIBLE REASONS FOR NEGATIVE FEELINGS, E.G. DEATH ANXIETY, CONCERN ABOUT THE FUTURE, DRUGS, ALCOHOL?

Manage as appropriate.

Fig. 9.4 *Continued.*

Breakthrough pain can be treated by adding a second opioid or by using an additional dose of morphine. Drugs such as Sevredol may be particularly useful in breakthrough pain. Opioids are available in long-acting and slow-release formulations to control background pain. Oral, buccal or sublingual opioids are useful for breakthrough pain or for use during procedures such as dressing changes.

Combining analgesics

Many patients with less severe pain will benefit from the use of simple analgesics. Paracetamol (acetaminophen) can be given alone or in combination with NSAIDs, codeine or morphine. Patients should take this 1–2 hours before a dressing change. NSAIDs are particularly useful at reducing the throbbing or aching pain associated with leg ulceration that is frequently exacerbated after dressing changes. It is important to remember that these drugs are associated with gastrointestinal side-effects such as gastric ulceration and renal and haematological disorders, particularly in those aged over 65 years (Wall & Melzack, 1999).

Controlling neuropathic pain

Due to the neuropathic element of chronic leg ulcer pain other forms of medication may be required. Tricyclic drugs such as amitriptyline may be useful (Monks & Merskey, 1999). They should be introduced in small doses and, due to their sedative action, be taken at night. Doses in excess of 30 mg may be required and it may take several weeks before the correct dosage is achieved. Anticonvulsant drugs such as gabapentin and carbamazepine may also relieve pain. Patients may benefit from combination therapy involving traditional analgesics and other therapies.

Self-management strategies

Patients should be taught how to manage their pain effectively. Analgesia should be used regularly rather than waiting until pain has developed. Practical strategies such as pill boxes and written instructions for carers can significantly improve pain relief.

Additional methods to control procedural pain

Appropriate planning and review of analgesia should effectively reduce the pain associated with procedures such as dressing changes. It is important to remember that these procedures may become more painful over time due to physiological changes in the central nervous system. The following factors should be considered:

Nursing issues
- Be aware of triggers that increase pain.
- Remember that a careful explanation is required for all procedures.
- Handle the wound as little as possible and with great care.
- Recognise that pain may extend some distance from the actual wound.
- Recognise that cleansing, soaking and the temperature of solutions may exacerbate pain.
- Avoid wound exposure, which can cause severe pain.
- Cover the wound with cling film to reduce pain if waiting for specialist opinion.
- Avoid draughts from windows or fans as they may also exacerbate pain.

Patient involvement
- Involve the patient in the procedure – this gives them a greater sense of control and will help to reduce pain and anxiety.
- Encourage deep rhythmic breathing, distraction through listening to music or visualisation.
- Allow patients to remove their own dressings if they wish.
- Allow patients to halt the procedure if it is becoming too painful – additional analgesia can then be administered.

Methods to reduce operative pain
Pain reduction during debridement
Topical application of a local anaesthetic can be used prior to sharp debridement. A systematic review of the use of Emla (a local anaesthetic containing lidocaine) in debridement demonstrated significant reductions in pain scores (Briggs & Nelson, 2001). Following the manufacturer's instructions, Emla should be applied to the ulcer and then covered with a semi-permeable film dressing or cling film. Pain relief should be achieved within 30 minutes and debridement should be undertaken promptly before the effect wears off.

- Sharp debridement of a wound should only be carried out by a skilled practitioner.
- Debridement of ischaemic ulceration should **only** be performed under the guidance of a vascular specialist, due to the risk of gangrene and infection.

Entonox (an analgesic gas) can also be used for debridement in hospital settings because of its rapid action, although it should not be used for prolonged periods or for general pain relief (Day, 2001). Pain levels should be assessed throughout a sharp debridement procedure. If pain control cannot be achieved adequately with a topical anaesthetic then the patient should be considered for a general anaesthetic or local injection of lidocaine (only administered by a member of the medical staff).

Pain may be severe following debridement and patients should be advised to take regular analgesia for a few days after this procedure. Reapplication of Emla to the debrided wound the following day has also been reported to be of clinical use, although this should not be repeated for prolonged periods. The appropriate choice of a non-adherent dressing, such as those containing soft silicone or cooling gel dressings, will also reduce the pain level following debridement (EWMA, 2002).

Non-pharmacological methods to reduce pain

Dressing choice and wound pain
Pain in leg ulceration may also occur because of the inappropriate choice of dressings or topical agents. Dressing selection is discussed in Chapter 13. Removal of adherent dressings causes severe pain and trauma. If soaking is required to remove a dressing it indicates an inappropriate choice or that the dressing has not adequately covered all exposed wound areas. Poor exudate management may also lead to wound trauma and pain. If the dressing is incapable of handling the degree of fluid, exudate dries into the secondary dressing or bandage causing trauma to the skin and wound on removal. This should be reviewed and a more suitable dressing applied.

Reducing pain with compression bandaging

Practitioners frequently report that patients do not adhere to compression therapy because of pain, despite them having an adequate arterial circulation (Moffatt, 2004b).

The main factors causing pain in these circumstances are due to:

- Inappropriate choice of compression bandage system.
- Lack of adequate padding over bony and tendinous areas.
- Failure to adapt the bandage to the limb size and shape.
- Over-tight bandaging around the ankle, foot and limb (Fig. 9.5).
- Over-extension of the bandage at calf level causing a tourniquet effect.
- Too many or too few layers of bandage causing a lack of graduated compression.
- Pressure damage to the skin (Fig. 9.6).

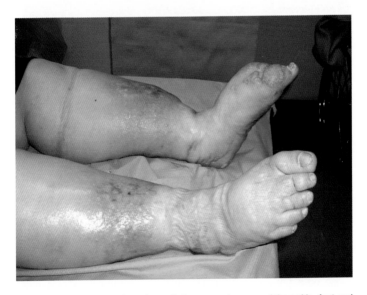

Fig. 9.5 Clinical picture of poorly applied compression around the ankle, foot and limb.

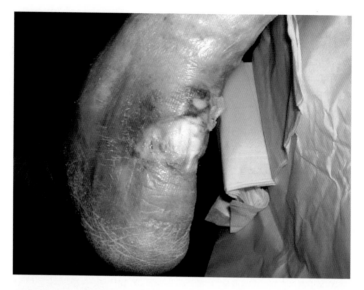

Fig. 9.6 Pressure damage to the skin.

- Bandage slippage causing trauma.
- Tight bandaging causing joint or muscle pain.
- Inability to wear shoes.
- Trauma from footwear over-bandaging.

The correct application and choice of bandaging can solve all the factors outlined above. This subject is dealt with more fully in Chapter 14.

Understanding the many factors that influence the development of pain in venous ulceration requires skill and experience. Traditional advice on walking, exercise and elevation may have varying effects: some patients experience pain while others gain relief. Many report pain from their venous ulcer at night and relief from getting up and walking about – a similar profile to those with peripheral vascular disease – while others find relief from going to bed. This reinforces the need for patient assessment that is:

- Continuing
- Comprehensive
- Individualised

Management of pain in mixed aetiology and ischaemic ulceration

Lower levels of compression (no more than 25 mmHg) are recommended for use in patients with mixed aetiology ulceration (venous and arterial element; ABPI 0.5–0.8) (see Chapter 14). Sudden severe pain with compression in this patient group requires rapid reassessment, including an ABPI recording. Increased pain may indicate a worsening of the arterial status, with a reduction in arterial perfusion to the limb when compression is applied. If in doubt seek vascular referral and discontinue compression therapy.

Amelioration of the pain associated with ischaemia is related to the ability to improve the blood supply to the limb by conservative, radiological or surgical methods. In addition to the use of powerful analgesics, relief can be achieved by careful positioning of the limb to avoid trauma and the use of foam gutters to prevent heel sores (see Fig. 9.7). High elevation should be avoided as this will

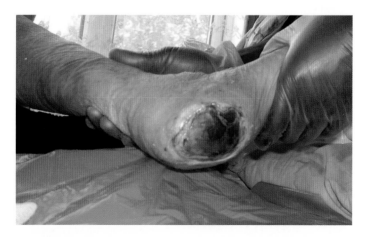

Fig. 9.7 Heel sore.

Table 9.2 Specialist pain management interventions.

- Electrical nerve stimulation
- Regional nerve blocks
- Steroid injections
- Cognitive–behavioural pain management
- Biofeedback
- Relaxation
- Hypnosis
- Family therapy

increase pain and reduce peripheral perfusion further. While many patients will find relief from keeping their limbs in a dependent position, some gentle elevation may be used to prevent dependency oedema, which may further exacerbate pain.

The role of pain management teams
All patients with poorly controlled pain, irrespective of the underlying aetiology, should be considered for a specialist pain management referral.

The role of the pain management team can be invaluable in achieving effective pain relief. Referral should be considered for all patients with inadequate pain relief or troublesome side-effects. Neuropathic pain or secondary depression may require more complex pharmacological options to be considered. Specialist advice is also required for patients with complex medical conditions that influence the appropriate choice of drug therapy. Specialist pain teams can offer a wide range of other interventions, as summarised in Table 9.2. Teaching patients skills in managing their pain can be of huge benefit and lead to improved quality of life as well as functional improvement.

SUMMARY

- Pain is a factor that affects 80% of patients with leg ulceration.
- Professionals frequently fail to assess or treat pain appropriately.
- Different physiological mechanisms lead to different pain manifestations.

Continued

- Different types of leg ulceration lead to different pain presentations.
- Pain is a complex, multi-factorial phenomenon that affects many dimensions of the patient's life.
- Comprehensive, ongoing assessment using validated pain assessment tools should be integrated into the assessment process.
- The layered approach to pain allows for assessment of background, incident and procedural pain.
- Appropriate analgesia may require a combination of different forms of medication.
- Self-management strategies may greatly assist patients in coping with their pain.
- Wound management procedures such as debridement are associated with significant pain and should only be undertaken by trained practitioners using a local or general anaesthetic.
- Appropriate choice and application of antiseptics and wound dressings can influence wound trauma and pain.
- Compression is the most frequent issue reported to cause pain in leg ulceration. An alternative choice of material and adaptation of the application technique can greatly reduce the level of pain experienced.
- Relief of pain is a key goal of treatment, irrespective of the underlying aetiology or prognosis for ulcer healing.
- Inadequate pain control should trigger referral to the pain specialist for a more comprehensive assessment and other interventions.

REFERENCES

Alison, J.H., Slater, M.A., Patterson, T.L., Grant, I. & Garfin, S.R. (1991) Prevalence, onset and risk of psychiatric disorders in men with chronic lower back pain: a controlled study. *Pain* **45**: 111–121.

Andrasik, F. (1999) The essence of biofeedback, relaxation and hypnosis. In: *Textbook of Pain*, 4th edn (P.D. Wall & R. Melzack, eds). Toronto, Churchill Livingstone.

Arathuzik, M.D. (1991) The appraisal of pain and coping in cancer patients. *Western Journal of Nursing Research* **13**: 714–731.

Briggs, M. & Hoffman, D. (1999) Pain management. Presented at the *9th European Conference in Advances in Wound Management*. Harrogate, 1999.

Briggs, M. & Nelson, E.A. (2001) Topical agents or dressings for pain in venous leg ulcers. Oxford, The Cochrane Library, Issue 1 (Update Software, online or CD-rom, updates quarterly), The Cochrane

Collaboration: www.cochrane.org and see The Cochrane Wounds Group: www.cochranewounds.org

Charles, H. (1995) The impact of leg ulcers on patients' quality of life. *Professional Nurse* **10**(9): 571–574.

Choniere, M., Melzack, R., Girand, N., et al. (1990) Comparisons between patients' and nurses' assessment of pain and medication efficiancy in severe burn injuries. *Pain* **40**: 143–152.

Day, A. (2001) Using Entonox in the community. *Journal of Wound Care* **10**(4): 1081.

Dworkin, R.H. & Breitbart, W. (eds) (2004) *Psychosocial Aspects of Pain: A Handbook for Health Care Providers*. Seattle, IASP Press.

Edmonds, M.E. & Foster A.V.M. (2000) *Managing the Diabetic Foot*. Oxford, Blackwell Science.

Embury, S.H. (1996) Sickle cell anaemia and associated haemoglobinopathies. In: *Cecil Textbook of Medicine*, 20th edn (J.C. Bennett & F. Plum, eds). Philadelphia, W.B. Saunders, pp. 882–893.

EWMA (2002) *European Wound Management Association Position Document: Pain at Wound Dressing Changes*. London, MEP.

Franks, P.J. & Moffatt, C.J. (1998a) Quality of life issues in patients with wounds. *Wounds* **10**(Suppl. E): 1E–9E.

Franks, P.J. & Moffatt, C.J. (1998b) Who suffers most from leg ulceration? *Journal of Wound Care* **7**: 383–385.

Franks, P.J., Moffatt, C.J. & Oldroyd, M. (1994) Community leg ulcer clinics: effect on quality of life. *Phlebology* **9**: 83–86.

Garafolo, J.P. (2000) Perceived optimism and chronic pain. In: *Personality Characteristics of Patients with Chronic Pain* (R.J. Gatchel & J.N. Weisberg, eds). Washington DC, American Psychological Association Press, pp. 203–217.

Geisser, M.E. (2004) The influence of coping styles and personality traits on pain. In: *A Handbook for Health Care Providers* (R.H. Dworkin & W.S. Breitbart, eds). Seattle, IASP Press.

Hofman, D. (1997) Assessing and managing pain in leg ulcers. *Community Nurse* **3**(6): 40–43.

Hollinworth, H. (1995) Nurses assessment and management of pain at dressing changes. *Journal of Wound Care* **4**(2): 77–83.

Houghton, A.D., Nicholls, G., Houghton, A.L., Saadah, E. & McCol, L. (1994) Phantom pain: natural history and association with rehabilitation. *Annals of the Royal College of Surgeons of England* **76**: 22–25.

Jayson, M.I.V. (1999) Rheumatoid arthritis. In: *Textbook of Pain*, 4th edn (P.D. Wall & R. Melzack, eds). Toronto, Churchill Livingstone, pp. 505–516.

Jenner, M., Turner, J., Romano, J. & Kardy, P. (1991) Coping with chronic pain: a critical review of the literature. *Pain* **47**(3): 249–283.

Jensen, T.S., Krebs, B., Nielson, J. & Rasmusen, P. (1984) Non painful phantom limb phenomena in amputees: incidence, clinical characteristics and temporal cause. *Acta Neurologica Scandinavica* **70**: 407–414.

Keeling, D.I., Price, P.E., Jones, E. & Harding, K.G. (1996) Social support: some pragmatic implications for health care professionals. *Journal of Advanced Nursing* **23**(1): 76–81.

Kitson, A. (1994) Postoperative pain management. A literature review. *Journal of Clinic Nursing* **3**: 7–18.

Krasner, D. (1998) Painful venous ulcers: themes and stories about living with the pain and suffering. *Journal of Wound/Ostomy/Continence Nursing* **25**, 158–168.

Low, S.M. (1984) The cultural basis of health, illness and disease. *Social Work in Health Care* **9**: 13–23.

McLain, R.F. & Weinstein, J.N. (1999) Orthopaedic surgery. In: *Textbook of Pain*, 4th edn (P.D. Wall & R. Melzack, eds). Toronto, Churchill Livingstone, pp. 1289–1306.

Moffatt, C.J. (2004a) Perspectives on concordance in leg ulcer management. *Journal of Wound Care* **13**(6): 243–248.

Moffatt, C.J. (2004b) Factors that affect concordance with compression therapy. *Journal of Wound Care* **13**(7): 291–294.

Monks, R. & Merskey, H. (1999) Psychotropic drugs. In: *Textbook of Pain*, 4th edn (P.D. Wall & R. Melzack, eds). Toronto, Churchill Livingstone, pp. 1155–1186.

Murphy, M.A., Joyce, W.P., Condon, C. & Bouchier-Hayes, D. (2002) A reduction in serum cytokine levels parallels healing of venous ulcers in patients undergoing compression therapy. *European Journal of Endovascular Surgery* **23**: 349–352.

Nikolajsen, L., Ilkajaer, S., Kroner, K, Christensen, J.H. & Jensen, T.S. (1997) The influence of preamputation pain on postamputation stump and phantom pain. *Pain* **72**: 393–405.

Phillips, T., Stanton, B., Provan, A. & Lew, R. (1994) A study of the impact of leg ulcers on quality of life: financial, social and psychologic implications. *Journal of the American Academy of Dermatology* **31**: 49–53.

Pohjolainen, T. (1991) A clinical evaluation of stumps in lower limb amputees. *Prosthetics and Orthotists International* **15**: 178–184.

Turner, J.A., Jensen, M.P. & Romano, J.M. (2000) Do beliefs, coping and catastrophising independently predict functioning in patients with chronic pain? *Pain* **85**: 115–125.

Twycross, R.G. (1999) Opioids. In: *Textbook of Pain*, 4th edn (P.D. Wall & R. Melzack, eds). Toronto, Churchill Livingstone, pp. 1187–1214.

Walker, J., Alcinsanya, J.A., Davis, B. & Marcer, D. (1990) The nursing management of elderly patients with pain in the community: Study and recommendations. *Journal of Advanced Nursing* **15**: 1154–1161.

Wall, P.D. & Melzack, R. (eds) (1999) *Textbook of Pain*, 4th edn. Toronto, Churchill Livingstone.

Williams, A.C. de C. (2004) Assessing chronic pain and its impact. In: *Psychosocial Aspects of Pain: A Handbook for Health Care Providers* (R.H. Dworkin & W.S. Breitbart, eds). Seattle, IASP Press.

World Health Organization (1996) *Cancer Pain Relief.* WHO Technical Report Series. Geneva, WHO.

World Union of Wound Healing Societies. (2004) *Principles of Best Practice: Minimising pain at wound dressing-related procedures.* A consensus document. London: MEP Ltd.

Psychosocial Factors in Leg Ulceration

10

LEARNING OBJECTIVES

Nurses involved in leg ulcer management should be able to demonstrate:

❏ An understanding of the impact that leg ulceration has on the emotional health and quality of life of patients.
❏ An understanding of the different ways patients cope with leg ulceration and adapt their lives.
❏ An understanding of the role of social factors in ulcer healing.
❏ The ability to describe how patients develop a new equilibrium when living with a leg ulcer.
❏ The ability to describe the psychological and social issues that must be considered within the assessment process.
❏ An understanding of the importance of the therapeutic relationship.
❏ The ability to describe the different interventions that may help the psychological health of patients.

INTRODUCTION

Since the 1980s, there has been a growing recognition of the psychological and social burden associated with leg ulceration (Lindholm et al., 1993; Krasner, 1998a, b). However, nurses frequently fail to assess and plan care that addresses these issues, relying solely on clinical information about the patient to inform their management decisions.

> Failure to understand the true impact of leg ulceration on patients and their families can lead to ineffective care and poor relationships between patient and professional.

THE EMOTIONAL IMPACT OF LEG ULCERATION

The emotional impact of wounding on a patient's life is poorly understood. A chronic non-healing leg ulcer may represent many different things to the patient and their family. As well as the very obvious loss of tissue integrity and symptoms such as pain and odour, the ulcer may also represent a continuous reminder of the loss of bodily integrity and potential frailty and vulnerability of life. Wells (1984, p. 95) acknowledged the profound psychological effect of tissue damage in a patient with a gangrenous limb:

'I am not dying, I am literally dropping to bits'

Leg ulceration and the associated smell may also lead to embarrassment and enforced social isolation (Neil & Munjas, 2000; Douglas, 2001). A study in the USA found that younger patients with leg ulceration reported feelings of frustration and negative self-image, leading to depression, anxiety and failed intimate relationships (Phillips et al., 1994). Tuckett suggests that stigmatisation is worse in visible conditions that affect patients' concept of themselves (Tuckett, 1976). Clearly, the social stigmatisation of leg ulceration may be an important factor in producing the embarrassment and alienation felt by many patients. Bernstein referred to the 'social death' that occurred in those who were visually deformed from facial burns: patients began an insidious withdrawal from society and the effects of social ostracisation (Bernstein, 1976). It is important to note that, while other aspects of health related, quality-of-life (HRQoL) issues improve with ulcer healing, levels of social isolation do not appear to change, suggesting that patterns of withdrawal from society may already be established (Franks & Moffatt, 1998).

HEALTH RELATED QUALITY-OF-LIFE (HRQOL) IMPACT

Research has shown that leg ulceration impacts on all aspects of the patient's life. Levels of pain and sleep deprivation, mobility, social isolation and emotional health are all significantly worse when compared to someone of a similar age and sex (Moffatt, 2004). While quality of life is poorest in very elderly ladies, there is evidence that young men suffer the most, although the reasons for this remain unclear (Franks & Moffatt, 1998). The most significant improvements in HRQoL are associated with complete ulcer healing; however, improvements, to a lesser degree, are also found in those who have not healed completely but have better control of symptoms (Franks et al., 1995). Very little is known about the long-term QoL issues for patients and the impact of recurrent periods of ulceration.

COPING WITH LEG ULCERATION

Professional views about how patients cope with a leg ulcer are often negative, although little research is available to support why these attitudes are held (Barrett & Teare, 2000; Rich & McLachlan, 2003). The literature refers to a lack of personal concern and care of their condition that leads to poor healing and frequent recurrence (Browse et al., 1988). Muir Gray (1983) described the 'social ulcer': a group of patients who had no significant symptoms but for whom healing was not sufficiently attractive to allow it to occur. Such patients were reported to deliberately interfere with their wound and prevent healing. Despite these negative attitudes there is little evidence to support such beliefs. Research suggests the opposite: patients will often go to extreme lengths to achieve healing and report frustration when they feel a lack of professional knowledge and care is inhibiting their progress (Charles, 1995).

Patients with leg ulcers may face a lifelong history of recurrent bouts of ulceration (Chase et al., 1997). This will require significant adaptation if the patient is to be able to lead a fulfilled life (Walshe, 1995).

Effective coping leads to adaptation, but patients need to make cognitive and behavioural changes to adjust positively to their new circumstances (Lazarus, 1966). This involves patients making decisions about how they will live their life in their new situation. The strategies people use to cope with chronic illness involve thought processes and actions, and a number of authors have grouped them in the following ways.

Monitoring and blunting

- **Monitoring** – constantly monitoring the illness and any changes, as well as seeking and processing information about the condition.
- **Blunting** – avoiding or distracting oneself from the stressors associated with the illness.

Excessive use of monitoring strategies may lead to anxiety as the patient continuously monitors minor changes in their signs and symptoms (Miller, 1987). Disproportionate use of blunting strategies may be associated with a failure to adhere to professional advice about treatment.

Approach and avoidance
- **Approach strategies** – trying to deal with the problem head-on.
- **Avoidance** – using distraction to avoid having to face the problems associated with the condition.

Patients who continuously use avoidance coping strategies will not make realistic or informed choices about their lives. However, patients who adopt approach strategies may become exhausted with their continuous drive to tackle the problem and their inability to disengage for relaxation time.

Problem and emotion focused coping
- **Problem focused** – dealing with the illness in a practical way.
- **Emotion focused** – dealing with the feelings associated with the illness.

Emotion focused coping is frequently the predominant coping strategy used in patients with chronic illness, particularly in situations in which the patient has little control. In this situation, emotion focused coping may still have practical value, allowing the patient to live well and to find a new level of emotional equilibrium.

Professionals frequently refer to 'good' or 'bad' coping; however, patients need to use a wide range of flexible coping strategies appropriately at different times during their illness (Lazarus, 1966). Flexible coping that responds to changes in the patient's health status is associated with good health outcomes. Nurses should be aware of the changing nature of coping strategies throughout the patient's illness as these are related to the individual's willingness to seek advice or support and their desire for information.

LIFE CHANGES WITH LEG ULCERATION

Krasner (1998a), in a phenomenological study involving 14 patients with painful venous ulceration, noted the frustration patients felt with many aspects of their lives. A number of patients had had to make major life changes, such as retirement, because they realised their ulcer was not healing as a consequence of their lifestyle. Patients experienced considerable guilt when they were facing choices between following healthcare providers' advice and continuing with an activity (e.g. work) that they felt was of greater importance. Professionals frequently used blaming behaviour that increased the emotional distress felt by patients, particularly if they were not healing. There was evidence, however, of patients' adjustment to their condition, with patients finding pleasure in new hobbies.

Walshe (1995) found that patients with chronic wounds coped by a process of 'normalisation', while Hyland et al. (1994) found that patients coped by spending time concentrating on their ulcer or considering ways that would improve their chance of healing. Practical coping strategies included avoiding crowds, children or pets that could damage the wound. Patients with leg ulceration were found to use fewer coping strategies overall than people without ulceration but of the same age and sex (Moffatt, 2004). Despite professional views that leg ulcer patients use maladaptive coping strategies, this was not supported by the research. Levels of alcohol and drug use were found to be very low.

Depression and anxiety

Research has shown that patients with leg ulceration frequently suffer with emotional problems such as depression and anxiety (Cole-King & Harding, 2001). Depression is often neglected in the elderly, with the cause often being unknown (endogenous). Ulceration may also be directly associated with the development of depression. It is unclear whether this is due to the symptoms such as pain and sleeplessness associated with the condition, the consequences of the ulcer not healing, or a combination of factors. Research has shown an association between patients with a clinical level of depression and delayed ulcer healing (Moffatt, 2004). A link between anxiety and healing has not yet been established. Clinicians frequently report that patients are anxious, but the true extent of the problem is unknown. The chronic illness literature shows that levels of anxiety are highest in the early stages of illness, particularly when the diagnosis or prognosis remains unclear, and in the late stages of illness where symptoms become pervasive and death impending (Dewar & Morse, 1995). It may be that anxiety levels are highest during the first episode of leg ulceration or during periods of deterioration. At other times, when treatment is progressing, albeit slowly, anxiety levels may be lower. Most leg ulcer research is cross-sectional in design and cannot therefore capture the experience of patients throughout their illness trajectory. Personality traits such as pessimism and optimism may also influence the psychological health of patients and their attitude to their condition and treatment. Screening for psychological health must be incorporated into a comprehensive leg ulcer assessment.

SOCIAL SUPPORT AND LEG ULCERATION

The HRQoL literature on leg ulceration has identified high levels of social isolation in these patients (Franks & Moffatt, 1998). A related concept to social isolation is that of social support. Thoits (1982, p. 147) defined social support as:

> 'the degree to which a person's basic social needs are gratified through interaction with others.'

This definition implies a transaction between individuals. House (1981) refers to a number of components that are essential to effective social support, these are:

- Emotional concern
- Instrumental help
- Provision of information
- Assistance in appraisal of a situation through a process of self-evaluation

The results of cardiovascular research have shown a strong association between social networks and access to social support and the morbidity and mortality of disease (Blazer, 1982; Cohen, 1988). Outcomes of chronic illness are also associated with levels of perceived social support (Schwarzer & Leppin, 1989).

Until recently, little research had examined the level of perceived social support available to patients with leg ulceration and the relationship it may play in ulcer healing and other outcomes such as depression and anxiety. A number of studies have now shown that patients with leg ulceration have low levels of social support and small social networks (Franks & Moffatt, 1998). Recent research has shown an association between the levels of social support available and ulcer healing. In this study the greatest chance of healing was found in those who reported the highest level of support, and the poorest healing in those with the least support (Moffatt, 2004). This strengthens the argument for ensuring that psychosocial dimensions are integrated within effective nursing management.

STRESS AND WOUND HEALING

There has been a limited amount of work examining the role of stress in the healing of chronic wounds. A number of authors have reported on the stressors associated with living with a wound. Walshe (1995) reported that key symptoms, such as pain, leakage of exudate, lack of mobility and odour, were particularly difficult. A number of authors have reported the importance of pain as a key stressor (Krasner, 1998a).

Research now suggests that these stressors may impact on the wound healing process. Kiecolt-Glaser et al. (1995) compared the healing rates of induced wounds in 13 women caring for demented relatives and 13 controls matched for age and sex (neither group had leg ulcers), and found that healing took significantly longer in the caregiver group. Patients frequently experience complex situations associated with stress that may influence their potential for healing as well as affecting their psychological health.

SOCIAL FACTORS AND LEG ULCERATION

In addition to the psychological factors that have been discussed, the social environment in which the patient lives may also play a role in whether healing will occur. While leg ulceration is frequently perceived as a problem of the elderly, it should be remembered that 20% of patients develop their first ulcer before the age of 40 and 50% before the age of retirement (Callam et al., 1985). A number of studies have examined the role of social class (economic status) and leg ulceration. The relationship with social status appears unclear; however, the duration of ulceration is often longer in those from the lower social classes with the lowest level of income. A qualitative research study in the USA found that, in the group of patients who were working, 50% were in manual jobs that required standing for protracted periods. In the group of patients who did not work, the leg ulcer had affected their decision to stop working in 42% of cases (Phillips et al., 1994). A number of other studies have found an association with socioeconomic status and wound healing, suggesting this may be an underestimated issue for patients (Franks et al., 2002).

Other social factors have been linked to delayed ulcer healing. Franks in a study of 168 patients with venous ulceration found that low social class, lack of central heating and being single were all associated with delayed healing (Franks et al., 1995). Other studies have reported that living alone and being male are associated with poor healing (Franks et al., 2002). While the underlying reasons for these factors are not yet fully explained they do support the need to consider these when caring for patients with leg ulceration.

THE ROLE OF ETHNICITY

Most leg ulcer studies have been undertaken in Caucasian populations. However, there is some research to suggest that ethnicity may affect the potential for ulcer development. Research has shown a reduced risk of venous ulceration in patients from South Asia, although this group has an increased risk of diabetes (Franks et al., 1997). A more recent study has confirmed these earlier findings and also reported a possible eightfold increased risk in Afro-Caribbeans (Moffatt et al., 2004). Many factors may influence our understanding of these findings. The low level of ulceration in people from South Asia may be due to their reluctance to present to a health professional and the use of traditional forms of medicine in these populations. Nurses must be sensitive to the religious and cultural belief systems and how they affect patients from these communities. It is also possible that diet, weight and genetic factors may influence whether these patients will develop ulceration and how they will progress with treatment.

A MODEL OF PSYCHOSOCIAL CARE

A model of psychosocial issues in leg ulceration has emerged from research and is diagrammatically presented in Fig. 10.1 (Moffatt, 2004). Nursing practice in leg ulceration has moved from ritualistic wound care to an emphasis on delivering evidence-based care. The major paradigm underpinning the nursing care of patients with leg

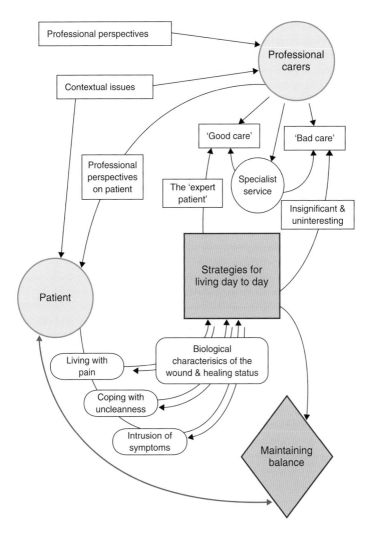

Fig. 10.1 A psychosocial model of care for patients with leg ulceration.

ulceration has been the traditional medical model. This approach has led to improvements in outcomes such as healing, but at the expense of a more holistic approach to patients.

There is evidence that the patients being cared for by nurses are becoming more complex (Moffatt et al., 2004). Such patients have multiple medical needs and may take protracted lengths of time to heal. Patients may be facing the reality of living with leg ulceration as a chronic condition rather than an acute episode of illness from which they will recover and return to a similar lifestyle. In this situation the priorities for daily living change. The emphasis is now placed on developing strategies for daily living that allow a balance in life to be maintained (Husband, 2001). The role of nurses in helping patients to achieve this is of critical importance. Issues such as symptom control are the priority. Nurses must focus on the importance of building a therapeutic relationship with patients who are experts in their own condition and treatment (Harker, 2000; Edwards, 2001; Moffatt et al., 2002).

INTEGRATING PSYCHOSOCIAL ISSUES INTO ASSESSMENT

The following sections consider the assessment of psychosocial issues in leg ulceration. While many of the recommendations can be successfully introduced by nurses, it is important to recognise when expert psychological opinion is required. Referral to psychiatric and psychology services can be of great value in such situations.

Psychosocial assessment

> The aim of assessment is to identify patients at risk of developing psychosocial problems and those with existing problems in order to develop strategies to improve their overall quality of care.

Patients should receive psychological screening at the time of referral and throughout the treatment period to:

- Assess their degree of psychological adjustment.
- Identify those who require help to cope with the condition.

- Identify those who require specialist psychological intervention.

The psychological assessment should consider:

- Levels of social support.
- Poor coping or maladaptive coping strategies (including reliance on alcohol and drugs).
- Poor understanding of health needs (beliefs about their condition).
- Lack of motivation.
- Signs of depression.
- Loneliness and isolation.
- Anxiety.
- Poor concordance with treatment (Moffatt, 2004).
- Psychological dependence on the ulcer (or professional visits for treatment).
- Withdrawal from society (feeling stigmatised or ostracised).

The National Institute for Clinical Excellence (NICE) has published very simple recommendations for the screening of depression by healthcare professionals that can be integrated into the assessment of patients with leg ulceration (Table 10.1):

Social assessment should consider the following:

- **Accommodation** – suitability, accessibility, general living standards, heating.
- **Care support** – involvement of carers.

Table 10.1 Screening for depression (Adapted from NICE, 2004).

Many patients with chronic illness can become depressed, and recognition of depression in this group can lead to improved outcomes.

Screening for depression should include the following 2 questions on mood and interest:

1. Have you often been bothered by feeling down, depressed or hopeless during the last month?
2. Have you often been bothered by having little interest or pleasure in doing things during the last month?

- **Employment** – whether the condition affects the patient's ability to work, how the current job affects their ulceration.
- **Financial status** – benefit entitlement, prescription charges.

Psychosocial support
The algorithm in Fig. 10.2 provides guidance on the role that general nurses can play in ensuring the psychosocial health of patients, and makes recommendations on the role of specialist referral and some of the interventions that may be successfully employed.

Generalist psychosocial intervention
Generalist psychosocial intervention involves planning and implementing psychosocial care strategies to help the patient and family/carers to:

- Take a positive role in the management of their leg ulceration, according to their capabilities.
- To achieve as good a quality of life as possible.

Recommended generalist interventions are set out in Fig. 10.2. It is important that if the identified psychosocial problems have not been resolved in 3 months then the patient should be referred for appropriate specialist intervention.

Specialist psychosocial intervention
Specialist psychosocial intervention may be accessed from a number of sources. These may range from psychiatric specialist treatment for depression and associated problems to social services tackling housing or financial problems. Often specialist intervention requires a combination of strategies to resolve the patient's psychological and social problems.

PRACTICAL SOLUTIONS FOR COPING WITH LEG ULCERATION
Research has shown that coping with leg ulceration requires appropriate care of the wound and symptom control. Table 10.2 outlines some of the common problems reported by patients and some solutions that can be successfully employed.

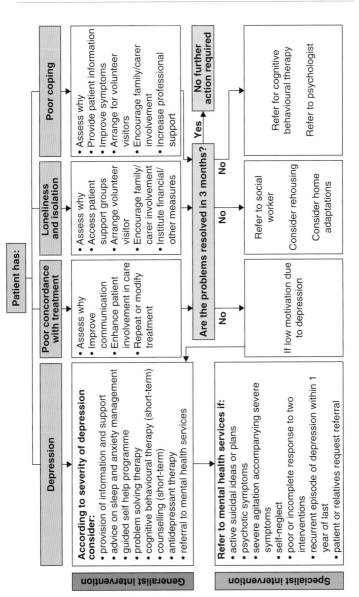

Patient has:

Generalist intervention

Depression

According to severity of depression consider:
- provision of information and support
- advice on sleep and anxiety management
- guided self help programme
- problem solving therapy
- cognitive behavioural therapy (short-term)
- counselling (short-term)
- antidepressant therapy
- referral to mental health services

Poor concordance with treatment
- Assess why
- Improve communication
- Enhance patient involvement in care
- Repeat or modify treatment

Loneliness and isolation
- Assess why
- Access patient support groups
- Arrange volunteer visitor
- Encourage family/carer involvement
- Institute financial/other measures

Poor coping
- Assess why
- Provide patient information
- Improve symptoms
- Arrange for volunteer visitors
- Encourage family/carer involvement
- Increase professional support

Are the problems resolved in 3 months?

Yes → **No further action required**

No

If low motivation due to depression

Refer to social worker

Consider rehousing

Consider home adaptations

Refer for cognitive behavioural therapy

Refer to psychologist

Specialist intervention

Refer to mental health services if:
- active suicidal ideas or plans
- psychotic symptoms
- severe agitation accompanying severe symptoms
- self-neglect
- poor or incomplete response to two interventions
- recurrent episode of depression within 1 year of last
- patient or relatives request referral

Fig. 10.2 Algorithm to address psychosocial problems.

Table 10.2 Practical solutions for coping with leg ulceration.

Symptom control	Solution	Comment
Smell from exudate	Increase the frequency of dressing changes	
	Control bacterial burden with antimicrobial agents	Check bacteriology
	Change to a dressing capable of handling large exudate volumes	
	Consider antimicrobial therapy, e.g. silver products	
	Use charcoal dressings	
	Introduce self-care regimens that allow more frequent dressing changes	
Pain control	Use principles discussed in Chapter 9	If not controlled refer to the pain team
Social isolation	Consider clinic or leg clubs; encourage the patient to socialise and not to allow the ulcer to dominate their lives	Mutual support may benefit the patient and relieve isolation
	Arrange professional ulcer care or teach self-care routines for holidays	Careful treatment planning by professionals will give the patient confidence to go away on holiday

SUMMARY

- Leg ulceration is associated with considerable emotional distress that reduces patients' quality of life and may lead to depression and anxiety.
- Prolonged periods of ulceration reduce patients' quality of life, leading to social isolation, reduced mobility, emotional disturbance, sleep problems and pain.

Continued

- Patients use different forms of coping strategies, which are influenced by their personality, stage of their illness and levels of support available.
- Assessment should include psychological and social issues.
- Patients with depression should be promptly identified and referred to their GP for treatment.
- Specialist interventions may be required if patients continue to suffer psychological problems, and referral to a psychologist should be considered.
- Social factors such as social isolation, low levels of social support, living alone and being male all lead to a reduction in ulcer healing.
- Nurses have a duty of care to understand and plan appropriate care for patients suffering psychological distress resulting from their condition.

CONCLUSION

Many of the issues discussed in this chapter are ignored during the treatment of leg ulceration. The research clearly portrays that living with a leg ulcer involves suffering and psychological distress. As our understanding of these issues increases it becomes clear that they may have a direct impact on whether healing will occur. Nurses have a professional duty to ensure that all patients receive the highest level of professional care. Attention to the issues described in this chapter will help patients to cope effectively with their leg ulcer by addressing the multitude of factors that can impact on their lives.

REFERENCES

Barrett, C. & Teare, J.A. (2000) Quality of life in leg ulcer assessment: patients' coping mechanisms. *British Journal of Community Nursing* **5**(11): 530–540.

Bernstein, N. (1976) *Emotional Care of the Facially Disfigured*. Boston, Little, Brown.

Blazer, D.G. (1982) Social support and mortality in an elderly community population. *American Journal of Epidemiology* **115**: 684–694.

Browse, N.L., Burnand, K.G. & Lea-Thomas, M. (1988) *Diseases in the Veins: Pathology, Diagnosis and Treatment*. London, Edward Arnold.

Callam, M.J., Ruckley, C.V., Harper, D.R. & Dale, J.J. (1985) Chronic ulceration of the leg: extent of the problem and provision of care. *British Medical Journal* **290**: 1855–1856.

Charles, H. (1995) The impact of leg ulcers on patients' quality of life. *Professional Nurse* **10**(9): 571–574.

Chase, S.K., Melloni, M. & Savage, A. (1997) A forever healing: the lived experience of venous ulcer disease. *Journal of Vascular Nursing* **15**(2): 73–78.

Cohen, S. (1988) Psychosocial models of the role of social support in the aetiology of physical disease. *Health Psychology* **7**(3): 269–297.

Cole-King, A. & Harding, K.G. (2001) Psychological factors and delayed healing in chronic wounds. *Psychosomatic Medicine* **63**: 216–220.

Dewar, A.L. & Morse, J.M. (1995) Unbearable incidents: failure to endure the experience of illness. *Journal of Advanced Nursing* **22**: 957–964.

Douglas, V. (2001) Living with a chronic leg ulcer: and insight into patients' experiences and feelings. *Journal of Wound Care* **10**(9): 355–360.

Edwards, L.M. (2001) Views of patients deemed non-compliant. *The Leg Ulcer Forum*: Spring Issue, p. 11.

Franks, P.J. & Moffatt, C.J. (1998) Who suffers most from leg ulceration? *Journal of Wound Care* **7**: 383–385.

Franks, P.J., Bosanquet, N., Connolly, M., Oldroyd, M.I., Moffatt, C.J., Greenhalgh, R.M. & McCollum, C.N. (1995) Venous ulcer healing: effect of socio-economic factors in London. *Journal of Epidemiology and Community Health* **49**(4): 385–388.

Franks, P.J., Morton, N., Campbell, A. & Moffatt, C.J. (1997) Leg ulceration. A study in West London. *Public Health* **111**(5): 327–329.

Franks, P.J., Doherty, D.C. & Moffatt, C.J. (2002) Are socio-demographic factors important in the development of chronic leg ulceration? *Ostomy/Wound Management* **48**: 73–74.

Harker, J. (2000). Influences on patient adherence with compression hosiery. *Journal of Wound Care* **9**(8): 379–381.

House, J. (1981) *Work, Stress, and Social Support*. Reading, Mass, Addison Wesley.

Husband, L. (2001). Shaping the trajectory of patients with venous ulceration in primary care. *Health Expectations* **4**: 189–198.

Hyland, M., Ley, A. & Thompson, B. (1994) Quality of life of leg ulcers patients: questionnaire and preliminary findings. *Journal of Wound Care* **3**(6): 294–298.

Kiecolt-Glaser, J.K., Marucha, P.T., Malarkey, W.B., Mercado, A.M. & Glaser, R. (1995) Slowing of wound healing by psychological stress. *Lancet* **346**: 1194–1196.

Krasner, D. (1998a) Painful venous ulcers: themes and stories about living with pain and suffering. *Journal of Wound/Ostomy/Continence Nursing* **25**(3): 158–168.

Krasner, D. (1998b) Painful venous ulcer: themes and stories about their impact on quality of life. *Ostomy/Wound Management* **44**(9): 38–50.

Lazarus, S. (1966) *Psychological Stress and the Coping Process*. New York, McGraw-Hill.

Lindholm, C., Bjellerup, M., Christensen, O.B. & Zederfeld, B. (1993) Quality of life in chronic leg ulcers. *Acta Dermato-Venereologica* **73**: 440–443.

Miller, S.M. (1987) Monitoring and blunting: validation of a questionnaire to assess styles of information seeking under threat. *Journal of Personality and Social Psychology* **52**: 345–353.

Moffatt, C.J. (2004) Perspectives on concordance in leg ulcer management. *Journal of Wound Care* **13**(6): 243–248.

Moffatt, C.J., Doherty, D.C. & Franks, P.J. (2002) Professional dilemmas of non-healing. Abstract presented at the *EWMA Conference*, Stuttgart, 2005.

Moffatt, C.J., Franks, P.J., Doherty, D.C., Martin, R., Blewett, R. & Ross, F. (2004) Prevalence of leg ulceration in a London population. *Quarterly Journal of Medicine* **97**(7): 431–437.

Muir Gray, J.A. (1983) Social aspects of peripheral vascular disease in the elderly. In: *Peripheral Vascular Disease in the Elderly* (S. McCarthy, ed.). London, Churchill Livingstone, pp. 191–199.

National Institute for Clinical Excellence (2004) *Depression: Management of Depression in Primary and Secondary Care*. London, NICE, www.nice.org.uk

Neil, J.A. & Munjas, B.H. (2000) Living with a chronic wound: the voice of sufferers. *Ostomy/Wound Management* **46**(5): 28–38.

Phillips, T., Stanton, B., Provan, A. & Lew, R. (1994) A study of the impact of leg ulcers on quality of life: financial, social and psychologic implications. *Journal of the American Academy of Dermatology* **31**: 49–53.

Rich, A. & McLachlan, L. (2003) How living with a leg ulcer affects people's daily life: a nurse-led study. *Journal of Wound Care* **12**(2): 51–54.

Schwarzer, R. & Leppin, A. (1989) Social support and health: a meta-analysis. *Psychology and Health* **3**: 1–15.

Thoits, P.A. (1982) Conceptual, methodological and theoretical problems in studying social support as a buffer against stress. *Journal of Health and Social Behaviour* **23**: 145–159.

Tuckett, D. (1976) *An Introduction to Medical Sociology*. London, Tavistock.

Walshe, C. (1995) Living with a venous leg ulcer: a descriptive study of patients' experiences. *Journal of Advanced Nursing* **22**(6): 1092–1100.

Wells, R. (1984) Wound Care. *Nursing Mirror* **158**(10): 94–96.

Improving Concordance

11

LEARNING OBJECTIVES

Nurses involved in leg ulcer management should be able to demonstrate:

❑ An understanding of the problems patients with leg ulceration have in adhering to professional instruction on treatment.
❑ The ability to describe the concept of compliance and concordance and how these have evolved over time.
❑ An understanding of how the attitudes held by professionals towards individual patients influences concordance.
❑ An understanding of how issues related to concordance should form part of the assessment process.
❑ An understanding of how effective negotiation with patients can influence their ability to adhere to treatment.

INTRODUCTION

Professionals often say that patients with leg ulcers are not concordant with therapy (Moffatt, 2004a). Little research has been undertaken to examine the credibility of such attitudes or to determine whether concordance is a major issue in leg ulcer management. It is possible that such negative attitudes reflect the complex interactions between professionals and patients whose ulcers do not heal as expected (Editorial, 1982).

In 1992, Blackwell reported that research had failed to identify common demographic or patient characteristics associated with poor concordance (Blackwell, 1992), and this is still the case today. Professionals are frequently judgemental in their attitudes to patients who do not 'comply' with professionally prescribed treatment. Fineman (1991, p. 15) states that:

'it is reasonable to suggest that non-compliance is not the neat, objective diagnostic label that biomedicine claims, rather it is better understood as a complex, subjective, provider created category of unacceptable behaviour.'

Concordance remains poorly understood and has largely been studied from the patient perspective, with little attention placed on the relationship between patient and professional (Koltun & Stone, 1986). The literature highlights the complexity surrounding our understanding of concordance. The patient's ability to 'concord' will be influenced by many factors, many of which will not be directly associated with their condition (Roberson, 1992). For example, a patient with leg ulceration may have been told to avoid standing for long periods, but be faced with an occupation that requires spending a considerable amount of time on their feet. Patients are constantly faced with competing demands and day-to-day situations that may require them to choose to compromise on the advice given by professionals (Stimson, 1974). Concordance is not a static event but may alter from hour to hour or on a daily basis according to the demands of life. Too little acknowledgement has been given to the potential role that symptoms such as pain or sleeplessness have on concordance with therapy (Farberow & Hehemkis, 1979; Nelson & Farberow, 1980; Franks & Moffatt, 1998).

DEFINITIONS OF COMPLIANCE AND CONCORDANCE

Since the 1980s, the negative views surrounding the use of the term 'compliance' have been challenged following the growing emphasis on patient autonomy and involvement in their own care. It also reflects a move away from the authoritarian, biomedical model to a biopsychosocial model that acknowledges the psychosocial issues that surround being ill and receiving treatment (Becker & Maiman, 1975).

In recent years the term 'compliance' has been replaced with definitions such as 'concordance' and 'adherence to therapy'. Despite these changes there is evidence that professionals continue to label patients 'non-compliant'. Terms used for such patients in the literature include: 'disobedient', 'deviant', 'irresponsible', 'negligent', 'failure to co-operate' and 'unreliable' (Blackwell, 1992).

Many of the techniques used to improve concordance fail to treat patients as responsible adults who are able to make informed decisions (Epstein & Masek, 1978).

HISTORICAL USE OF THE TERM 'COMPLIANCE'

The historical use of the term 'compliance' in healthcare emerged from a professional perspective of how patients are expected to behave towards their illness and professionally prescribed treatment. A widely used definition of compliance (Haynes, 1979) is:

'the extent to which a person's behaviour (in terms of taking medications, following diets, or executing life style changes) coincides with medical or health advice.'

This definition places the responsibility for successful treatment on the patient, who must not deviate from what the clinician tells him/her to do. Such an attitude abdicates professional responsibility for treatment failure. Success or failure is professionally judged, and frequently takes no account of the circumstances facing the patient or the fluctuations in concordance that may occur over time. Inherent within this definition is the assumption that all medical advice is good and that the rational patient should follow clinical advice precisely (Zola, 1981; Roberson, 1992). A meta-analysis of 153 studies that addressed 'compliance' failed to identify a single strategy that was more effective at improving 'compliance' than others, although approaches that had included educational, behavioural and affective components were likely to be the most effective (Roter et al., 1998).

THE DISADVANTAGES OF GOOD CONCORDANCE

There are instances when the benefits of concordance have been challenged (Blackwell, 1992). For example, patients with hypertension have demonstrated good blood pressure control at the expense of an increased sense of vulnerability, leading to adoption of illness behaviour and absenteeism from work (Becker & Maiman, 1975). There are occasions when following professional advice may not be helpful to a patient with a leg ulcer. This may reflect poor professional knowledge and an inappropriate choice of treatment that exacerbates symptoms such as pain.

CONCORDANCE AS A SOCIALLY CONSTRUCTED CONCEPT

Fineman (1991) found that 'compliance' was socially constructed by professionals, and was defined as the extent to which a patient's behaviour deviated from what was considered to be appropriate, reasonable patient behaviour. Such labelling influenced professionals' interactions with these patients. Professional attitudes and behaviour towards patients considered 'non-compliant' include: anger, anxiety, labelling, distancing, resentment, lack of respect and a failure to treat the patient as an equal.

CRITERIA FOR BEING A PATIENT

Professionals define the norms for expected patient behaviour and make judgements if patients deviate from these ideals. 'Good' patients have been defined as those who comply with treatment, whereas 'bad' patients are non-compliant and are seen as wasting staff time and contributing to their own lack of progress (Lorber, 1975). Compliant behaviour has been characterised as:

- Following treatment
- Being helpful to professionals
- Expressing gratitude
- Using pleasant behaviour

Those who question professional decisions, demand attention or are generally troublesome are often labelled as 'non-compliant'. Research has failed to identify demographic, personality or health belief characteristics that are consistent with 'non-compliant behaviour'. To a limited extent the literature has highlighted features which can be viewed as 'risk factors' for increased or decreased compliance (Becker & Maiman, 1975; Blackwell & Gutmann, 1985).

Concordance can be enhanced if:

- A therapeutic relationship is established with the patient who feels the professional has a sustained interest and understanding of their problems.
- The patient perceives their condition to be serious and that treatment can control symptoms.
- Treatment can be moulded into everyday life without too much disruption.

- If a family member shares an interest in the patient's progress (Becker & Green, 1975).

Concordance may be poorer in:

- Diseases with few symptoms. For example, where patients with healed ulceration are told to wear hosiery when they no longer consider themselves to have a health problem.
- Conditions requiring complex treatments with unpleasant side-effects.
- Patients living alone who are at risk of developing depression and anxiety.
- Patients who do not have confidence in a health professional or who feel they are not progressing. For example, Charles (1995) found that patients with intractable ulceration no longer believed that professionals knew how to treat them, which led to feelings of hopelessness and helplessness. In some cases, professionals show poor understanding and lack of motivation to take the trouble to consider other treatment options that may achieve a better patient outcome.

ASSESSMENT ISSUES AFFECTING CONCORDANCE

Careful assessment remains the most important priority in leg ulcer management (Moffatt & Harper, 1997) (see Chapter 3). Without accurate knowledge of both the underlying ulcer aetiology and the wider factors affecting the patient, effective treatment cannot be ensured and factors influencing concordance adequately addressed. A number of key clinical and psychosocial issues are summarised in Tables 11.1 and 11.2. The importance of assessment and management of pain in influencing concordance with leg ulcer treatment cannot be underestimated, and this is discussed further in Chapter 9 (see also Gillmore & Hill, 1981).

PSYCHOSOCIAL ISSUES INFLUENCING CONCORDANCE

Clearly, patients are influenced by numerous issues including lay beliefs and the influence of those within their social network (Roberson, 1992). Sherbourne et al. (1992) found that avoidant coping strategies, poor physical heath and reduced role functioning

Table 11.1 Clinical assessment issues influencing patient concordance (reproduced from Moffatt (2004a) with permission of Emap Healthcare).

Clinical issues	Comments	Professional considerations
Correct diagnosis	Mild peripheral vascular disease may cause pain with compression	Seek clarification if diagnosis is in doubt
Concurrent illness	General poor health may prevent full concordance with therapy	Set realistic treatment goals in patients with poor health which may affect progress
Level of mobility	Reduced general mobility and fixed ankle joint are associated with delayed healing	Consider interventions such as physiotherapy to improve mobility. Identify whether poor mobility is linked to depression
Level of bodily pain	Bodily pain may reduce tolerance to treatment	Assess pain regularly and also the effectiveness of analgesia
Ulcer pain	Present in around 80% of patients	Identify what factors influence ulcer pain; consider use of pain diaries and refer to pain specialists
Size and state of wound	Pain associated with a wound is a common problem and underestimated	Debridement, clinical infection, uncontrolled oedema and overtight compression exacerbate ulcer pain

were associated with reduced concordance. Aspects of the patient/ professional relationship also affected concordance (Ley, 1982; Sherbourne et al., 1992).

Charles (1995), in a phenomenological study involving four patients with ulceration, noted a number of psychological effects of ulceration including hopelessness, helplessness and lack of control. Of these, three patients had an internal locus of control and showed evidence of looking for other ways to cope with the ulcer. Only one patient had an external locus, and was resigned to the fact that the ulcer would not heal and made no attempts to influence the situation. Following ineffective treatment, the three

Table **11.2** Assessment of psychosocial issues affecting concordance.

Psychosocial issues	Comments	Professional considerations
Clinical depression	May be a result of failed ulcer treatment or be unrelated	May predict delayed healing
Anxiety	Levels of anxiety may be high in patients with their first ulcer who have not adapted to their illness	Understand the issues causing anxiety and seek practical intervention
Social isolation	Common in patients with ulceration	Consider community clinics, leg clubs or increasing social support
Perceived social support	Very low levels of support in ulcer patients	Shown to be associated with ulcer healing
Health beliefs/internal and external locus of control	Influences patients' perceptions of how they can influence their own health	Health beliefs influence the desire and use of health information by different patients
Lay beliefs/understanding of condition	Many patients do not understand their condition or treatment	Professionals should not assume understanding; patients now have greater access to electronic information
Previous treatment experience	Major factor in influencing future treatment experiences	Wound pain at dressing changes is common and should be avoided

Patient expectations of care	Influenced by past experiences and their belief in whether healing can occur	Development of a therapeutic relationship influences these issues
Impact of leg ulceration on HRQoL	Leg ulceration is associated with a major impact on all aspects of quality of life	Effective treatment improves the quality of life in patients who either heal completely or partially
Sleep disorder	Sleep disorders are a common problem and are associated with pain	Professionals rarely address this issue adequately
Coping strategies/illness adjustment	Little research on how leg ulcer patients cope with their condition	Problem-based coping useful if the situation is solvable (the ulcer will heal). Emotion-based coping used when the situation cannot be solved and the patient must learn to live with their ulcer
Patient/professional conflict	The true extent of this problem remains unknown	Labelling and blaming are used in patients perceived as difficult, which includes those who will not concord with treatment
Manipulative behaviour	Patients whose needs have not been met may engage in manipulative behaviour, whereby they favour individual practitioners over others	Better communication and understanding may lessen the 'difficult' behaviour that is linked to unmet need

patients also gave up and believed they could not influence the situation.

In a case-control study of 88 patients and 60 community controls using the health locus of control, Roe et al. (1995) found that patients were more externally orientated than the controls, supporting the view that patients with leg ulcers often feel they have little control over factors influencing their health.

Charles (1995) also noted that nurses were often not interested in the patients' condition and did not explain procedures to them. Patients stated that nurses lacked knowledge about the treatments and were resistant to their comments. In a recent study (Moffatt, 2004a), patients described themselves as 'insignificant and uninteresting' to professionals caring for them, particularly when admitted to hospital where the knowledge and interest was often poorest. Patients reported that they had to instruct nurses on which materials to use and how to dress their ulcers, a situation that was often resented. Nurses, however, often resent this intervention and may view the patient as manipulative.

Edwards et al. (2002) found that patients' knowledge of their condition was poor, with little understanding of the underlying pathology delaying healing. Providing information to patients is complex and influenced by the types of coping strategies that patients employ. Styles of coping, such as monitoring and blunting which were examined in Chapter 10, have been linked to concordance with therapy and satisfaction with treatment (Lazarus, 1985; Steptoe & O'Sullivan, 1986). Patients who use denial as a major coping strategy may be particularly challenging. While denial has been shown to be a useful coping strategy in acute situations, in long-term conditions, such as leg ulceration, this may lead to poor concordance and a refusal to actively engage in treatment (Soloff, 1980). The impact on professionals can be considerable.

CONCORDANCE AND ADJUSTMENT

Krasner (1998) noted the frustration that patients felt with many aspects of their lives. Many had had to make major life changes such as retirement because they realised their ulcer was not healing as a consequence of their lifestyle. Patients experienced considerable guilt when faced with a choice between following professionals' advice and continuing with an activity they felt was of greater importance. Professionals often used blaming behaviour, increasing the patients' emotional distress, particularly if they were not healing.

THE ROLE OF CONCORDANCE
IN LEG ULCER MANAGEMENT

Cullum & Last (1991) examined whether patients perceive an active benefit to having a leg ulcer. In a study involving 301 patients receiving district nursing care for a leg ulcer, nurses were asked to subjectively grade the patient's 'compliance' with treatment. Only 11% were described as non-compliant. While no attempt was made to clarify this assessment, the findings do suggest that professionals exaggerate the issue of non-concordance in this patient group, or perhaps attribute non-healing to patient behaviours considered non-concordant.

A recent study, which followed 113 patients prospectively for 48 weeks of treatment, found no evidence that professional descriptions of concordance were predictive of ulcer healing (Moffatt, 2001).

Little attention has been paid to methods of improving concordance in leg ulcer management. Brooks et al. (2004) found that a structured, nurse-led concordance programme run over one year was associated with a reduction in leg ulcer recurrence rates. Jull et al. (2004) highlighted two factors associated with the use of hosiery in patients whose leg ulcer healed: a belief that hosiery was beneficial and that it was uncomfortable.

- Increase continuity of care – same nurse to attend.
- Listen to patient concerns.
- Introduce level of compression slowly.
- Do not dismiss patients' knowledge of what suits them.
- Retain flexibility in planning care.
- Demonstrate commitment to solving the patients' issues.

Professional reactions to non-concordance

The dilemmas of 'non-healing' have generally been studied from a patient perspective, with little attention paid to the impact that 'non-healing' has on professionals. Since the 1990s, improvements in assessment and treatment have led to heightened expectations of healing. Healing rates are considered the most important outcome of leg ulcer care, but little is known about the factors that influence ulcer healing or recurrence (Franks et al., 1995a, b). Professionals who are unable to heal a wound often feel impotent and may become anxious when faced with increasing pressure from the patient and family.

It has long been recognised that professionals have great difficulty containing their anxiety when observing suffering and death (Menzies, 1959). This may be partly because professional practice frequently fails to adequately deal with patient suffering.

Perceived professional failure, such as failing to heal a patient's leg ulcer, may lead to defensive behaviour. Menzies (1959) described how professionals developed defensive routines such as task allocation and ritualistic practice to protect them from the anxiety generated from caring for the sick and dying. Such beliefs act as a defence against acknowledging the 'failure' of professional care.

Recent research explored patient and professional reactions to 'non-healing' and 'non- compliance' in leg ulceration. In-depth qualitative interviews were carried out with five patients described as both 'non-compliant' and 'non-healing'. After the patient interviews, focus groups were held with the corresponding nursing teams (Moffatt, 2001). The research found that professionals struggled with the realities of the situation. The effects of continuously dealing with emotionally distressed patients appeared to be overwhelming. This led to social defences such as withdrawal of visits, avoidance of continuity of care, labelling, blaming, distancing and blunting of emotional responses to patient suffering. Non-healing was largely blamed on non-concordance. The study supported previous research in other areas, which identified that such patients are perceived as 'difficult' or 'unpopular' thus leading to deterioration in relationships.

Patient attitudes to treatment and ulcer healing

Little attempt has been made to examine the impact of patients' attitudes and behaviour on healing and concordance. Salaman et al. (1995) investigated a group of 45 hospital patients with venous ulcers of whom 16 (36%) were considered to be failing to make satisfactory progress.

Patients were questioned about their knowledge and attitude to their ulcer and its treatment. Of the sixteen whose ulcers were not improving, only eight (50%) claimed to have received explanations about its cause and treatment. However, 75% of the patients appeared to understand the importance of compression, but 62% felt that it was not effective in healing their ulcer. Only seven (44%) patients believed their ulcer would ever heal.

While this study was small and focused on a highly refractory group of patients, nevertheless it raises issues about the impact of patient beliefs on ulcer healing, and the effectiveness of patients' coping strategies. Questions must arise about patients' ability to tolerate and follow treatment modalities that they do not believe will help them.

Patient control

Patient control over treatment is a major factor (Conrad, 1987). Professionals often appear unaware of, or unwilling to acknowledge, the expertise the patient has developed about their condition, and their need to exercise control over areas of their care they consider important. English & Morse (1988) suggested that controlling behaviour is likely to increase passive, dependent behaviour.

English & Morse (1988) discussed the 'difficult' patient and concluded that this type of behaviour frequently emanates from patients' perceived unmet needs and from poor communication. They postulated that improved communication gives patients a greater sense of control, and that withdrawal of information leads to increasingly 'difficult' behaviour. Professionals reported that patients used manipulative behaviour by favouring practitioners who were easier to influence and rejecting others. This led to a lack of team cohesion. Nurses reported a sense of catharsis in being able to discuss issues generally considered taboo.

Improving patient concordance requires a sensitive, therapeutic relationship to be developed between professional and patient and a willingness to comprehend the difficulties the patient experiences on a day-to-day basis (English & Morse, 1988).

Treatment issues affecting concordance with leg ulcer treatment

Despite the lack of research evidence about the most effective methods for improving concordance in leg ulcer management, clinical experience suggests that these issues can often be resolved by appropriate treatment choices. At commencement of therapy it is important to consider the following:

- The overall health status of the patient including co-morbidities and mobility.
- The patients' knowledge and beliefs about their condition.
- Their understanding of treatment.
- How actively they wish to be involved in their care.
- The social pressures, such as work, that impact on treatment.
- Their desire to use self-care treatment regimes.
- Their cognitive ability and skills to manage the condition.
- The general patient and family attitude to treatment.
- Previous bad treatment experiences that are influencing their outlook on care and its effectiveness.
- The role of family and friends in care provision.
- Compounding social and psychological factors.

Research has shown that professionals fail to understand how different aspects of leg ulcer treatment affect the daily lives of patients. A number of issues are presented in Table 11.3 and discussed further.

Improving concordance through appropriate treatment

Improving concordance requires nurses to pay close attention to the factors above when deciding on treatment methods. This may require engaging the help of the family or significant others, and paying attention to practical problems such as immobility or isolation.

Control of symptoms such as pain and sleep disorder are essential factors in improving concordance and are discussed in Chapter 9. The impact of odour on the lives of patients is frequently underestimated by professionals, but is one of the most important issues for both the patient and their family and friends.

Problems with inappropriate bandage selection and poor application technique are the commonest reasons why patients with

Table 11.3 Factors influencing patient concordance with compression therapy.

Comprehensive assessment	
Goal:	
Seek to identify the real issues affecting adherence to compression	Identify the aetiology
	Identify the patient's attitude to their ulcer and compression therapy
	Identify the patient's previous experience with compression therapy
	Identify symptoms such as pain, sleep deficit, depression, anxiety and social isolation
	Identify concurrent illness, reduced mobility, inability to go to bed at night
	Assess the patient's knowledge and involvement in their own care
Relationships	
Goal:	
Establish a therapeutic relationship	Avoid judgemental attitudes and do not blame the patient
Treatment	
Goal:	
Apply an appropriate compression system according to the patient's needs	Ensure that skin care regimes and dressings are appropriately used to avoid irritation, odour, maceration, etc.; apply padding to protect the limb and absorb exudate
	Apply compression, taking account of the shape of the limb
	Continuously evaluate the compression and address the patient's issues
	Ensure all staff are skilled in the application of compression

venous ulceration cannot tolerate compression therapy (Moffatt, 2004b). Table 11.4 outlines how different compression regimes may be used for specific issues affecting concordance. (Chapter 14 examines compression therapy.) Other useful strategies include

Table 11.4 Choosing compression systems to enhance concordance.

Inelastic compression regimens	Particularly useful for patients who experience pain at rest or during the night due to the low resting pressure.
Cohesive inelastic compression systems	These greatly reduce slippage and are effective in immobile patients for whom elastic compression has previously been the first line of treatment.
Multi-layer elastic compression systems	May be of value to patients who experience pain. The padding and number of layers gives good protection and the application of layers can be built up gradually as the patient's tolerance increases.
Single-layer elastic bandages	These can apply very high levels of pressure that some patients with severe venous disease find reduce their symptoms. May also be associated with increased pain.
Compression hosiery	A number of two-layer systems with a washable under-sock and stocking are available. The incorporation of a zip in some products makes application and removal easier. Invaluable for those who wish to self-care.
Intermittent pneumatic compression	A useful system for patients with severe oedema or immobile patients who find elevation difficult. Can be combined with compression bandaging.

slowly introducing compression over a number of weeks until the patient can tolerate high compression (40 mmHg). It is important to remember that any level of compression is better than no compression (Cullum et al., 1999). Little research has been undertaken to evaluate factors that influence the experience of patients with compression. It is likely that psychological and social factors influence concordance with compression as well as the many complex clinical conditions affecting these patients.

Case study

Mrs X, a 67-year-old active lady who still worked as a dinner lady in the local primary school, presented to her nurse with a large leg ulcer on her right medial malleolus that she had been dressing herself for a number of weeks. Although it was clean and granulating, it was exuding copious amounts of clear serous fluid and not improving. On presentation, she had gross varicosities in her thigh and calf and a previous history of venous ulceration 5 years ago. She had no isch-aemic symptoms and her ABPI was 1.1. She admitted wearing support hosiery for some months after her initial ulcer, but had not worn any for the past few years. The ulcer was extremely painful and the sur-rounding area bright red and inflamed.

The nurse diagnosed the ulcer as being venous in origin, and applied full high compression (multi-layer elastic bandaging), and arranged for a course of antibiotics. By that evening Mrs X could no longer bear the pressure of the bandaging and was in agony with the pain. She removed the bandages and returned to the nurse a week later, refusing to have the leg bandaged again. After 2 weeks of anti-biotics and foam dressings there was no improvement, and the pain had become so bad that Mrs X was forced to take time off work. She was referred to a specialist – the referral read: 'Mrs X has an infected venous ulcer that is failing to heal as she is non-compliant with compression'.

The first time she saw the leg ulcer specialist she was in tears with the pain. A full assessment – including a comprehensive pain assess-ment – was completed. Mrs X described the pain as 'sharp and stab-bing, as if someone kept driving needles into my leg. Sometimes it's a bit easier, then suddenly – bam – the pain shoots up my leg. It's worse when I'm standing, but it can come on at any time.' This sug-gested a typical neuropathic pain, and what the nurse had diagnosed as local cellulitis was, in fact, acute painful lipodermatosclerosis and atrophie blanche. The wound was clean, and there was no malodour or clinical signs of infection. It was no surprise that Mrs X was unable to tolerate compression, and she should never have been labelled as non-compliant.

The specialist took time to explain to Mrs X that the pain was related to venous congestion, and that, although she needed compression to treat it, there was no point even beginning compression until the pain was controlled. Mrs X was very reluctant to take regular painkillers, although she had recently started taking ibuprofen, and found it gave her some relief. She agreed to take the maximum dose of ibuprofen

Continued

regularly for a period of 2 weeks, plus 10 mg of amitriptyline at night. The wound was dressed with a hydrogel sheet (designed to reduce pain), padding and a retention bandage.

Within just 2 weeks the pain had subsided so much that she was ready to start compression bandaging. An inelastic bandage was chosen because it gave a lower pressure at rest and would help her sleep better. She continued taking her analgesia for a further week as she got used to the compression, then slowly weaned herself off it. The ulcer healed within 2 months.

SUMMARY

- There are no common demographic or personality factors that define whether patients will 'comply' with treatment.
- Definitions of compliance have been replaced in recent years with terms such as 'concordance' that imply a more equal partnership between professional and patient.
- Research has identified characteristics that professionals use to judge whether patients are considered 'good', 'bad', 'difficult' or 'non-compliant'.
- Many factors within patients' social lives influence their ability to adhere to treatment regimes.
- Poor control of symptoms, such as pain, influence adherence to therapy.
- Many patients report difficulty managing compression therapy. A change in compression regime or the method of application can significantly improve concordance.
- The literature reports that a group of patients do not wish their leg ulcer to heal because they perceive some secondary gain from having the wound. This has been described as the 'social ulcer' and may relate to social isolation, loneliness and reliance on professionals to give support. Little research evidence exists to support this belief.
- Many problems with concordance can be solved by better communication and the avoidance of labelling patients.

CONCLUSION

While a robust research basis for improving concordance in leg ulceration is lacking, nevertheless there is much that a professional can do to help patients come to terms with their condition. It is essential that nurses develop skills in reflective professional practice, and consider how their attitudes and behaviour may be exacerbating the suffering of patients and contributing to poor concordance with therapy. It is also important to understand how poor relationships and negative attitudes to patients affect the emotional health of both the patient and professional (Ley, 1982). Patients need to have confidence that nurses are knowledgeable about their condition and will quickly identify those nurses who lack knowledge and skills.

For a small group of patients healing cannot be achieved, and in these cases the priorities of treatment may change. While it is acknowledged that a small proportion of patients interfere with their compression to prevent healing, the numbers are likely to be very small and indicate that wider issues such as loneliness may be behind this behaviour (Muir Gray, 1983). Table 11.5 provides

Table 11.5 Reflection on concordance.

Key questions

Do you believe you are at fault if a patient's leg ulcer does not heal?
- If you do, how does this make you feel?
- How does it affect your relationship with the patient?
- How does it influence the way in which you organise their care?

What should you do?
- Check your assessment – is the aetiology of the leg ulcer correct?
- Consider getting expert advice if you are unsure
- Select a treatment that the patient can manage to live with
- Make sure **all staff** employ the treatment correctly
- Control **all** symptoms
- Seek expert advice if you cannot control pain or other symptoms
- Be sensitive to the emotional impact of non-healing on the patient as well as yourself

What should you avoid doing?
- Blaming the patient for the situation – it is unlikely to be their fault
- Labelling the patient – this can lead to poor care – distancing, denial of symptoms, etc.
- Recognise that many factors influence healing
- Acknowledge that a small percentage of patients with leg ulcers do not heal but can live 'well' if their symptoms are controlled

Note: If you do not believe you are at fault in causing delayed wound healing, are you certain that you have addressed every issue, including control of the patient's symptoms?

---

questions that nurses should consider when facing concordance problems with any patient who has a leg ulcer. At the centre of the concordance debate is the ability to develop a therapeutic, non-judgemental relationship with patients struggling to live with leg ulceration.

REFERENCES

Becker, M.H. & Green, L.W. (1975) A family approach to compliance with medical treatment – a selective review of the literature. *International Journal of Health Education* **18**, 1–11.

Becker, M.H. & Maiman, L.A. (1975) Sociobehavioral determinants of compliance with health and medical care recommendations. *Medical Care* **XIII**(1): 10–24.

Blackwell, B. (1992) Compliance. *Psychotherapy Psychosomatics* **58**: 161–169.

Blackwell, B. & Gutmann, M. (1985) Compliance. In: *Handbook of Hypertension*, Vol. 6 (C.J. Bulpitt, ed.). New York, Elsevier.

Brooks, J., Ersser, S.J., Lloydd, A. & Ryan, T.J. (2004) Nurse led education set out to improve patient concordance and prevent recurrence of leg ulcers. *Journal of Wound Care* **13**(3): 111–116.

Charles, H. (1995) The impact of leg ulcers on patients' quality of life. *Professional Nurse* **10**(9): 571–573.

Conrad, P. (1987) The noncompliant patient in search of autonomy. *Hastings Center Report* **17**: 15–17.

Cullum, N.A. & Last, S. (1991) The prevalence, characteristics and management of leg ulcers in Wirral Health Authority. (Unpublished report.)

Cullum, N., Nelson, E.A., Fletcher, A.W. & Sheldon, T.A. (1999) *Compression Bandages and Stockings for Leg Ulcers. Systematic Review.* Cochrane Wounds Group. Cochrane database of Systematic Reviews, Issue 4. http://www.cochrane.org (General address: http://www.cochrane.org)

Editorial (1982) Diagnosis and treatment of venous ulceration. *Lancet* **2**(8292): 247–248.

Edwards, L., Moffatt, C.J. & Franks, P.J. (2002) An exploration of patient understanding of leg ulceration. *Journal of Wound Care* **11**: 33–39.

English, J. & Morse, J.M. (1988) The 'difficult' elderly patient: adjustment or maladjustment? *Journal of Nursing Studies* **25**(1): 23–29.

Epstein, L.H. & Maseck, B.J. (1978) Behavioural control of medical compliance. *Journal of Applied Behaviour Analysis* **11**: 1–9.

Farberow, N.L. & Hehemkis, A.M. (1979) Indirect self-destructive behaviour in patients with Beurger's disease. *Journal of Personality Assessment* **43**: 86–96.

Fineman, N. (1991) The social construction of noncompliance: a study of health care and social service providers in everyday practice. *Sociology of Health and Illness* **13**(3): 14–27.

Franks, P.J. & Moffatt, C.J. (1998) Who suffers most from leg ulceration? *Journal of Wound Care* **7**(8): 383–385.

Franks, P.J., Bosanquet, N., Connolly, M., Oldroyd, M., Moffatt, C.J., Greenhalgh, R.M. & McCollum, C.N. (1995a) Venous ulcer healing: effect of socio-economic factors in London. *Journal of Epidemiology and Community Health* **49**: 385–388.

Franks, P.J., Oldroyd, M.I., Dickson, D., Sharp, E.J. & Moffatt, C.J. (1995b) Risk factors for leg ulcer recurrence: a randomized trial for two types of compression stocking. *Age and Ageing* **24**: 490–494.

Gillmore, M.R. & Hill, C.T. (1981) Reactions to patients who complain of pain: Effects of ambiguous diagnosis. *Journal of Applied Social Psychology* **11**: 14–22.

Haynes, R.B. (1979) Introduction. In: *Compliance in Health Care* (R.B. Haynes, D.W. Taylor & D.L. Sackett, eds). Baltimore, John Hopkins University Press.

Jull, A.B., Mitchell, N., Arroll, J., Jones, M., Waters, J., Latta, A., Walker, N. & Arroll, B. (2004) Factors influencing concordance with compression stockings after venous leg ulcer healing. *Journal of Wound Care* **13**(3): 90–92.

Koltun, A. & Stone, G. (1986) Past and current trends in patient noncompliance: focus on diseases, regimens–programs, and provider disciplines. *Journal of Compliance in Health Care* **1**(1): 21–32.

Krasner, D. (1998) Painful venous ulcers: themes and stories about their impact on quality of life. *Ostomy and Wound Management* **44**(9): 38–49.

Lazarus, R.S. (1985) Coping theory and research: past, present and future. *Psychosomatic Medicine* **55**: 237–247.

Ley, P. (1982) Satisfaction, compliance and communication. *British Journal of Clinical Psychology* **21**: 241–254.

Lorber, J. (1975) Good patients and problem patients. Conformity and deviance in a general hospital. *Journal of Health and Social Behaviour* **16**: 213–225.

Menzies, I.E.P. (1959) The functioning of social systems as a defence against anxiety. *Human Relations* **13**: 95–121.

Moffatt, C.J. (2001) Patient and professional dilemmas in non healing. Abstract presented at the *Symposium on Advances in Wound Care and Medical Research Forum on Wound Repair*. Las Vegas.

Moffatt, C.J. (2004a) Factors that affect concordance with compression therapy. *Journal of Wound Care* **13**(7): 291–294.

Moffatt, C.J. (2004b) Perspectives on concordance in leg ulcer management. *Journal of Wound Care* **13**(6): 243–248.

Moffatt, C.J. & Harper, P. (1997) *Leg Ulcers*. Singapore, Churchill Livingstone.

Muir Gray, J.A. (1983) Social aspects of peripheral vascular disease in the elderly. In: *Peripheral Vascular Disease in the Elderly* (S. McCarthy, ed.). London, Churchill Livingstone, pp. 191–199.

Nelson, F.L. & Farberow, N.L. (1980) Indirect self-destructive behaviour in the elderly nursing home patient. *Journal of Gerontology* **35**(6): 949–957.

Roberson, M.H.B. (1992) The meaning of compliance: patient perspectives. *Qualitative Health Research* **2**(1): 7–26.

Roe, B., Cullum, N. & Hamer, C. (1995) Patients' perspectives on chronic leg ulceration. In: *Leg Ulcers: Nursing Management* (N.A. Cullum & B. Roe, eds). Harrow, Scutari Press, pp. 125–134.

Roter, D.L., Hall, J.A., Merisca, R., et al. (1998) Effectiveness of interventions to improve patient compliance: a meta-analysis. *Medical Care* **36**(8): 1138–1161.

Salaman, R.A., Salaman, J., Baragwanath, P. & Harding, K. (1995) Patient factors in the poor outcome of venous ulceration. Presented at the *5th European Conference on Advances in Wound Management*, Harrogate. London, Macmillan, pp. 79–80.

Sherbourne, C.D., Hays, R.D., Ordway, L., DiMatteo, M.R. & Kravitz, R.L. (1992) Antecedents of adherence to medical recommendations: results from the Medical Outcomes Study. *Journal of Behavioural Medicine* **15**(5): 447–468.

Soloff, P.H. (1980) Effects of denial on mood, compliance, and quality of functioning after cardiovascular rehabilitation. *General Hospital Psychiatry* **2**: 134–140.

Steptoe, A. & O'Sullivan, J. (1986) Monitoring and blunting coping styles in women prior to surgery. *British Journal of Clinical Psychology* **25**: 143–144.

Stimson, G. (1974) Obeying doctor's orders: a view from the other side. *Social Science and Medicine* **8**: 97–101.

Zola, I.K. (1981) Structural constraints in the doctor patient relationship: The case of non compliance. In: *The Relevance of Social Science for Medicine* (L. Eisenberg & A. Kleinman, eds). Boston, D. Reidel, pp. 241–252.

Part IV
Clinical Management

Part IV of this book relates to phase 2 of the leg ulcer care pathway – planning and implementing care. The critical elements of successfully treating a patient with a leg ulcer (after a thorough assessment and management of the psychosocial factors) are to manage the underlying disease/s causing the ulcer, addressing the wider factors that can delay wound healing and managing the condition of the wound bed.

It is anticipated that practitioners will be dealing with patients who have numerous health related problems that require more consideration than just choosing the correct dressing and bandaging. Due to the complex nature of leg ulcer management, a number of different health professionals will probably need to be involved in order to ensure that a holistic approach is taken.

All practitioners must recognise and acknowledge both their skills and their limitations. It would be wise to ask yourself: 'Is there anyone else I should be involving in the management of this patient?'. Chapter 12 considers the potential members of the multi-disciplinary team, taking into account that the requirements of each patient will vary according to the problems associated with their ulcer. It is a misconception to think that just because leg ulcer patients tend to receive the bulk of their care in the community setting that only primary care nurses can provide it. Referring a patient on for further specialist assessment or specific medical or surgical management is not a sign of inadequacy, though this attitude is not uncommon. The real problems tend to arise more so when patients are not referred on, with practitioners blindly carrying on providing treatment that is just not appropriate – alarmingly, this can go on for months and years.

Dressings and wound treatment choices have exploded since the 1980s and 1990s. Nowadays the challenge more often than not becomes 'which one to choose?' Customarily, this quest for the perfect dressing becomes the obsession when, in the majority of cases, it is not the most crucial element of treatment. An extensive number of features are expected of the ideal dressing, but, in regards to individual requirements, this will always vary from patient to patient. The TIME framework helps to make the dressing decision-making process a little easier and is utilised for this purpose in Chapter 13. A few key features need to be considered, namely the condition of the wound bed, the levels of bacteria present – including how vulnerable the patient is to infection – the amount of exudate produced, the condition of the wound edges and if healing is being observed. Of course, there are some other very important considerations to take into account relating to patient comfort, the research or development behind a product and its cost-effectiveness.

Compression therapy remains the cornerstone of venous ulcer management. It is a treatment that has notable effects on the haemodynamics of the body and is capable of healing venous ulcers. Nevertheless, its mechanisms remain somewhat of a mystery and when applied to the wrong person the consequences can be disastrous. The one thing compression definitely is not is just a bandage to hold a dressing in place. Knowing how to apply compression is not just about knowing how to complete a task, it is about understanding what is trying to be achieved, the effect of the treatment and how to troubleshoot problems. Both a theoretical understanding and practical skills are vital to the art of being capable of applying therapeutic compression. The theory underlying the application of compression is covered in considerable depth in Chapter 14, with the addition of some practical tips to aid the practitioner in really being able to apply theory in day-to-day practice. Nevertheless, inexperienced practitioners should seek further guidance and identify opportunities to practise their skills under the supervision of an experienced and trained colleague.

Involving the Multi-disciplinary Team

12

LEARNING OBJECTIVES

Nurses involved in leg ulcer management should be able to demonstrate:

❏ A recognition of the importance of involving the multi-disciplinary team in the management of patients with leg ulceration.
❏ A consideration of the various appropriate members of the multi-disciplinary team in regards to individual patient needs.
❏ An appreciation of the benefits and complexities of multi-disciplinary teamwork.
❏ A familiarisation of the possible options available for patients in relation to specific ulcer types (venous/arterial/and multifactorial)

INTRODUCTION

It is true that with the accessibility of national and international guidelines for best practice together with effective compression therapy and nursing education programmes, the standards of care for leg ulcer patients should improve and prevalence levels reduce, as demonstrated by Moffatt et al. (2004). The complex nature of leg ulceration can never be underestimated and, despite the above-mentioned improvements to practice, some ulcers will prove to be intractable and additional measures will need to be taken to enable healing, or even to stabilise a patient's condition.

In reality, there are few clinical situations in relation to leg ulceration that cannot be regarded as being complex – be it in regards to the diagnosis, treatment or prevention of recurrence – and thus patients often require referral to other health professionals, aside from GPs and district or practice nurses. Yet this approach to multi-disciplinary management can be quite variable in practice. There are many possible explanations for this:

- The leg ulcer is perceived as just a wound that can be managed with dressings.
- A lack of understanding as to the additional possibilities for treatment, or just not knowing who to refer on to.
- Restrictions on general nurses of being unable to make direct referrals to hospital services.
- Limited availability of certain services or procedures.
- Patient choice (though this may come back to the patient being poorly informed).
- Pride – practitioners not wanting to appear as though they cannot manage on their own.

Frequently, referrals to other services or health professionals are seen as an afterthought, only actioned when problems arise. It is because of this issue that referral comes before treatment in the Wandsworth tPCT leg ulcer pathway (see Fig. 2.2a in Chapter 2). The referral pathways are there to trigger a reminder, most often to the nurse managing the patient, that it is right to consider involving other practitioners – ultimately, because certain tests and procedures just cannot be done or met by one person or one specialty.

Best practice

- Patients with complex/chronic wounds should undergo comprehensive holistic assessment.
- The assessment process and management options may involve more than one healthcare professional or discipline. Ideally, this would take place in one location to ensure a holistic approach; however, the most crucial element is effective communication between all practitioners involved – not forgetting the patient.
- Regardless of where patients receive their care, the service provided should be seamless and standardised.

NURSE-LED WOUND MANAGEMENT

Wound care has customarily been considered a nursing task. More recently, however, this area of nursing has developed into a significant role, with nurses leading the way in making decisions, prescribing treatments and monitoring outcomes. General medical practitioners often recognise their nursing colleagues' expertise in this field; though whether this is recognition of a lack of sufficient involvement to develop the necessary expertise or just a general lack of interest is possibly quite variable. With advances in medical technology and treatments the human lifespan has significantly increased, but along with an increasing lifespan the burden of chronic disease has also increased. Chronic wounds are frequently associated with chronic diseases, such as diabetes mellitus and rheumatoid arthritis, though the wounds can themselves become the dominating problem. As a result, wound management has developed into a separate discipline frequently led by a nurse in a specialist role (Baxter, 2002). This is certainly one of the key features of the Wandsworth tPCT model and has demonstrated good outcomes for patients (Moffatt et al., 2004).

When it comes to the management of complex chronic wounds nurses, however, cannot and should not be the only participants in a patient's care. One of the key nursing responsibilities is to know whom to refer on to and when. This is especially the case in regards to leg ulceration, where a more complex process of assessment is involved than just finding the right dressing. In these situations, the multi-disciplinary team (MDT) is essential in correctly identifying and managing the underlying condition (Moore & Cowman, 2005). The specialist nurse can often take a lead role as a part of the MDT, acting as the link between acute and primary care and between the different disciplines involved, so ensuring open lines of communication are maintained.

THE MULTI-DISCIPLINARY TEAM

A team approach can help to ensure that any assessment covers the full spectrum of a holistic assessment, taking into account the physical, mental and social factors potentially contributing to the ulcer. The results of such an assessment then allow for the appropriate treatments and interventions to make healing possible.

One only has to reflect on the level of care many patients received prior to the introduction of specialist leg ulcer clinics or wound healing centres (Franks & Gottrup, 2004) to see the problems associated with allowing practitioners who have inadequate knowledge of chronic wound management to continue to work autonomously. Even after such centres have been established there is room for improvement, and a realisation that specialist practitioners, diagnostic tests and surgery are perhaps still not used to their full potential (Kjaer et al., 2005).

Along with their wound, a patient may also be dealing with numerous potential problems or issues. These other factors may contribute to the cause or may be a result of the wound; nevertheless, they need to be addressed and, if possible, resolved (Baxter, 2002). For this reason no single health professional has all the necessary skills to help manage a patient with a complex chronic wound (Franks, 1999). Table 12.1 lists the potential problems and who might need to be involved, but it is by no means exhaustive and many other health professionals may also be involved.

It is also worth acknowledging the role of researchers and industry in the wider context of the MDT. Both contribute to the care

Table 12.1 Involvement of the multi-disciplinary team (MDT).

Requirement for MDT involvement	MDT members
Mobility issues	Physiotherapists, podiatrists, specialist footwear departments
Nutritional status	Dieticians, psychologists, exercise co-ordinators/facilitators
Equipment provision	Occupational therapists (OTs), physiotherapists, community nurses
Pain control	Chronic pain teams, hospice care
Diabetic management	GP, specialist nurse, diabetologist, podiatrist
Skin problems	Dermatologist
Vascular insufficiency	Vascular surgeon, vascular technician, specialist nurse
Home environment issues	OTs, social services
Social problems	Social worker, other independent agencies
Psychological issues	Psychologist, counsellors, expert patient programmes
Medical problems	Geriatricians, haematologist, infectious disease teams, rheumatologists, microbiologist, GP

of patients by publishing, presenting and disseminating findings to guide best practice, and by developing products that reflect the needs of patients (Baxter, 2002).

WOUND HEALING CENTRES
Specialised wound centres or teams are gradually being formed in various settings around the world (Granick & Ladin, 1998; Ghauri et al., 2000; Gottrup et al., 2001; Collier & Radley, 2005). Some centres focus on specific wound types, i.e. leg ulcers, diabetic foot wounds or pressure sores, others offer a service to anyone with a chronic or complex wound. Some are purely nurse-led but with relatively easy access to other health professionals, while others comprise large teams of various specialised practitioners with access to both inpatient and outpatient facilities.

Benefits
Operating specialised wound care centres offers numerous benefits, including (Franks & Gottrup, 2004):

- Greater availability of diagnostic tools.
- Accurate diagnosis.
- Highly skilled specialised practitioners to guide and standardise practice.
- Equality in the provision of innovative treatments.
- Opportunities for education and research.
- Improved patient outcomes in terms of ongoing care, healing and prevention of recurrence.

Drawbacks
The problems related to multi-disciplinary working and wound care tend to revolve around legitimising the need for the service, cost issues and team dynamics.

Chronic wound care has never been high on any political agenda: it does not feature frequently in the media, tugging at our heartstrings. Although it is not recognised as a major cause of mortality, this is incorrect as many patients die as a consequence of the complications of their condition, such as septicaemia. The experience for those people and their loved ones who live with a chronic wound and its effects can be devastating. It is now well documented that chronic wounds have a significant impact on quality of life (Lindholm et al., 1993; Charles, 1995; Franks & Moffatt, 1998), and it is time that this problem was suitably acknowledged by commissioners of services.

Chronic wound management is costly in both human and financial terms. In 2004 the cost of dressings alone was around £229.2millon (NHS Purchasing and Supply Agency, 2004), but this does not account for a whole raft of other related costs such as nursing or medical time, antibiotic therapy, hospital admission, etc. The reality of finite resources of course means that every effort should be made to find the most cost-effective means of providing the level of care any patient would expect to receive in the twenty-first century. The implementation of standardised, evidence-based care in specialised leg ulcer clinics has consistently demonstrated that cost reductions and improved outcomes for patients are achievable (Franks & Gottrup, 2004).

Team dynamics can be tricky when professional egos or misunderstandings about other health professionals' roles get in the way of the overall aims of such a venture. Providing those involved do have a clear role to play and the opportunity to be involved, the potential for a successful and rewarding collaboration is achievable.

The key elements of an effective MDT are (Moore & Cowman, 2005):

- Good teamwork
- Standardised care
- Strategic approach
- Should cross the boundaries of primary and secondary care

The remainder of this chapter will look more specifically at the role of particular teams in relation to ulcer aetiology and additional adjuvant therapies or treatments that may be considered by the MDT.

VENOUS ULCERATION

Essentially, the most important element of healing a venous leg ulcer is to improve the venous return and overcome the effects of chronic venous hypertension. At present, the primary means of achieving this is with compression therapy, and this is covered in considerable depth in Chapter 14. There are, however, some additional measures that can be considered; some of which are quite general and appropriate for most ulcer types, while others are of particular benefit to patients with venous leg ulcers. When deciding upon the best management approach to take, always take into account a patient's overall medical condition and any other underlying disorders that may complicate treatment options – and seek further advice if you are unsure.

Some additional things patients with uncomplicated venous leg ulcers should be advised and encouraged to do include:

- Walking
- When not walking or when unable to walk, rest with their legs above heart level.
- Avoid standing or sitting with their legs dependent for any significant length of time.
- Perform ankle exercises (Figs 12.1a, b and 12.2).
- Maintain a normal weight (by having a balanced diet and taking regular physical activity).
- Consider elevating the foot of the bed (assuming they are sleeping in their bed, which if not is a priority to address).

While compression therapy remains the cornerstone of managing patients with uncomplicated venous ulceration, the vascular surgeon also has a role to play. Recent studies suggest that while surgery may not have a significant impact on venous ulcer healing, it is beneficial in regards to the prevention of ulcer recurrence. Both Ghauri et al. (1998a) and Barwell et al. (2004) demonstrate improved reduction in ulcer recurrence (up to a 12-month follow-up) following surgery where only superficial venous disease or superficial and deep venous disease is detected, compared to compression therapy alone. As yet, deep venous corrective surgery is not routinely performed. There does seem to be some potential for deep venous surgery for patients with mild to moderate deep venous incompetence due to primary valvular failure. However, the indications for its application to patients with more severe disease or venous disease resulting from an obstruction, such as DVT, are less clear (Hardy et al., 2004). Prosthetic valve replacement has been experimented with, though due to the associated

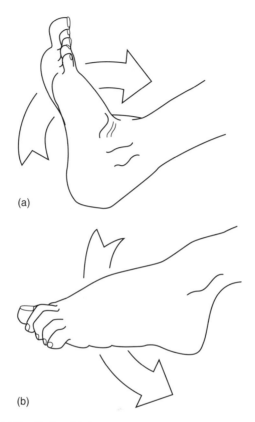

Fig. 12.1 (a) Dorsiflexion, (b) plantar flexion.

post-operative high mortality rates this intervention is likely to be some way off in the future.

As a part of managing the patient with venous ulceration and, in particular, those patients who have no known history of DVT, there should be some discussion between nurse and patient revolving around the consideration of the prospect of more detailed venous assessment with a view to corrective surgery. While referral to a vascular team is recommended on the pathway in the case of

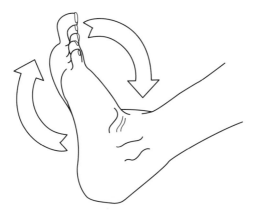

Fig. 12.2 Ankle rotation.

uncomplicated venous ulceration, this is a less urgent situation in comparison to an arterial problem. Surgery is not routinely performed while there is an open wound, so patients do not need to feel pressured when thinking about the possibility of undergoing such intervention. The patient should be reminded that the first step will be more 'non-invasive' assessment, following which, options can then be discussed with the vascular surgeon.

Drug therapies such as pentoxifylline have been identified as having potential benefits in improving the effects of chronic venous hypertension. Following a Cochrane review (Jull et al., 2004), pentoxifylline (400 mg tds) appears to offer benefits as an adjuvant treatment to compression therapy. The authors of the review highlight that because no work has been done on the cost-effectiveness of this treatment, its use in mainstream practice may therefore not be supported by healthcare commissioners. Hence, its use may be limited to those patients with severe venous disease and venous ulcers that prove difficult to heal with the recommended high levels of compression. Clinical impression suggests that it may also be useful in patients with severe pain from atrophie blanche.

For numerous reasons a certain percentage of venous ulcers will fail to respond to high compression therapy and optimal wound bed management. Providing other rarer aetiologies have been ruled out, a plastic surgeon may be able to help resolve these situations. A combination of shave therapy, a process of effectively slicing off the upper layers of the wound bed including some of the surrounding sclerosed tissues, followed by skin grafting essentially returns these chronic recalcitrant ulcers back to an acute wound state.

This procedure is also indicated for other ulcer types; however, the important point to remember is that this procedure has no effect on the underlying problem causing the ulcer. This means that, in the case of venous ulceration, compression therapy must be recommended following surgery (before the patient begins mobilising). The success of the skin graft will very much depend upon the ability to resolve or at least manage the underlying disease/s, in addition to the other factors that lead to the ulcer not healing in the first instance. The preparation work leading up to the graft taking place is very important – ensuring there is a good arterial blood supply, that bacterial levels are under control and the wound bed is in the best possible state (free from devitalised tissue) – in order to maximise successful skin graft take.

Skin grafting can be carried out alone; however, the wound bed is unlikely to be healthy after months or years of ulceration. The combination of shave therapy and skin grafting has been shown to be a more effective therapy than skin grafting alone (Bechara et al., 2006).

Follow-up care for a skin graft should include:

- Prevention of wound infection. Pseudomonas and haemolytic streptococcal infections are both associated with early- and late-onset graft rejection. Prophylactic antibiotics may be required for those at risk for a prolonged period. Antimicrobials may also be used if early signs of infection and graft rejection are seen.
- Compression remains the most important element. This should be applied immediately the patient gets out of bed to prevent movement of the graft and haematoma development.

New developments that involve tissue expansion include keratinocyte grafts, allografts and cultured human epidermis. Further research is required to assess their effectiveness in the treatment of venous leg ulcers. Allografts have been shown to stimulate wound healing, although the grafts themselves are eventually rejected. There is limited evidence that artificial skin used in conjunction with compression bandaging increases the chances of healing compared to compression therapy alone (Jones & Nelson, 2000). Essentially, further research is required into this area and hence the availability of these products is extremely limited.

Alternative adjuvant therapies

There are numerous innovative treatments proposing improvements to venous leg ulceration and other chronic wounds, including: hyperbaric oxygen, ultrasound, laser and electromagnetic therapy. Each work in slightly differing ways to improve the condition of the local wound bed and influence the wound healing process.

Based on the premise that the common factor shared by most chronic wounds is the problem of tissue hypoxia, hyperbaric oxygen therapy (HBOT) aims to improve healing by intermittently increasing the oxygen level within haemoglobin, hence elevating oxygen tissue tension at the wound site. The administration of HBOT promotes fibroblast replication, reduction of inflammatory cytokines, enhanced collagen formation, increased presence of growth factors and improved leucocyte function enabling an antibacterial effect (Kranke et al., 2004).

Ultrasound has been used regularly by physiotherapists for the past 50 years to treat soft tissue injuries, and more recently it has been used in specialist centres for the management of chronic wounds. The cellular effects of ultrasound can be divided into thermal and non-thermal. As low intensities are used the beneficial effects are likely to be due to non-thermal mechanisms (Dyson, 1987). These effects include modification of the permeability of certain cells, acceleration of the inflammatory phase, increasing fibroblast motility, faster rate of angiogenesis, increased collagen secretion and wound contraction.

All these treatments have been subject to systematic reviews. HBOT (Kranke et al., 2004) does seem to offer some benefits in preventing amputation in patients with diabetic foot ulceration. However, the benefits for leg ulcers as a result of PAOD are less obvious: most likely due to the fact that the blood supply to the wound bed is already restricted by an occlusion and increased levels of oxygen in the blood do not compensate for this. In practice, HBOT is rarely recommended for treating venous disease, except when there is real tissue anoxia or a limb is threatened, such as in cases of gas gangrene. Aside from the evidence to recommend the use of HBOT and cost considerations, one of the biggest issues in utilising HBOT is the availability of this service.

The evidence around the use of ultrasound therapy does suggest a benefit in the healing of venous leg ulcers. Though due to the poor quality of the studies reviewed, the results need to be interpreted with caution, and there is insufficient evidence to give clear direction for practice (Flemming & Cullum, 2000). There is insufficient data to recommend the use of laser (Flemming & Cullum, 1999) and electromagnetic therapies (Ravaghi et al., 2006) at this time.

ARTERIAL ULCERATION

If peripheral arterial occlusive disease (PAOD) is recognised or suspected as being a contributing cause then the patient should be referred to a vascular surgeon for further assessment. Possible options for treatment to be considered include drug treatments to promote arterial perfusion (e.g. clopidogrel, cilostazol and prostanoids), angioplasty or reconstructive surgery. The urgency of this referral will depend upon the severity of the disease, which will be guided by ABPI readings (see Chapter 5), and the symptoms experienced by the patient.

Risk factor management will also play an important part in overall patient management. For those patients presenting with PAOD, certain reversible risk factors will most likely have been identified during the initial assessment. These may include obesity, hypertension, hyperglycaemia, hypercholesterolaemia, smoking and a lack of exercise. Not only are these factors detrimental to good arterial health but most will also have a negative impact on wound healing. Most of these factors are interlinked, and improvements in some areas will lead to improvement in others and can ultimately effect the progression of PAOD (Aronow, 2005). Patients may require further input or support from the wider MDT, such as dieticians, physiotherapists, specialist clinics for diabetes, hypertension, vascular rehabilitation and smoking cessation, in order to help manage these problems. In some instances and with further information, advice and support, patients can start to make some changes to their lifestyle themselves; though the success of this will largely depend upon the patient's understanding of the problem, the changes that need to be made and how willing the patient is to make those changes.

Information regarding smoking cessation, healthy eating and active lifestyle programmes are now readily available from many different sources, including the internet, health centres and surgeries, pharmacies, libraries and even in supermarkets. Some patients may just require pointing in the right direction, but in reality most people (health professionals included) have probably already struggled to make a change with one of these three factors at some stage in their life. Ultimately, awareness is important: even if patients are only able to make some small change, it may encourage them to attempt bigger changes in the future.

It is sometimes helpful to think of Prochaska and DiClemente's (1983) model of change when trying to help patients make health-related changes such as quitting smoking, getting active and losing weight. In order to offer the most suitable advice it is important to assess where the patient is in relation to their physical and psychological readiness in making a commitment to the necessary lifestyle changes (Fig. 12.3). Patients with severe or unstable medical conditions should be assessed by their GP before making any significant changes to their diet or activity pattern.

Surgical and interventional radiological treatment

Surgical intervention is usually reserved for critical ischaemia situations (i.e. acute episodes) that threaten a limb. This may occur in conjunction with chronic ischaemic disease (i.e. an acute or chronic situation), or when the severity of ischaemic pain becomes intolerable (Murray, 2001).

Percutaneous transluminal angioplasty (PTA) is the more commonly performed procedure for patients presenting with claudication (which is not improving on an exercise programme) or rest pain, ulceration and where a stenosis (blockage) is threatening a bypass graft. Angioplasty involves the insertion of a balloon catheter passed over a guide wire (under X-ray control) to the point where the balloon sits within the stenosis. The balloon is then

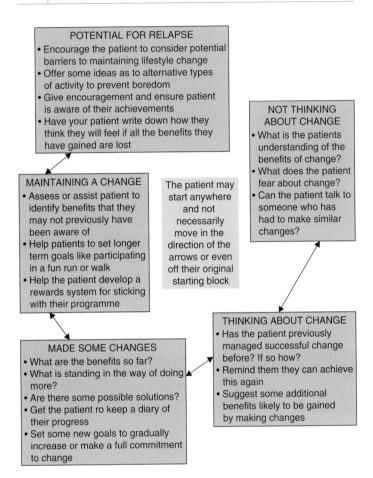

Fig. 12.3 Using Prochaska and DiClemente's model of change as a guide to advising patients to make health-related changes, for example increasing exercise (adapted from Marcus & Forsyth (2003)).

inflated for varying lengths of time and pressures according to the size and site of the stenosis, thereby compressing the atheromatous plaque within the vessel (Fig. 12.4). Hence the lumen of the vessel becomes patent again. This procedure is performed under a local

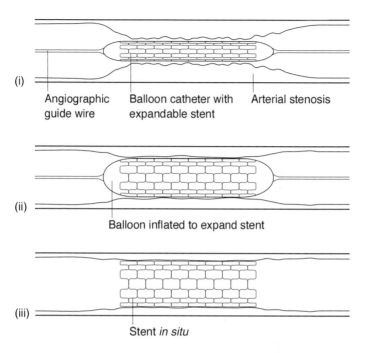

(i)

Angiographic   Balloon catheter with   Arterial stenosis
guide wire   expandable stent

(ii)

Balloon inflated to expand stent

(iii)

Stent *in situ*

Fig. 12.4 Angioplasty and placement of mesh stent.

anaesthetic and can actually be performed at the same time as a diagnostic arteriogram, providing there is a skilled radiologist to hand. Following angioplasty, intraluminal stents (these are made from a fine metal mesh) can, in some instances, be inserted into the lumen at the site of the stenosis to help improve the long-term patency of the vessel (Murray, 2001).

Where PTA is not a suitable option for a patient (for example, if there are very large or numerous occlusions, where there is severe rest pain, ulceration or gangrene and when the risks associated with performing surgery outweigh the risks associated with preserving life and limb and no surgery), reconstructive bypass surgery may be necessary. This essentially means grafting a new vessel to the artery above and below the occlusion allowing blood to effectively bypass the blockage. A number of surgical techniques can be used to revascularise different parts of the leg, e.g. aortobifemoral graft, femoral–popliteal bypass (Fig. 12.5). The type of operation obviously varies according to the site of the obstructed vessel. Revascularisation can be performed using either autologous vessels (a vein harvested from the patient and then stripped of its valves) or an artificial prosthesis. Choice will largely depend upon the size of the vessel needing to be bypassed and the availability of a suitable vein (Murray, 2001).

Surgery may improve the arterial blood supply and so promote ulcer healing, but there are no controlled studies to underpin the strategy.

It is worth bearing in mind that post-operative lower limb oedema is a potential problem. This may be due to a number of reasons, be it an inflammatory-related oedema due to the surgery, reperfusion oedema due to the sudden rise in hydrostatic pressure

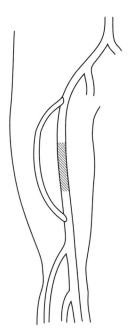

Fig. 12.5 Femoral–popliteal bypass.

following the opening of the artery (Herbert, 1997), or a venous-related oedema if a vein has been harvested for use as a graft. Management with supportive or reduced levels of compression bandaging will depend upon the success and site of the surgery. If such bandaging is not safe to apply then more conservative means of treatment, such as gentle exercise and leg elevation, may be the only option.

MIXED VENOUS AND ARTERIAL ULCERATION

The combination of venous and arterial disease is not uncommon, and frequently in various epidemiology studies (Scriven et al., 1997; Ghauri et al., 1998b; Moffatt et al., 2004) around 15% of ulcers are identified as having this clinical picture. In light of the ageing population and the link between increasing age and peripheral arterial occlusive disease, this occurrence is only likely to increase. Vowden and Vowden (2001) suggest that, for the majority of cases, it is perhaps wrong to refer to these ulcers as 'mixed'. They say the ulcer is not so much a result of dual aetiology, but rather that the ulcer is most likely due to venous disease that is then complicated by progressive arterial insufficiency.

Managing patients with a combination of both arterial and venous disease can be very challenging. Ultimately, it revolves around optimising both conditions without compromising one or the other. In its simplest form, management will primarily involve surgically correcting the underlying arterial problem and then addressing the venous element with compression therapy. Unfortunately, in reality things are rarely this straightforward. Some patients may be suitable for surgery, but there may be concerns about the use of compression and its potential to compromise a graft/bypass thereafter. In addition, some individuals will be inoperable (either due to the site/extent of the occlusion or to other health problems, therefore increasing the risks of a general anaesthetic) and more conservative measures may be the only option. Patient choice is also likely to have a significant effect on the approach taken.

The options discussed in the specific venous and arterial sections in this chapter are also obviously relevant, though the options need more careful weighing up in regards to the benefits for both the venous and arterial components.

Case study

Albert, a 77-year-old gentleman, lives alone; he has never married. He has been attending the leg ulcer clinic for treatment reviews on a 2- to 3-monthly basis for the past 18 months because of his slow-healing, bilateral venous leg ulcers. His community nurse team attends to him twice a week for his regular treatment. Albert has superficial venous disease affecting both legs, plus a history of DVT affecting his left leg following a left knee replacement 10 years ago. His general mobility is somewhat restricted, in that he has to use a walking frame to walk about indoors and his ankle mobility is limited. He is over-weight and spends much of his day seated in his chair with his legs dependent. His ulcers were initially quite large, but had been showing signs of healing and reducing in size.

On his most recent visit he reported that he had been experiencing more pain from the left leg ('the leg aches constantly') and had been unable to have his usual multi-layer elastic compression bandaging, only just tolerating padding and a crepe bandage. The ulcer was getting larger.

His ABPI was rechecked and there had been a significant drop in the left leg reading, from 0.86 just 2 months ago to 0.69 at this time. The right leg reading was virtually unchanged at 0.91. Albert was then seen by the vascular team who arranged for him to have an angiogram. The angiogram showed an occlusion in the popliteal artery and, as a result, Albert underwent bypass surgery.

The surgery has been successful at improving the arterial perfusion; his ABPI is now 0.84, but the vascular team have advised against high levels of compression due to the site of the arterial graft. Reduced levels of compression bandaging are recommenced using elastic bandages, while ensuring the limb is well padded and protected from the potential for excessive levels of compression just below the knee.

The importance of leg elevation is much more critical now for Albert. After much discussion with his community nurses, some additional measures are taken to ensure he is able to elevate his legs more – his television is moved into his bedroom so he can lie on the bed instead of sitting in his chair, and he now receives meals on wheels so does not have to stand to prepare his dinner.

Albert is encouraged to do his ankle exercises while resting on the bed. In the meantime, his nurses are exploring the options of obtaining a flowtron machine to combine some intermittent compression therapy with his bandaging.

Exercise

Keeping mobile is important for everyone and national guidelines (Department of Health, 2000) recommend that we all should undertake at least 30 minutes of activity at least five times a week. Walking in particular has benefits for both the arterial and venous circulation. It promotes the formation of collateral vessels to improve arterial perfusion to the limb and it works the calf muscle pump so enhancing venous return.

Patients with symptomatic arterial disease (intermittent claudication) may benefit from a specific exercise rehabilitation programme. As most walking programmes encourage patients to walk until pain is experienced, many will need reassurance that exercise is unlikely to cause them any harm and that not exercising is likely to be far more detrimental to their health. A Cochrane review (Leng et al., 2000) exploring the benefits of walking to improve intermittent claudication, found that walking three times a week offered notable benefits in improving the distance that patients could walk before they experienced pain (maximal walking time) plus improved general walking ability. Studies have also been undertaken to explore the benefits of walking on calf muscle activity; Padberg et al. (2004) found that patients on a structured exercise programme aimed at strengthening the calf muscle pump could make notable improvements within a 6-month time frame. Although these findings do not indicate that healing times will be improved, in theory if the underlying condition (be it venous or arterial disease) can be made better then this should have a positive effect on healing.

AMPUTATION

With more advanced surgical techniques and improved prevention and management of infection, the incidence of amputation is decreasing. Nevertheless, it is a distressing, major life-changing surgical operation with the potential for unknown outcomes (in the event that phantom limb pain becomes a new problem for the patient). Patients undergoing amputation are prime examples of a situation where multi-disciplinary teamwork is vital to achieve the best outcomes. Community nurses can play a large role in ensuring patients are physically, emotionally and mentally prepared for their surgery.

To many patients and practitioners this may be seen as the worst possible outcome for the management of any type of leg ulcer. For some, however, it is the beginning of a new life free from pain, discomfort, bandaging, unpleasant odour and social isolation.

Peripheral vascular disease and diabetes are the main causes of amputations nowadays. The type or extent of the amputation will depend upon several factors, including the degree of arterial obstruction, the presence and site of any wounds, the presence of infection, the general condition of the surrounding skin and the possibility for mobilising and fitting of a prosthesis following surgery. Fig. 12.6 shows an amputation of the great toe and metatarsal (this procedure is referred to as a 'Ray amputation') following a failed femoral–popliteal bypass graft. It is a decision often made when no other options remain, and usually at a point where there are several factors contributing to a severely compromised limb, where pain is intolerable and infection is putting the patient's life at risk. Unfortunately, leaving this decision to the final stages often leaves patients and their families in a crisis situation trying to make informed decisions and prepare mentally and emotionally for such an operation. Ensuring patients have

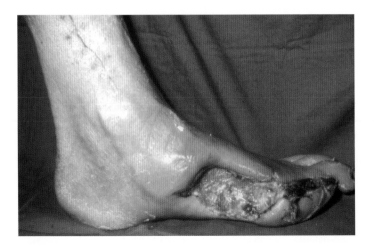

Fig. 12.6 Ray amputation after a failed femoral–popliteal bypass.

adequate pain relief prior to such an intervention is vital. Not only will this better enable them to prepare themselves psychologically for the surgery and the effect on their life, but there is evidence to suggest that successful pain management pre-surgery will help prevent problems post-surgery with phantom limb pain (Donohue & Sutton-Woods, 2001).

OTHER ULCER AETIOLOGIES AND MULTI-FACTORIAL ULCERATION

For the other rarer causes of ulceration (for example, inflammatory, haematological and infectious disorders), the fundamental elements of treatment and who should be involved in the management of these patients has been addressed in Chapters 6 and 7. There are, however, some basic principles that can be applied to this group of patients to enable healing; these relate to:

- Oedema management.
- Ensuring that any drug therapies prescribed are administered and monitored accordingly, with any problems reported to the prescriber.
- Maintaining some regular activity such as walking.
- Leg elevation when resting.
- Maintaining a normal weight and ensuring a balanced diet and adequate hydration.
- Further health promotion advice appropriate to the patient's condition, depending upon the underlying cause/s of the ulcer.

Oedema management

The first step in the management of oedema will be to understand its cause; if this is unknown then the patient will initially require further assessment by their GP. Referral may also be required to a vascular team, cardiac or general medical team for those more complex patients.

Depending upon the cause and the severity of the problem, oedema management may well be managed relatively simply with some form of support or compression bandaging; in some cases an even more conservative approach (i.e. leg elevation) may only be suitable. Some patients may require medication (e.g. diuretics) or a review and change in medication if peripheral oedema is a known side-effect (e.g. some calcium-channel blockers). Drug therapy is not indicated in cases of lymphoedema; instead a more conservative approach combining compression, exercise and manual lymphatic drainage is considered most appropriate (Jenns, 2000). For patients with severe lymphoedema, particularly where there is limb shape distortion or where the level of oedema extends to the genitalia or trunk, referral on to a specialist lymphoedema therapist for more intensive treatment is recommended (Doherty et al., 2006).

Nutrition

The importance of an adequate nutritional intake in the wound healing process and how practitioners can assess this has already been addressed in Chapter 3. A patient's nutritional state can have wide-reaching effects on their general state of health, specific disease management and overall wound healing potential.

The ideal solution would be that, with some simple advice, the majority of patients could boost their present dietary intake by making some small changes to their normal eating habits. In effect, those all-important macronutrients (protein, carbohydrates and fat) and micronutrients (vitamins and minerals) vital to successful wound healing are readily available from a normal varied diet (Trodorvic, 2002; Williams, 2002): though it is acknowledged that many potential barriers can stand in the way of achieving this.

Where these barriers prove difficult to address, or for patients with numerous medical problems and very large, heavily exuding wounds, further specialist nutritional assessment and management may be required from a dietician. Other people who may be involved in an indirect manner include carers: helping with tasks such as shopping and preparing food could effectively improve a patient's nutritional state.

CONCLUSION

When managing patients with leg ulcers, practitioners need to always remember that the wound is in essence a symptom of an underlying disorder and therefore managing the underlying condition is vitally important. While the nurse will play a major role in the assessment and management of these patients, the decisions about care and further specialist assessment should not lie with one individual but within the remit of the MDT. The Wandsworth tPCT leg ulcer pathway (see Fig. 2.2) gives basic guidance and recommendations regarding referrals for each ulcer type, though this present chapter has highlighted a multitude of other potential members of this team. It is important to bear in mind that the MDT will vary from patient to patient according to their problems and needs. All healthcare professionals have different skills and limitations and it is each individual's professional responsibility to recognise these. No one person can be all things to all people, but we can be good team players who are able to communicate effectively and work together towards achieving the best outcome for the patient.

REFERENCES

Aronow, W.S. (2005) Management of peripheral arterial disease. *Cardiology in Review* **13**(2): 61–68.

Barwell, J.R., Davies, C.E., Deacon, J., et al. (2004) Comparison of surgery and compression with compression alone in chronic venous ulceration (ESCHAR study): randomised controlled trial. *Lancet* **363**: 1854–1859.

Baxter, H. (2002) How a discipline came of age: a history of wound care. *Journal of Wound Care* **11**(10): 383–392.

Bechara, F.G., Sand, M., Sand, D., Stucker, M., Altmeyer, P. & Hoffmann, K. (2006) Shave therapy for chronic venous ulcers: A guideline for surgical management and post-operative wound care. *American Society of Plastic Surgical Nurses* **6**(1): 29–34.

Charles, H. (1995) The impact of leg ulcers on a patient's quality of life. *Professional Nurse* **10**: 571–572.

Collier, M. & Radley, K. (2005) The development of a nurse-led complex wound clinic. *Nursing Standard (Tissue Viability Suppl.)* **19**(32): 74–84.

Department of Health (DH) (2000) Reducing heart disease in the population. Chapter 1, pp. 41–2. Appendix C – Effectiveness of physical activity programmes. In: *NHS our Healthier Nation: Modern Standards and Service Models. Coronary Heart Disease National Service Frameworks*. London, DH.

Doherty, D.C., Morgan, P.A. & Moffatt, C.J. (2006) Role of hosiery in lower limb lymphoedema. In: *EWMA Position Document: Lymphoedema Framework. Template for Practice: Compression Hosiery in Lymphoedema*. London, MEP, pp. 10–21.

Donohue, S. & Sutton-Woods, P. (2001) Lower limb amputation. In: *Vascular Disease Nursing and Management* (S. Murray, ed.). London, Whurr, pp. 313–342.

Dyson, M. (1987) Mechanisms involved in therapeutic ultrasound. *Physiotherapy* **73**: 116–120.

Flemming, K. & Cullum, N. (1999) Laser therapy for venous leg ulcers. *The Cochrane Database of Systematic Reviews*, Issue 1. Art. No.: CD001182 DOI: 10.1002/14651858.CD001182. http://www.mrw.interscience.wiley.com/cochrane/clsysrev/articles/CD001182/pdf_fs.html

Flemming, K. & Cullum, N. (2000) Therapeutic ultrasound for venous leg ulcers. *The Cochrane Database of Systematic Reviews*, Issue 4. Art. No.: CD001180 DOI: 10.1002/14651858.CD001180. http://www.mrw.interscience.wiley.com/cochrane/clsysrev/articles/CD001180/pdf_fs.html

Franks, P.J. & Gottrup, F. (2004) Outcomes and structure of care: the European perspective. *Wounds: a Compendium of Clinical Research and Practice* **16**(5).

Franks, P.J. & Moffatt, C.J. (1998) Who suffers most from leg ulceration? *Journal of Wound Care* **7**: 383–385.

Franks, Y. (1999) Healthy alliances in wound management. *Journal of Wound Care* **8**(1): 13–17.

Ghauri, A.S.K., Sullivan, J.G., Whyman, M.R., Farndon, J.R. & Poskitt, K.R. (1998a) Prevention of leg ulcer recurrence: a role for the vascular surgeon? *British Journal of Surgery* **85**: 562.

Ghauri, A.S., Nyamekye, I., Grabs, A.J., Farndon, J.R. & Poskitt, K.R. (1998b) The diagnosis and management of mixed arterial/venous leg ulcers in community based clinics. *European Journal of Vascular and Endovascular Surgery* **16**(4): 350–355.

Ghauri, A.S.K., Taylor, M.C., Deacon, J.E., Whyman, M.R., Earnshaw, J.J., Heather, B.P. & Poskitt, K.R. (2000) Influence of a specialized leg ulcer service on management and outcome. *British Journal of Surgery* **87**: 1048–1056.

Gottrup, F., Holstein, P., Jorgensen, B., Lohmann, M. & Karlsmark, T. (2001) A new concept of multidisciplinary wound healing centre and a national expert function of wound healing. *Archives of Surgery* **136**: 765–777.

Granick, M.S. & Ladin, D.A. (1998) The multidisciplinary in-hospital wound care team: two models. *Advances in Wound Care* **11**(2): 80–88.

Hardy, S.C., Riding, G. & Abidia, A. (2004) Surgery for deep venous incompetence. Cochrane Database of Systematic Reviews 2004, Issue 3. Art. No.: CD001097. DOI: 10.1002/14651858.CD001097.pub2. http://www.mrw.interscience.wiley.com/cochrane/clsysrev/articles/CD001097/pdf_fs.html

Herbert, L.M. (1997) *Caring for the Vascular Patient*. Edinburgh, Churchill Livingstone.

Jenns, K. (2000) Management strategies. In: *Lymphoedema* (R. Twycross, K. Jenns & J. Todd, eds). Abingdon, Oxon, Radcliffe Medical Press, pp. 97–117.

Jones, J.E. & Nelson, E.A. (2000) Skin grafting for venous leg ulcers. Cochrane Database of Systematic Reviews 2000, Issue 2. Art. No.: CD001737. DOI: 10.1002/14651858.CD001737.pub2. http://www.mrw.interscience.wiley.com/cochrane/clsysrev/articles/CD001737/pdf_fs.html

Jull, A.B., Waters, J. & Arroll, B. (2004) Pentoxifylline for treating venous leg ulcers. *The Cochrane Database of Systematic Reviews*, Issue 2, Art. No.: CD001737. DOI: 10.1002/14651858.CD001737.pub2. http://www.mrw.interscience.wiley.com/cochrane/clsysrev/articles/CD001733/pdf_fs.html

Kjaer, M.L., Sorensen, L.T., Karlsmark, T., Mainz, J. & Gottrup, F. (2005) Evaluation of the quality of venous leg ulcer care given in a multidisciplinary specialist centre *Journal of Wound Care* **14**(4): 145–150.

Kranke, P., Bennett, M., Roeckl-Wiedmann, I. & Debus, S. (2004) Hyperbaric oxygen therapy for chronic wounds. *The Cochrane Database of Systematic Reviews*, Issue 1. Art. No.: CD004123. DOI: 10.1002/14651858.CD004123.pub2. http://www.mrw.interscience.wiley.com/cochrane/clsysrev/articles/CD004123/pdf_fs.html

Leng, G.C., Fowler, B. & Ernst, E. (2000) Exercise for Intermittent Claudication. Cochrane Database of Systematic Reviews 2000, Issue 2. Art. No.: CD000990. DOI: 10.1002/14651858.CD000990 http://www.mrw.interscience.wiley.com/cochrane/clsysrev/articles/CD000990/pdf_fs.html

Lindholm, C., Bjellerup, M., Christensen, O.B. & Zederfeld, B. (1993) Quality of life in chronic leg ulcers *Acta Dermato-Venereologica* **73**: 440–443.

Marcus, B.H. & Forsyth, L.H. (2003) Using the stages model in individual counselling. In: *Motivating People to Be Physically Active: Physical Activity Intervention Series* (S. Blair, series ed.). Champaign, ILL, Human Kinetics, pp. 107–138.

Moffatt, C.J., Franks, P.J., Doherty, D.C., Martin, R., Blewett, R. & Ross, F. (2004) Prevalence of leg ulceration in a London population. *Quarterly Journal of Medicine* **97**: 431–437.

Moore, Z. & Cowman, S. (2005) The need for EU standards in wound care: an Irish survey. *Wounds UK* **1**(1): 20–27.

Murray, S. (2001) Chronic ischaemia. In: *Vascular Disease Nursing and Management* (S. Murray, ed.). London, Whurr, pp. 238–269.

NHS Purchasing and Supply Agency (2004) *NHS Supply Chain Excellence Programme: National Contracts Sourcing Project, 2004.* www.pasa.nhs.uk

Padberg, F.T., Johnston, M.V. & Sisto, S.A. (2004) Structured exercise improves calf muscle pump function in chronic venous insufficiency: a randomised trial. *Journal of Vascular Surgery* **39**: 79–87.

Prochaska, J.O. & DiClemente, C.C. (1983) The stages and processes of self-change in smoking: towards an integrative model of change. *Journal of Consulting and Clinical Psychology* **51**: 390–395.

Ravaghi, H., Flemming, K., Cullum, N. & Olyaee Manesh, A. (2006) Electromagnetic therapy for treating venous leg ulcers. *The Cochrane Database of Systematic Reviews*, Issue 2. Art. No.: CD002933. DOI: 10.1002/14651858.CD002933.pub3.

Scriven, J.M., Hartshorne, T., Bell, P.R., Naylor, A.R. & London, N.J. (1997) Single-visit venous ulcer assessment clinic: the first year. *British Journal of Surgery* **84**(3): 334–336.

Trodorvic, V. (2002) Food and wounds: nutritional factors in wound formation and healing. *British Journal of Community Nursing* **7**(9) (Suppl.): S43–54.

Vowden, K. & Vowden, P. (2001) Mixed aetiology ulcers. *Journal of Wound Care* **10**(1): 52.

Williams, L. (2002) Assessing patients' nutritional needs in the wound-healing process. *Journal of Wound Care* **11**(6): 225–228.

Management of the Wound Bed and Surrounding Skin

13

LEARNING OBJECTIVES

Nurses involved in leg ulcer management should be able to demonstrate:

❏ An understanding of acute versus chronic wound healing.
❏ An understanding of TIME as applied to wound bed preparation.
❏ An understanding of what constitutes an optimal wound environment, what factors can help create the optimal wound environment and the properties of dressings that may help to achieve this.
❏ The ability to identify the properties of the various wound dressings, and the impact they have on the wound bed.

INTRODUCTION

Chronic wounds such as leg ulcers do not follow the normal pattern of repair (Enoch & Harding, 2003) (see Chapter 8). The tightly controlled and well-ordered cellular and biochemical processes seen in acute wounds become disordered, causing the wound to become 'stuck' in the inflammatory or proliferative stages of healing. This is largely due to underlying medical problems that require accurate diagnosis and treatment if the wound is to heal. However, local barriers at the wound site can also slow or prevent wound closure, specifically: necrotic or sloughy tissue; bacterial imbalance; and altered exudate levels and composition (Enoch & Harding, 2003).

This chapter will introduce the reader to the concept of wound bed preparation – those things that practitioners can do to remove these barriers and introduce positive factors to assist healing (Douglass, 2003). It will show how the TIME framework – introduced in Chapter 8 – can be used to guide the practitioner through this process, and how best practice in dressing choice, wound cleansing and skin care can contribute to faster healing.

Best practice

- Wound bed preparation, cleansing and dressing choice should be based on:
  — the ulcer aetiology
  — the TIME assessment (Falanga, 2004)
  — a thorough understanding of the dressing or wound treatment properties.
- Routine swabbing of wounds should be avoided. Swab only if clinical infection is suspected.
- Judicious use of antimicrobial dressings – if a raised bacterial count is suspected or if the patient is at increased risk of infection – may reduce the risk of spreading infection and minimise antibiotic use (Cooper, 2004). Avoid long-term use. Over-use may encourage the development of resistant strains of bacteria (Vowden & Cooper, 2006).
- Infection should generally be treated with a 14-day course of systemic antibiotics, in accordance with the swab result.
- Patients with leg ulceration are at an increased risk of developing allergic contact dermatitis due to breaks in their skin and exposure to multiple wound care products. Keep cleansing and dressing regimes as simple and bland as possible, and avoid the use of latex gloves (Cameron, 1998a).

A WORD OF CAUTION

It should be clear by now that the key to effective leg ulcer management lies in diagnosing and treating the main barrier to healing – the underlying medical condition(s). Wound bed preparation is almost always of secondary importance, and much time and money will be wasted on wound bed preparation if diagnosis and treatment of the ulcer aetiology is neglected. Where adequate treatment of the underlying disease is possible – as in the case of uncomplicated venous ulceration – relatively little attention will need to be given to wound bed preparation, since correction of the underlying cause will almost always suffice to achieve healing. However, much more effort will need to be made in the area of wound bed preparation where adequate control of the underlying cause is more difficult, such as in the case of complex multi-factorial ulcers.

WOUND BED PREPARATION AND DRESSING CHOICE USING THE TIME FRAMEWORK

Most practitioners, especially those new to leg ulcer care, find the wide range of dressing choice somewhat baffling. Apart from anything else, it is very hard to remember all their names, let alone what sizes and shapes they come in! To make life simpler, some practitioners often opt for a range of 'favourite' dressings, for no other reason than that they have 'seen them work' on other patients and feel familiar with them.

The problem with this way of managing wounds is that it tends to place too much emphasis on the dressing, and not enough emphasis on what is actually happening at the wound bed. It also means that practitioners will keep trying different dressings to find out which one will 'work' on their patient. However, it is important to note that:

- This only introduces the patient to multiple products, each one increasing the patient's chances of developing a contact allergy.
- The fact that a dressing appeared to 'work' or 'not work' on a previous patient may have nothing to do with the dressing, but more to do with the underlying cause of that ulcer and how it was being treated, e.g. the patient was put into compression, or started sleeping in their bed at night.

Using the TIME framework (Falanga, 2004) will help shift practitioners' attention from the dressing back to the wound bed. It focuses thinking on exactly what the problems at the wound bed are, and from there the priorities of management soon become clear. Once these priorities are established, the whole issue of dressing choice is made much easier, because it is then just a matter of matching the properties of a dressing to the priority. It is important to remember that the priorities of management usually include other interventions in addition to dressing choice. Many practitioners remain convinced that successful healing is a matter of finding the 'right' dressing and are surprised when, after a TIME assessment, they discover the reason for poor healing may have little to do with the dressing choice.

The TIME framework for wound bed preparation involves:

- Tissue management
- Inflammation and infection control
- Moisture balance
- Epithelial (edge) advancement

Tissue management

The harmful effects of devitalised tissue in a wound have already been described in Chapter 8. Removal of this tissue not only takes away the physical barrier to healing, but also lowers bacterial burden, with the aim of progressing the wound from a state of prolonged inflammation to one of proliferation. Some chronic wounds may require repeated or maintenance debridement, since the underlying pathological processes contributing to the ulcer may still be at work (Falanga, 2004).

There are five main methods of debridement: autolytic; enzymatic; larval (biosurgery); mechanical; and sharp or surgical (Enoch & Harding, 2003). The choice of method will depend on the wound characteristics, patient attitude, available skills and resources, pain, exudate levels and risk of infection (Vowden & Vowden, 2002; Enoch & Harding, 2003).

> Not all wounds are considered 'safe' for debridement, and the treatment goals should be based on a realistic assessment of the 'healability' of the wound. Attempts to debride dry necrotic tissue in patients with a poorly vascularised limb (as in patients with diabetes or arterial disease) are likely to result in a moist, limb- or life-threatening gangrene.
>
> The priority here is urgent vascular referral (or in the case of diabetic foot ulceration, urgent referral to a specialist diabetic podiatry unit). Where re-vascularisation of the limb is carried out successfully, debridement can proceed.

Autolytic debridement

Autolytic debridement, or autolysis, is the body's natural means of selectively removing devitalised tissue through the activity of endogenous proteolytic enzymes. It is part of the normal inflammatory stage of healing and requires a moist environment. The problem for a chronic wound is either that the environment is not conducive to autolysis, or that autolysis is too slow to keep pace with the underlying processes causing tissue destruction.

If it is possible to achieve adequate control of the underlying disease process, successful autolysis will ensue with very little effort. Venous ulcers are a good example of this principle: in these wounds slough is usually a direct result of venous hypertension, and the application of adequate compression to aid venous return as well as using a simple low-adherent dressing is generally all that is required. Venous ulcers tend to produce sufficient exudate to ensure a moist environment without the need for more complex dressings. With more complex wounds, where the wound bed may be too wet or too dry, more advanced dressings may be required:

- Amorphous or sheet hydrogels to rehydrate dry slough or necrosis.
- Manuka honey to provide a moist environment (Enoch & Harding, 2003).
- Hydrocolloids to promote moisture retention.
- Calcium alginates or hydrofibre dressings to absorb exudate and create a moist 'gel' that is in contact with the wound.

For ulcers that are wet (rather than simply moist), control of the source of exudate is required, and dressings such as calcium alginates and hydrofibres may simply expose the wound bed to prolonged contact with harmful exudate. In such cases it may be better to use a simple non-absorbent dressing or a capillary action dressing, which allow excess exudate to pass away from the wound into the bandage layers, and to ensure frequent dressing changes.

Where autolytic debridement is slow or ineffective, other methods of debridement must be considered.

Enzymatic debridement
Use of an exogenous enzymatic preparation applied directly to the wound can promote rapid debridement. Examples of these agents

include: streptokinase/streptodornase; bacterial collagenase; papain/urea; fibrinolysin/DNAs; trypsin; and subtilisin (Enoch & Harding, 2003). The availability of these products varies world-wide, and in some areas is decreasing due to reduced demand. These products generally require daily application. However, caution must be taken not to allow the enzyme to come into contact with healthy tissue – something that can be quite difficult to achieve with leg ulcers. The enzyme may be inactivated by metals (zinc, silver) and detergents, and can cause an allergy.

Larval therapy (biosurgery)

Now available on drug tariff in the UK, the use of sterile maggots is a particularly successful treatment for persistent slough in leg ulcers. The maggots rapidly and selectively digest sloughy tissue, and there is some evidence that they also reduce bacterial burden and stimulate healing (Enoch & Harding, 2003). No toxicity or allergic reaction has been reported, though it may be an unacceptable choice for some patients, and can increase pain (Vowden & Vowden, 2002).

The treatment is available through hospital and community pharmacies, and is generally applied every 3–4 days. A hydrocolloid or zinc paste is applied to the surrounding skin and the larvae sealed in place with a thin porous sheet. Dampened gauze is placed on top and a light retention bandage on top of this, taking care not to squash the maggots or restrict the air supply (Fig. 13.1). Daily observation and changing of the gauze are both required to ensure that the maggots neither dry out nor drown. Once removed, the maggots are disposed of using standard clinical waste procedures.

Mechanical debridement

Mechanical debridement is the use of non-discriminatory physical force. Although potentially rapid and effective, this method is generally discouraged because of the risk of damage to granulation tissue and the wound edges and because of the associated pain.

Examples include: the wet-to-dry dressing technique; pressure irrigation; whirlpool therapy; and ultrasound (Enoch & Harding, 2003). Topical negative pressure therapy, such as VAC (vacuum-assisted closure) can be used as a more controlled form of mechani-

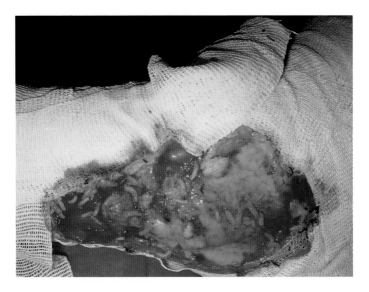

Fig. 13.1 Larval therapy for wound management.

cal debridement, exposing the wound to a predetermined negative pressure (usually 125 mmHg) and removing exudate, slough and bacteria, as well as increasing local tissue perfusion (Enoch & Harding, 2003). However, it is ineffective on dry eschar and may be slow to remove large areas of sloughy tissue.

Sharp or surgical debridement

Although possibly the fastest method of removing dead tissue, sharp/surgical debridement requires the use of a local or general anaesthetic and may not be readily available to patients in the community. Because it requires a good knowledge of anatomy, access to suitable sterile equipment and carries the risk of damage to underlying structures, it should therefore **only be carried out by professionals trained and competent in the technique**. Some damage to viable tissue may occur and bleeding is likely, but this can actually be beneficial in converting a chronic wound back into a state of acute wound healing (Enoch & Harding, 2003) particularly where cell senescence has occurred.

Inflammation and infection control

All chronic wounds contain bacteria – generally the same bacteria found in skin flora. This is normal, and does not necessarily create a barrier to wound healing. However, an increase in bacterial levels – or the presence of particularly virulent bacteria, such as beta-haemolytic streptococci – can significantly slow healing, and may result in tissue breakdown if allowed to proceed to infection. Effective wound bed preparation therefore includes measures to achieve bacterial balance as well as management of infection (Enoch & Harding, 2003).

Certain micro-organisms can be particularly detrimental or problematic in leg ulceration, and can result in considerable anxiety for the patient:

- **MRSA**. It is not uncommon for leg ulcers to be colonised with methicillin-resistant *Staphylococcus aureus* (MRSA) in the absence of infection. Management should be aimed at good infection control and reassuring the patient that healing can still progress normally in the absence of infection. Routine use of antibiotics in the absence of clinical signs of infection is not recommended due to the increased risk of resistance. Local protocols on MRSA should be adhered to. Antimicrobial therapy should be commenced if the wound shows signs of bacterial imbalance.
- **Streptococci**. Beta-haemolytic streptococci can be particularly problematic in leg ulceration and even at low levels they can delay healing. Therefore, treatment, often in the form of systemic antibiotics, is required to achieve healing. Haemolytic streptococci should be suspected if exudate is haemoserous.
- **Pseudomonas aeroginosa** (see Fig. 13.2). This Gram-negative pathogen frequently colonises leg ulcers causing delayed healing, increased levels of exudate and giving a characteristic green discoloration to the wound and/or exudate (Caple, 2003). Since it is a pathogen that survives well in moist environments (Reynolds, 2000), care must be take to ensure that the bowl or bucket used to wash the leg in is lined with a fresh plastic liner and cleansed and dried thoroughly between treatments. Alternatively, it may be easier to avoid the problem altogether by using warmed sterile saline and an aseptic technique.

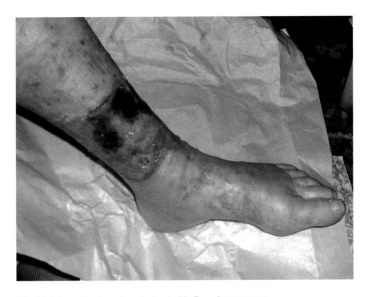

Fig. 13.2 Leg ulcer heavily colonised with *Pseudomonas* spp.

Using a clean or aseptic technique

Wounds can become contaminated with bacteria from the environment or from another patient via a practitioner's hands. Good infection control procedures are essential if this is to be avoided and the risk of infection reduced.

A clean technique is generally advised for the management of leg ulcers (Royal College of Nursing, 1998). The rationale behind this is that leg ulcers are not sterile wounds and therefore it is pointless trying to maintain complete sterility; thus the use of sterile dressing packs and sterile gloves for chronic wounds simply represents a waste of resources. Moreover, research suggests that better cleaning of the wound bed and surrounding skin occurs when patients are allowed to soak their legs in a bucket of clean tap water rather than when the wound is cleansed with sterile saline. However, an aseptic technique may be preferred where deeper underlying structures such as bone and tendon are visible, where there is a deep sinus, or where the patient is particularly vulnerable to infection (for example, if the patient is severely immunosuppressed). Use of sterile saline for wound cleansing is also recommended in patients susceptible to pseudomonal infection, since *Pseudomonas aeruginosa* is a water-borne pathogen. Table 13.1 summarises clean and aseptic techniques.

Unfortunately, the move away from strict asepsis in leg ulcer care has led some practitioners to adopt a careless approach, resulting in not a clean but a dirty technique. Examples include:

- Failure to change gloves once they become contaminated from an external source such as the patient's footwear, the outer layer of bandaging, dressing packaging, patient notes, or even the floor. Always consider the last thing that has been in contact with the gloves. Open all packaging prior to applying the gloves, and change gloves whenever necessary. Avoid removing ointments from a tub with a gloved hand that has been in contact with the leg: instead use a spatula or a clean gauze swab.
- Failure to place the patient's leg on a clean towel/plastic sheet, resulting in transfer of bacteria from the environment into the wound.
- Secondary usage of single-use only equipment, such as disposable plastic forceps for removing dry skin plaques.
- Failure to keep wound care products (e.g. packets of gloves or gauze) clean in-between dressing changes.
- Sharing of dressing materials between patients. This can be a particular problem in the hospital, clinic or nursing-home setting, but is unacceptable practice. Once a dressing has been opened for one patient, it cannot be cut and shared with another patient.

Removal of debris

The presence of foreign bodies and devitalised tissue can increase the risk of infection. Good tissue management, as already discussed, is essential, as well as efforts to ensure that no debris is left in the wound. Avoid the use of cotton wool and other products that may leave behind insoluble particles. Use forceps to remove any dry skin plaques.

Table 13.1 Summary of clean and aseptic techniques.

	Aseptic technique	Clean technique
Hand cleansing	Wash with an antiseptic detergent and dry thoroughly. Where adequate washing facilities are not available and hands are physically clean, use an alcohol hand gel.	Wash with liquid soap or antiseptic detergent and dry thoroughly. Where adequate washing facilities are not available and hands are physically clean, use an alcohol hand gel.
Apron	Disposable plastic. Change between patients and if soiled.	Disposable plastic. Change between patients and if soiled.
Gloves	Sterile: change if contamination occurs, and between removal of soiled dressings and application of new dressings.	Non-sterile, e.g. box of non-sterile vinyl gloves: change if contamination occurs and between removal of soiled dressings and application of new dressings.
Dressing field	Sterile dressing pack on which to lay out dressings. Sterile sheet under patient's leg to prevent transfer of bacteria between the leg and stool/couch/floor.	Clean sheet/paper towel on which to lay out dressings. Clean towel, or disposable plastic sheet/apron placed under patient's leg to prevent transfer of bacteria between the leg and stool/couch/floor.
Technique	Non-touch	Non-touch
Wound cleansing	Sterile normal saline/sterile water. Pat dry with sterile gauze/sterile paper towel.	Wash the legs in a clean bucket or bowl, lined with a clean plastic bin-liner. The bowl should be cleaned with a general purpose detergent and dried thoroughly after use. Clean gauze can be used to sluice water over the leg. Pat dry with clean gauze/paper towel.
Dressings	Sterile: sterile gauze/pad where required as secondary dressing.	Sterile: non-sterile gauze/pad where required as a secondary dressing.
Forceps/scissors	Sterile or sterile single-use forceps for removing dry skin plaques/debris.	Single-use or clean, re-useable implements cleansed with alcohol wipe.
	Sterile or sterile single-use scissors for cutting dressings.	Clean, re-usable bandage scissors to remove outer bandage layers.

Using larvae to achieve bacterial balance

Bacterial balance can also be achieved in sloughy wounds with the use of larvae. A number of studies have found that larvae are effective at removing bacteria, particularly Gram-positive bacteria (Vowden & Cooper, 2006).

Using topical antimicrobials

Topical antimicrobials should not be used routinely in wound management (Moffatt, 2006) since they can cause pain, damage new tissue and promote bacterial resistance. They should be reserved for patients where progress towards an overt infection is suspected or where healing is stalled, and long-term use should also be avoided (Vowden & Cooper, 2006). A recommended algorithm for managing wound infection, including the use of antimicrobials, has been produced by the European Wound Management Association (Fig. 13.3), and suggests the use of topical antimicrobials for wounds where signs of infection are limited to the wound only, as well as those showing spreading infection.

There is much debate about the best topical antimicrobials to use, and the literature remains inconclusive. Factors to consider when selecting an antiseptic dressing include the specificity and efficacy of the agent, potential damage to tissue, risk of development of resistant strains and its potential to induce an allergy (Vowden & Cooper, 2006). In addition, practitioners should take into account the individual wound characteristics and the dressing's ability to manage exudate, its effect on pain levels, cost and frequency of dressing changes required, as well as its ability to conform to the size and shape of the wound so as to ensure maximum efficacy (Jones et al., 2005). The use of topical antibiotics should be avoided due to the high incidence of contact allergies in leg ulcer patients. Other topical antimicrobial agents include:

- **Silver**. This has been shown to be effective against both Gram-negative and Gram-positive bacteria, but there is some evidence of the development of silver-resistant strains (Vowden & Cooper, 2006). Some patients experience increased pain. It is particularly effective against *Pseudomonas aeruginosa*. Due to its non-specific action some damage to healing tissue is thought to be inevitable (Maillard & Denyer, 2006).

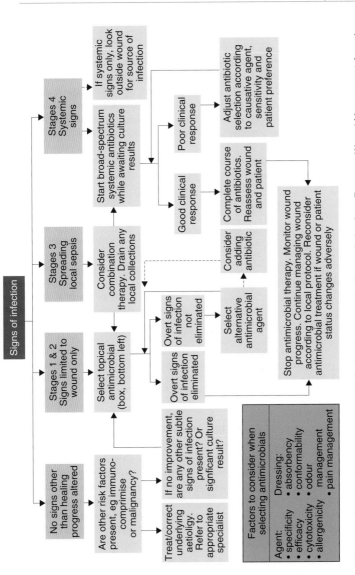

Fig. 13.3 Algorithm for managing wound infection (reproduced with permission from European Wound Management Association (EWMA). Position document: Management of wound infection. London: MEP Ltd, 2006).

- **Iodine**. Also effective against Gram-negative and Gram-positive bacteria, and to date no evidence of resistance has been recorded (Vowden & Cooper, 2006). Iodine is available as long-acting (cadexomer–iodine) and short-acting (povidone–iodine) dressings. Care should be taken due to the risk of iodine toxicity, particularly in individuals with thyroid function disorders. The manufacturer's instructions on dosage and contraindications must be strictly adhered to. Some patients experience increased pain.
- **Manuka honey**. Now available on prescription in the UK, it is effective against both Gram-negative and Gram-positive bacteria, and to date no evidence of resistance has been recorded (Vowden & Cooper, 2006). However, it can cause increased pain, as well as maceration of surrounding skin.
- **Chlorhexidine**. Effective against both Gram-negative and Gram-positive bacteria (Vowden & Cooper, 2006), but due to evidence of resistance it is not generally recommended in leg ulcer management.

Using systemic antibiotics

Generally, antibiotic use should be reserved for the treatment of spreading infection (see Table 8.2). Over-use of antibiotics leading to increased bacterial resistance can be a problem where practitioners lack a good understanding of leg ulceration and assume that all leg ulcers are infected, or mistake acute lipodermatosclerosis for cellulitis (see Chapter 4). Use of antibiotics should be considered:

- If spreading cellulitis is present or the patient is particularly susceptible due to arterial disease, diabetes, immunosuppression or some other reason. Take a wound swab and commence broad-spectrum antibiotics immediately. Adjust them in accordance with the swab result. Otherwise, take a wound swab and await the swab result to guide the choice of antibiotic therapy.
- The practitioner whose clinical judgement leads him/her to take a wound swab is responsible for ensuring the results are followed through. This is a particular issue in the primary care setting where swab results tend to be sent directly to the GP and not to the community nursing team treating the patient. Close liaison with the GP and transfer of the results into the nursing notes are essential.

- Generally, treatment with oral antibiotics for a leg ulcer-related infection should last for 14 days. A 7-day period is usually only sufficient to destroy the 'weaker' bacteria, leaving the 'stronger' ones to mutate and develop antibiotic resistance.

Improving the patient's ability to fight infection

A patient's susceptibility to developing an infection is largely related to their level of defence. Since their main defence – their skin – is broken, all leg ulcer patients are vulnerable to infection. However, those who are particularly vulnerable are those with arterial disease, diabetes, reduced immunity, or poor nutrition and poor general health. Measures should be taken to address and manage any of these problems.

Managing inflammation due to other causes

See Chapter 7 for particular guidance on the management of those rarer conditions of vasculitis and pyoderma gangrenosum.

It should go without saying that antibiotic therapy will be ineffective for treating inflammatory conditions that are unrelated to infection. Nevertheless, inflammation can present the clinician with a perplexing clinical picture. In light of the possibility of missing an aggressive infection, which may lead to far more serious implications, it may be sensible to err on the side of caution and commence antibiotic therapy for those patients who are particularly vulnerable. See page 190 (Chapter 8) for a list of factors affecting a patient's defence against infection. Patients should be followed up and reviewed before the completion of antibiotic treatment: if there has been no notable effect then further assessment in relation to the above should be undertaken. It should always be borne in mind that: a cellulitis may have been present in conjunction with another inflammatory condition; there may be an ongoing immunological response, although bacteria levels have been reduced; or it may also be the case that oral antibiotic treatment was ineffective, though this is likely to be matched by worsening symptoms of increasing, unrelieved pain and spreading cellulitis.

For inflammation related to chronic venous hypertension (CVH), the most effective means of calming the inflammatory process is to resolve the CVH using compression therapy. It is important to note, however, that high compression may aggravate the patient's pain during the initial stages, so begin with reduced levels of compression (15–25 mmHg). As the pain subsides, gradually increase the level of compression according to the patient's needs and taking into account any other underlying problems. Consider the use of non-steroidal anti-inflammatory drugs (NSAIDs) to help alleviate the pain and discomfort.

Moisture balance

Leg ulcers that lack sufficient moisture may be covered with a dry eschar or slough, slowing or preventing autolytic debridement. Appropriate dressings should be chosen that rehydrate or occlude the wound (see the section on autolytic debridement above). A lack of moisture can also lead to failure of a granulating wound to epithelialise, since epithelial cells require moisture to migrate across the surface and because dressings may adhere to and 'strip off' delicate epithelial tissue. Very low adherent dressings that promote a moist environment, such as lipocolloid or silicone dressings, may be beneficial.

The majority of leg ulcers, however, tend to be too wet rather than too dry, usually due to underlying oedema (Fig. 13.4).

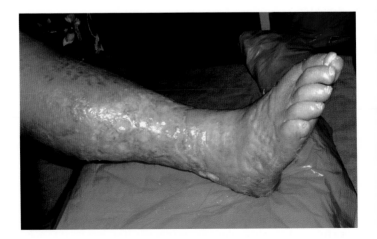

Fig. 13.4 Leg ulceration producing copious exudate.

Large wounds or skin conditions that result in the formation of papules and vesicles are also likely to exude heavily. Chronic wound exudate differs markedly from acute wound exudate – rather than being beneficial to the wound, it can cause substantial damage to both the wound bed and surrounding skin. It is also an excellent culture medium for bacterial growth, and results in loss of protein to the patient. Grossly oedematous legs and heavy exudate levels can place an increased demand on nursing time and dressing costs, as well as reducing the patient's quality of life through discomfort, malodour, embarrassment, social isolation, reduced mobility, damage to clothing and shoes, possible safety problems if the floor becomes wet, increased risk of infection and increased pain. Cellulitis or erysipelas can develop rapidly and occur repeatedly where oedema remains uncontrolled (Anderson, 2003a).

When treating wet ulcers, it can be tempting to simply 'pad up' the leg with absorbent dressings and wadding, to avoid frequent dressing changes. Note, however, that this strategy is likely to simply delay healing by:

- Exposing the wound to the harmful effects of wound exudate over a prolonged time, including destruction of growth factors and granulation tissue.
- Exposing the wound edges to the harmful effects of wound exudate, causing maceration, excoriation and increased ulcer size.
- Possibly distorting the shape of the limb with excess padding, thus preventing adequate levels of compression or support due to an abnormally large ankle and distorting the graduation of the pressure (so that the pressure increases towards the knee, thus forcing fluid back down to the ankle and foot). This in turn will lead to an increase in oedema and exudate.

Effective management of excess exudate is governed by the following principles:

- Identifying and controlling the source of excess exudate.
- Matching the absorbency or moisture properties of the dressing to the wetness of the wound.
- Ensuring adequate frequency of dressing changes.

Identifying and controlling the source of exudate

This is the most important intervention when trying to manage excess wound exudate. Simply mopping up wound exudate with absorbent dressings is a waste of time if the source of the excess exudate is not controlled. Potential sources that should be considered include:

- **Venous oedema**. Check that the patient is in the correct bandage system for the size of their ankle, and where possible increase the level of compression. Ensure the patient is going to bed at night. During the day, advise the patient to elevate their feet – ideally to heart level – when sitting, and to exercise. **Caution**: first check for any contraindications to high compression.
- **Lymphoedema**. Work closely with a specialist lymphoedema team to ensure correct management with bandaging, exercise and possibly manual lymphatic drainage (Board & Harlow, 2002).
- **Cardiac/renal oedema**. Liaise with the GP to review the patient's medication and, where necessary, to arrange for a review by the cardiac/renal team. In may be necessary to introduce or increase diuretics to treat cardiac oedema; patients with poor mobility may need practical assistance managing the resulting increased frequency of urination, such as provision of a commode. High levels of compression are contraindicated as a sudden return of fluid to the heart and kidneys could be fatal. Reduced compression or light support may be introduced with caution once the patient's cardiac/renal oedema is stabilised. Begin with one leg at a time and monitor closely for adverse effects.
- **Dependent oedema**. Excellent communication with the patient and carers is essential in understanding the reasons behind the patient's failure to elevate their legs, and for exploring possible solutions. Reasons for sleeping in a chair can vary considerably, from ischaemic pain, concerns about soiling bedding with exudate, uncontrolled backache, difficulty transferring in and out of bed, and habit. Involvement of multi-disciplinary team members such as the GP, vascular team, physiotherapists, occupational therapists and the pain team should be considered. Note that diuretics are ineffective in managing dependent oedema and should not be used.

- **Bacterial burden**. Any infection or increase in bacterial load will tend to result in increased exudate production. If suspected, treat with antiseptics or antibiotics. There is some evidence that the use of antiseptic potassium permanganate soaks can help to dry up exudate (Hollinworth & Quick, 1995), and can be particularly effective where skin folds and cracks prevent antiseptic dressings from coming into direct contact with the skin. However, on its own, potassium permanganate is unlikely to resolve the problem, and a full investigation into all factors contributing to excess exudate is essential (Anderson, 2003b). The manufacturer's instructions should be closely adhered to in order to ensure adequate soaking time, correct dosage and to prevent irritation or burning of the skin (Anderson, 2003b). Patients should be informed that temporary discoloration of skin and nails will occur.
- **Side-effects of medication**. Some drugs such as amlodipine can cause peripheral oedema. While changing the patient's medication should not be the first line of action, if all else fails it may be necessary to liaise with the GP to review the patient's medication.

Choosing appropriate dressings

When dealing with a very wet wound it can be tempting to use absorbent dressings such as calcium alginates or hydrofibres, and in some instances these are a good choice. However, bear in mind that chronic wound exudate is harmful to the wound bed, and these dressings may simply create a soggy 'mess'. Similarly, foam dressings – though designed to be semi-permeable – struggle to be as effective under bandaging when exudate levels are high, tending to trap fluid close to the wound bed. In these instances it is preferable to choose a dressing that allows fluid to 'wick right away' from the wound bed into the bandaging layers:

- Knitted viscose coated in silicone (e.g. N-A Ultra) or – if bacterial levels are high – povidone–iodine (e.g. Inadine) are both excellent options, as they do not hold fluid close to the wound bed. Provided that the source of exudate has been identified and managed, and the level of compression/support and frequency of dressing changes are adequate, exudate levels should fall without the need for more absorbent dressings. If there are problems with the dressings adhering to the wound, consider the more expensive low-adherent dressings such as a silicone sheet (e.g. Mepitel), a lipocolloid (e.g. Urgotul) or a silver-impregnated lipocolloid (e.g. Urgotul SSD) where an antiseptic is required.

- Where more absorbency is required, choose a dressing that will 'wick' fluid away. A good option would be a capillary action dressing (e.g. Vacutex). Note that this cannot be placed directly against the wound bed, but needs to be used in conjunction with a low-adherent dressing. Note also that to be effective it is important to ensure good contact with the wound – if necessary, cut it to the shape of the wound and cut slits into it so that it conforms to the contours of the wound bed. Some patients experience a 'drawing' sensation with these dressings, which may make them difficult to tolerate.

- Where a stronger antiseptic is required, cadexomer–iodine (e.g. Iodoflex, Iodesorb) can provide high levels of absorbency. To avoid iodine toxicity, the manufacturer's dosage instructions must be strictly adhered to, and it should not be used in patients with thyroid disorders.

- Avoid adhesive dressings on oedematous legs, due to the risk of tearing taut skin.

Frequency of dressing changes

When deciding on the frequency of dressing changes, it is important to bear in mind the harmful nature of chronic wound exudate. Although it may seem a waste of resources to change the dressing three or four times a week, temporarily increasing dressing frequency until exudate levels are under control will save time and money in the long run by preventing wound breakdown and delayed healing. It is unacceptable to leave a wet nappy on a baby for a prolonged period – and in the same way it should be unacceptable to leave wet dressings in place over several days.

Note too that wet dressings and bandages can have a significant impact on:

- The patient's quality of life. Their appearance and malodour can cause severe embarrassment and add to social isolation.

- Financial pressures, if shoes and furniture becomes spoilt.
- Pain levels. Many patients experience a direct link between their level of pain and how wet their dressings are.

> If exudate levels remain uncontrolled, advice should be sought from a specialist team for further assessment and management options.

Epithelial (edge) advancement

It is not always easy to identify why some ulcers fail to epithelialise, and all possible factors should be considered, which may include:

- The underlying aetiology has not been adequately diagnosed or managed.
- Infection or heavy colonisation – consider using an antiseptic dressing or, if infection is suspected, take a wound swab and treat with antibiotics.
- Wound too dry – consider dressings that retain or donate moisture, such as a hydrogel sheet.
- Wound too wet, causing maceration or excoriation of the wound edges – ensure good moisture balance and consider using a barrier film.
- Trauma from dressing removal – consider using a very low adherent dressing such as a silicone sheet or lipocolloid, and avoid adhesive dressings such as hydrocolloids.
- Hyperkeratosis or callous at the wound edge – use emollients to soften the area, such as 50% liquid paraffin and 50% white soft paraffin.

Maceration and excoriation

These occur when wound exudate is left in contact with the wound edges for a prolonged period. Maceration and excoriation are evidence of the harmful effect of chronic wound exudate, will slow or prevent epithelialisation and often cause the ulcer to enlarge. Maceration is seen as white 'soggy' epithelium, whereas excoriation appears as red and raw due to 'stripping off' of the top layer of epithelium (see Fig. 8.7).

A barrier spray (e.g. Cavilon non-sting barrier film) may be used to help protect the wound edges. However, if the wound edges are becoming damaged from wound exudate, it is likely that the wound bed is too, and measures must be taken to improve moisture balance.

Advanced therapies

> Before commencing an advanced therapy, it is essential that: the underlying ulcer aetiology has been diagnosed and managed as far as possible; good wound bed preparation has been implemented; and the wound bed is clean and free from slough, necrosis or infection. Advanced therapies are an expensive option, and if used inappropriately could represent a waste of resources. Advice should first be sought from a specialist team.

Where wounds fail to close due to biochemical imbalance and cell senescence, leading to a disordered healing response, more advanced therapies may be required. Research into this area of wound care is ongoing, and increasing numbers of wound care 'treatments' aimed at optimising the wound environment are becoming available. The problem for practitioners is that there is no easy way of telling what defect may be affecting a particular ulcer. Exudate testing kits to analyse the chemical make-up of wound exudate may be a welcome advance in the future, but are currently not available in practice. Practitioners must therefore make a decision based on what can be known about the wound, and seek advice from a specialist team. Biopsy may be required.

Examples of advanced therapies include:

- **Skin grafting** (Fig. 13.5). Close liaison with the plastic surgery team is essential if the skin graft is to 'take'. Surgical debridement or 'shaving' of the wound by a plastic surgeon prior to the graft can improve healing by reverting the wound back into an acute stage of healing. VAC therapy prior to and following grafting can also enhance chances of success. Grafts will not 'take' where tissue perfusion is poor due to ischaemia or oedema. Patients with venous or other oedemas must have the oedema tightly controlled immediately post-operatively and on

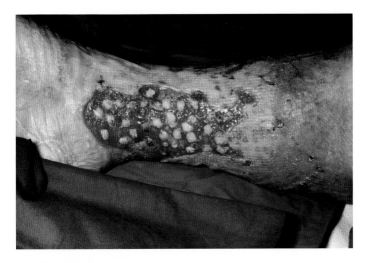

Fig. 13.5 Pinch skin graft.

an ongoing basis. This may involve compression bandaging, and requires close liaison between the primary and acute sectors to ensure the same level of compression that was used prior to grafting is continued in hospital.

- **Tissue engineering**. Autologous or allogeneic cells taken from donors can be cultured in vitro and used as a substitute for skin grafting. Access to these products is limited and currently not available on prescription in the UK.

- **Wound treatments**. A number of wound treatments are currently available that have been developed in an attempt to address biochemical imbalance and localised disordered healing responses. These are normally applied directly to the wound prior to the primary dressing, and dissolve into the wound bed. Care must be taken to follow the manufacturer's instructions to ensure the greatest chance of success. Examples of wound treatments include:
  — *growth factors*: at present platelet-derived growth factor is the only product to be licensed for topical application, and only for diabetic ulcers.

— *protease inhibitors*: a protease-modulating matrix, available on prescription in the UK, has been designed to stimulate healing by inactivating excess proteases and protecting growth factors. Further research into highly selective protease inhibitors is ongoing.

— *hyaluronic acid*: several products have been developed that deliver multi-functional hyaluronic acid to the wound bed.

— *collagen*: a collagen-based powder is now available and is thought to aid healing by promoting re-establishment of a collagen matrix. It is applied directly to the wound either dry, or as a paste.

SKIN CARE

Some patients with leg ulcers will experience no problems with the skin on the rest of the leg, while achieving and maintaining healthy skin can seem almost impossible for others. As a minimum, most patients experience some dryness and flaking, often as a result of bandaging. At worst, others develop acute wet or dry eczema that can become infected and flare up repeatedly, or large areas of hyperkeratosis that seem impossible to soften. Maceration and excoriation of the wound edges have already been discussed, but if left to progress can extend far beyond the area of ulceration.

The causes of eczema and other chronic skin conditions have been discussed in Chapter 8. The key to management is to try to prevent problems developing in the first place, as follows:

• To reduce the risk of the patient developing allergies, keep all cleansing and dressing products as simple and bland as possible, avoid exposure to multiple products, and avoid the use of latex gloves.

• To reduce the risk of irritant eczema, avoid the use of adhesives and adhesive dressings, apply a cotton stockinette dressing under the first layer of padding when applying bandaging, and avoid prolonged exposure to wound exudate.

• Moisturise the leg using a bland ointment – such as 50/50 paraffin (50% liquid paraffin and 50% white soft paraffin). Where possible, avoid creams as these contain preservatives and emulsifiers that can cause allergies and irritation.

- Apply ointment to the leg using downward strokes. Avoid using circular movements or upwards strokes as this can cause hair follicles to become blocked or irritated, which may result in folliculitis.
- Gently remove any loose skin plaques to avoid a build-up of moisture and bacteria.

Managing allergic, irritant or varicose eczema

It can be very difficult to distinguish between these three types of eczema. Although it is important to try to identify the cause, it is often best initially to assume that all three may be playing a part.

Eliminate potential allergens and irritants

Start by reviewing all products that are currently coming into contact with the patient's leg, and eliminate any potential allergens. Common allergens include (Cameron, 1998a):

- **Latex** – found in latex gloves and some bandages.
- **Emulsifiers and preservatives** – such as cetostearyl alcohol, parabens and hydroxybenzoates – found in creams, some emulsifying ointments and paste bandages.
- **Adhesives** – such as colophony and ester gum resin – found in adhesive-backed dressings.
- **Topical antibiotics** – such as neomycin, framycetin and bacitracin – found in medicated tulle dressings, medicated powders and some fungal and cream preparations.
- **Lanolin** – found in some creams, bath additives and emollients.
- **Perfume** – found in some creams and bath additives.

In addition to true allergens, some products can simply irritate the skin causing a potentially severe eczema. A common culprit is orthopaedic wool (cotton/synthetic padding bandage) directly applied to the skin. Although this is unlikely to cause a true allergy, many patients say they are allergic to these products. This is because the friction of the fibres against the skin can set up an irritant dermatitis. Use cotton stockinette as a protective layer. Other causes of irritant eczema include a bandage or hosiery slipping and rubbing on the skin, or prolonged contact with wound fluid.

Consider referral for patch testing

If an allergy is suspected, consider referring the patient to a dermatologist for patch testing. This usually involves a series of three visits within the space of a week to an outpatient clinic. At the first visit, a series of small adhesive discs will be applied to the patient's back, each containing a small dose of a potential allergen. These will be removed several days later and any reaction recorded. Patch tests are applied in 'batteries' – each battery being a set of potential allergens. It is important that the person making the referral specifies that the patient has a potential leg ulcer-related allergy, and requests testing with the 'Standard' and the 'Leg ulcer/medicaments' batteries. In addition, it can be useful if patients take samples of the suspected allergen with them to their first appointment, particularly if it is a new or unusual product.

Consider and treat any venous hypertension

If the patient is known to have venous disease, check whether this is being adequately controlled. Poor control through an inadequate level of compression could be causing a varicose eczema. Check that the patient's bandage regime is suitable for their ankle circumference. Good control with compression therapy and the use of a simple ointment, such as 50/50 paraffin, are often sufficient.

Consider the use of topical corticosteroids

Severe or acute eczema require treatment with a topical corticosteroid (Cameron, 2004). Practitioners should use the following principles:

- Topical steroids are universally classified according to their potency. The potency of the steroid should match the severity of the eczema (Cameron, 1998b). If in doubt about a steroid's potency, consult the manufacturer's instructions, a pharmacist or a formulary such as the *BNF* (*British National Formulary*).

  Corticosteroid potency:
  — *very potent* – e.g. clobetasol propionate 0.05% (Dermovate)
  — *potent* – e.g. betamethasone (as valerate) 0.1% (Betnovate)
  — *moderately potent* – e.g. clobetasone butyrate 0.05% (Eumovate)
  — *mildly potent* – e.g. hydrocortisone 1%

- Use a steroid ointment, and not a steroid cream which may itself contain allergens such as cetostearyl alcohol (Cameron, 1998a).
- The dosage should be measured and recorded in fingertip units (Long & Finlay, 1991). One fingertip is the length from the tip of the finger to the first joint (Fig. 13.6) – approximately 2.5 cm: six fingertips are recommended for a leg and two for a foot.
- When treating acute or severe eczema, begin with the maximum dosage, then wean down over the course of several weeks, by reducing the frequency of application, potency of steroid and/ or number of fingertips applied. Although daily treatment may not be realistic long-term, there is no point in applying a topical steroid only once or twice a week to severe eczema; in addition, the frequency of dressing changes may need to be increased temporarily in the initial stages. Never stop the treatment suddenly without weaning it down, as this is likely to trigger a recurrence (rebound) of the eczema.
- Long-term use of topical corticosteroids should generally be avoided. Occasionally, however, chronic eczema may require

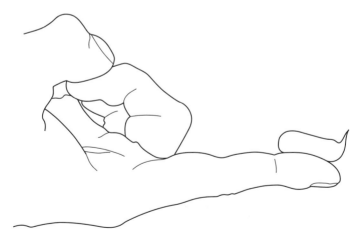

Fig. 13.6 One 'fingertip' unit.

maintenance therapy and a moderately potent steroid should be used (Cameron, 1998b). Mild steroids such as hydrocortisone are unlikely to be effective and may themselves cause an allergic reaction.

Managing hyperkeratosis

Hyperkeratosis is a thick scaling of the skin, and is often found in association with venous disease or lymphoedema. Keeping the area well hydrated with 50/50 paraffin will help to loosen the plaques. Application of a hydrocolloid dressing can also be beneficial – the hydrocolloid softens the area and when removed lifts off some of the hyperkeratosis with it (Cameron, 2004). Use of Whitfield's ointment (benzoic acid ointment) can be beneficial in some patients, particularly if an associated fungal infection is suspected.

CONCLUSION

This chapter has addressed the complex issues of managing the wound bed and surrounding skin. Too often decisions about issues such as dressings and the use of antimicrobials are made on an *ad hoc* basis. Using the TIME framework described in this chapter can help to introduce a more methodical approach to identifying and treating the many factors that influence wound healing. Issues such as poor exudate control and uncontrolled eczema are also major problems that reduce the ability of the patient to 'live well' with their ulcer.

REFERENCES

Anderson, I. (2003a) The management of fluid leakage in grossly oedematous legs. *Nursing Times* **99**(21) (Suppl.): 54–56.

Anderson, I. (2003b) Should potassium permanganate be used in wound care? *Nursing Times* **99**(31) (Suppl.): 61.

Board, J. & Harlow, W. (2002) Lymphoedema 3: the available treatments for lymphoedema. *British Journal of Nursing* **11**(7): 438–450.

Cameron, J. (1998a) Contact sensitivity in patients with venous leg ulcers. *British Journal of Dermatology Nursing* Winter Edition: 5–7.

Cameron, J. (1998b) Skin care for patients with chronic leg ulcers. *Journal of Wound Care* **7**(9): 459–462.

Cameron, J. (2004) What I tell my patients about eczema and venous leg ulcers. *British Journal of Dermatology Nursing* **8**(2): 12–13.

Caple, S. (2003) Managing pseudomonas wound infection and colonisation in patients with chronic leg ulcers. *Leg Ulcer Forum Journal* **17**: 31–35.

Cooper, R. (2004). A review of the evidence for the use of topical antimicrobial agents in wound care. *World Wide Wounds* February.

Douglass, J. (2003) Wound bed preparation: a systematic approach to chronic wounds. *British Journal of Community Nursing Wound Care.* June (Suppl.) S26–34.

Enoch, S. & Harding, K. (2003) Wound bed preparation: the science behind the removal of barriers to healing. *Wounds: A Compendium of Clinical Research and Practice* **15**(7): 213–229.

Falanga, V. (2004) Wound bed preparation: science applied to practice. In: *European Wound Management Association Position Document: Wound Bed Preparation in Practice.* London, MEP, pp. 2–5.

Hollinworth, H. & Quick, A. (1995) Using potassium permanganate for wound cleansing. *Journal of Wound Care* **4**(2): 194.

Jones, S., Bowler, P.G. & Walker, M. (2005) Antimicrobial activity of silver-containing dressing is influenced by dressing conformability with wound surface. *Wounds* **17**(9): 263–270.

Long, C.C. & Finlay, A.Y. (1991) The finger-tip unit – a new practical measure. *Clinical and Experimental Dermatology* **16**: 444–447.

Maillard, J.-Y. & Denyer, S.P. (2006) Demystifying silver. In: *European Wound Management Association Position Document: Management of Wound Infection.* London, MEP, pp. 7–10.

Moffatt, C.J. (2006) Management of wound infection. In: *European Wound Management Association Position Document: Management of Wound Infection.* London, MEP, p. 1.

RCN Institute (1998) *Clinical Practice Guidelines. The management of patients with venous leg ulcers.* London, Royal College of Nursing.

Reynolds, P. (2000) Understanding *Pseudomonas aeruginosa. Nursing Times Plus* **6**(23): 7–8.

Vowden, P. & Cooper, R.A. (2006) An integrated approach to managing wound infection. In: *European Wound Management Association Position Document: Management of Wound Infection.* London, MEP, pp. 2–6.

Vowden, P. & Vowden, K. (2002) Wound bed preparation. *World Wide Wounds* http://www.worldwide-wounds.com

Bandaging and Compression Therapy

14

LEARNING OBJECTIVES

Nurses involved in leg ulcer management should be able to demonstrate:

- ❏ An understanding of the haemodynamic effects of compression therapy.
- ❏ An understanding of how to achieve graduated compression therapy.
- ❏ An understanding of bandage classification.
- ❏ The ability to holistically assess their patient and, in conjunction with the patient, decide on the most appropriate means of compression, including adapting compression systems to meet the individual needs of patients.
- ❏ The ability to apply compression safely and effectively.

INTRODUCTION

Compression therapy forms the cornerstone of venous ulcer management. Its use as a treatment dates back to Egyptian times, though even to this day the effects of this therapy on the body's underlying vessels and structures remain, to a certain extent, a mystery. It has only been in very recent times (since the 1980s) that the variety or means of applying compression therapy has truly expanded to allow some real choices and offer improvements in healing rates.

Interestingly, few patients recognise or accept bandaging as a modern treatment. Despite the development of new materials, an improved awareness of the effects of compression and a number of randomised controlled trials demonstrating its benefits, the perception still is that (compression) bandaging is an old-fashioned remedy.

Although this is not a treatment to be taken lightly by patients or practitioners, the notion that compression is just about putting on a bandage does not do justice first to its benefits and second in appreciating the potential for serious harm to arise when applied to the wrong patient. Yes, an assessment can be done to ensure compression is safe and appropriate to be commenced, but assessment should never just happen once, but at each patient review or visit.

Numerous associated issues related to the impact of such a treatment on a patient's life also need to be taken into account. What effect will the bandaging have on the patient's ability to work, put on shoes and walk, bathe or shower; could it make their pain and discomfort worse? These are very important issues to patients about to undergo compression therapy and they cannot be brushed aside just because healing is the all-important goal (at least to the practitioner). It is perhaps for these reasons that concordance with this treatment is so often an issue.

This chapter will hopefully allow the practitioner to develop their understanding of how compression therapy helps to heal venous leg ulcers, and how to minimise some of the potential problems through comprehensive patient assessment, an open and collaborative approach with the patient and by developing a good application technique.

THE EFFECTS OF COMPRESSION THERAPY

Compression is, as it suggests, a therapy that affects the venous, arterial and lymphatic systems. It is capable of causing a series of complex physiological and biochemical changes to the body's vascular structures. Compression:

- Reduces the distension of the blood vessels, thereby increasing the velocity of blood flow within the vessels.
- Enables absorption of fluid back into the veins and lymphatic vessels.
- Facilitates the action of the calf muscle pump.
- Influences endothelial function and affects cell mediators involved in the local inflammatory response.
- Relieves the symptoms associated with venous disease and improves the healing rate of venous ulcers.

- May help to increase arterial flow by the hyperaemic response and reduction in oedema.

The most effective way to achieve these therapeutic results is by applying sustained graduated compression. Graduated meaning that **the highest pressure is at the ankle and that this gradually reduces towards the knee**. The amount of pressure required at the ankle to cause a significant effect on the blood flow in the limb of a mobile person is 40–50 mmHg (Partsch, 2003).

Best practice

- High compression therapy is the recommended treatment for venous ulcers.
- Prior to the application of compression, patients need to be assessed for the presence of peripheral arterial disease.
- Venous disease should be confirmed.
- High levels of compression should not be applied to patients who have an ABPI below 0.8 (unless under the guidance of a specialist team).
- Compression therapy should only be applied by trained healthcare professionals.

(RCN, 1998; SIGN, 1998; Marston & Vowden, 2003)

HOW GRADUATED COMPRESSION WORKS

The amount of compression applied to a limb is governed by numerous interacting factors (Clark, 2003). Understanding the principles that underline the application of compression is vital to being able to choose and apply the appropriate amount of compression required for the patient. This includes an in-depth knowledge of: the variety of bandages available and their individual properties; the patient (e.g. the degree of venous disease present, the size of the limb, the patient's ability to mobilise, etc.); and the practitioner's own ability to apply compression bandaging.

Bandage pressure (at the time of application) is largely governed by a law of physics – Laplace's law, which essentially describes the relationship between the internal and external pressure of a vessel, the diameter of the vessel and the resulting tension produced in the vessel wall. Laplace's law has been adopted in relation to the application of compression therapy (Thomas, 2003a) and is represented by the following equation (see Table 14.1 for a further explanation of the terms used in the equation):

$$\text{Pressure}\,(\text{mmHg}) = \frac{\text{Tension} \times \text{Number of layers} \times 4620\,(\text{constant})}{\text{Circumference of limb} \times \text{Bandage Width}}.$$

Therefore the pressure applied is directly proportional to the tension, but inversely proportional to the size of the limb. In other words:

The tighter the bandage is applied, the higher the pressure
The larger the limb, the lesser the pressure
(and vice-versa: the smaller the limb, the greater the pressure).

Other important factors that affect the level of compression applied include (Clark, 2003):

Table 14.1 Explanation of the components of Laplace's law.

P = Pressure	The amount of pressure exerted by the bandage on to the limb, expressed as mmHg.
T = Tension	Tension relates to the amount of force required or used to apply the bandage. Tension is directly proportional to bandage pressure. The bandage's ability to retain that tension depends on the elastomeric properties of the bandage.
N = Number of layers	The more bandages applied (of a similar type), the higher the pressure will be. The number of layers not only relates to the number of bandages used, but the application of the bandage using either a spiral or figure-of-eight technique, and the degree of overlap.
C = Circumference of the limb	Sub-bandage pressure is inversely proportional to limb circumference, i.e. the smaller the limb the higher the pressure. It is imperative to measure the ankle circumference (at the thinnest point, just above the malleolous) as this measurement will help to determine the appropriate bandage choice.
W = Width of the bandage	The narrower the bandage the greater the pressure, and vice-versa. For a 'normal' adult-sized leg a 10-cm bandage is usually the most appropriate.

- Other properties of the bandage, such as its power and elasticity.
- The skill and technique of the person applying the bandage.
- The amount of exercise undertaken by the patient – affecting changes in the limb circumference.

Compression may be applied using bandages, hosiery or intermittent pneumatic compression pumps (ICP). Many bandages are available, but not all provide high levels of compression.

Bandage classification

At present, there is no international or even European consensus of bandage classification, hence compression therapy practice can vary quite significantly depending upon geographical location. Different bandage systems are commonly used in different parts of the world: Unna's boot (a combination of a zinc paste impregnated bandage and an elastic or tubular support bandage) is often referred to in north American literature; inelastic bandaging in western Europe; and elastic bandaging in the United Kingdom. However, with the advent of new technologies – enabling the development of innovative materials that offer alternatives to existing products and an international approach to sharing and disseminating information – a gradual change in practice is reflected in the different systems being adopted.

A wide variety of compression systems are presently available (Moffatt, 2004a):

- Inelastic bandages
  — non-cohesive
  — cohesive
- Elastic bandages
  — single-layer
  — multi-layer
  — vari-stretch
- Hosiery/stockings (two-layer systems)
- Intermittent pneumatic compression

However, the terminology often used to describe different compression systems can sometimes be quite confusing and may lead to ambiguity. For example, terms such as 'four-layer bandaging' or 'three-layer paste bandaging' may mean something to experienced practitioners, working in the same geographical area. However, for inexperienced practitioners or where patients might be receiving 'shared care' (across two different sectors) there is a risk of mis-understandings, which may lead to inconsistencies, or poor and inappropriate treatments.

Bandage classification is currently being reviewed by the Leg Ulcer Advisory Board, and hopefully this will help to clarify some of the issues practitioners currently face when making decisions about compression therapy. For example, knowing what bandages are appropriate for what situations and what are the options for applying varying levels of compression are particularly important when managing patients with multi-factorial ulceration.

Classifications are available for compression hosiery, though there are differences between European and British standards (Coull & Clark, 2005) and only the UK has previously had a bandage classification (Partsch, 2005a). The aim is to have a more universal standard when referring to light, moderate and strong compression (Table 14.2).

The present UK bandage classification covers all bandages, not just compression bandages, within three different types with four

Table **14.2** Compression hosiery classifications (Adapted from Coull & Clark, 2005).

	UK class (British Standard)	European class	Ulcer care hosiery kits (British Standard)
Class 1	14–17 mmHg	18–22 mmHg	Liner stocking 10 mmHg
Class 2	18–24 mmHg	23–33 mmHg	
Class 3	25–35 mmHg	34–46 mmHg	+ Secondary stocking Class 3 (~30 mmHg)
Examples	Activa Credalast Duomed/Medi Scholl	Activa Credenhill Medi Jobst Sigvaris Venosan	Activa Bauerfeind Convatec Jobst

subgroups for type 3 (elastic) bandages. To some extent, the classification is quite useful, though for type 2 (inelastic) bandages the classification may be somewhat confusing for practitioners, as there is considerable variation between the bandages in this group, and it could possibly benefit from further sub-grouping as is the case for type 3 bandages. Thomas (1998) describes the bandage classification according to their performance and ability to produce sustained levels of compression, and divides them accordingly.

The classification is based on application of the bandage on an average sized limb (ankle circumference 23 cm) in a spiral configuration with 50% overlap between turns, producing a double layer of bandage at any point on the limb.

> All bandages, regardless of type, should be applied toe to knee.

Type 1 bandages

This group includes retention bandages. These apply little or no pressure and are generally used to hold dressings in place. Even though these bandages apply virtually no pressure if they are applied very tightly, or numerous layers are wrapped around the same area on a limb, the resulting tourniquet can cause oedema either side of the bandage.

Examples of type 1 bandages include: Slinky (SSL), Easyfix (BSN) and K Band (Urgo).

Type 2 bandages

Bandages in this category are capable of applying light support to moderate levels of compression. They are used for the management of sprains, to prevent and treat oedema and for the treatment of venous ulcers. Thus there is considerable variation in the levels of pressure the bandages in this group can apply. It is this variation that can cause some confusion for practitioners and lead to potential problems regarding appropriate bandage choice.

Examples of bandages that provide:

- Light support – Crepe, Profore#2 (S&N) and K-lite (Urgo)
- Moderate support – Elastocrepe (BSN)

- Moderate to high level of compression – Actico and Actiban (Activa), Comprilan (BSN) and Rosidal K (Vernon-Carus)

Application: All bandages **must** be applied toe to knee. Inelastic bandages are generally made of cotton, so they are only capable of stretching 70–90% of their original length. These bandages are applied at full stretch, keeping the bandage short and near to the limb to ensure consistent pressure, in a simple spiral (see Figs 14.7a–h) with 50% overlap, from toe to knee with adequate padding to protect the limb. European practitioners may employ more complex application techniques, but unless this is usual practice it is best to follow the manufacturer's instructions. Depending on the size of the limb, more layers can be used to increase the level of compression. For example, the manufacturer of Actico (Activa) bandaging recommends that: for a patient with an ankle circumference between 18 and 25 cm, one layer of Actico (applied in a spiral) is adequate; and for an ankle over 25 cm in circumference, a second layer of Actico should be incorporated – to be applied from ankle to knee in the opposite direction as the first, i.e. either clockwise or counter-clockwise.

Because these bandages are inelastic they are less able to provide sustained compression over long periods (i.e. a week) due to their inability to react to changes in the limb circumference. So as oedema in the limb reduces (as it should), the bandaging, due to its inelastic nature, will be unable to adjust in accordance with the size and shape of the limb and will therefore need to be reapplied. Over the course of treatment as the oedema reduces and stabilises, the issues related to sustainability will be less of a problem.

How pressure is applied: Inelastic bandages work by forming a firm, almost rigid, wall around the leg. The bandage will feel firm and very supportive and following initial application will be applying quite a high level of compression (similar to elastic bandages). However, over the course of wear-time, and in particular the first 24 hours (due most likely to changes in limb size/shape), the pressure will gradually reduce, by approximately 40% while the patient is in a resting state (Brouwer et al., 2005). This loss of pressure is somewhat compensated for when the person wearing the bandage is active. Due to the rigidity (or stiffness) of the bandage, when the calf muscle expands during exercise the force produced by the calf muscle on to the bandage is effectively reapplied back onto the vessels within the leg. So, although the bandage has not become tighter, the size of the leg increases (during activity), which effectively results in an increased sub-bandage pressure during activity (Charles, 2001).

High working and low resting pressures: Because of the action described above, inelastic bandages are said to offer high working pressures and low resting pressures. This resulting fluctuation of pressures experienced by the patient during work or active periods, as opposed to during rest periods, may be seen as being more appealing to a patient than wearing a bandage that applies high levels of compression, with only very minor fluctuations, at all times. This feature is particularly relevant for those patients with mixed (venous and arterial) disease, where inelastic bandages may be a suitable choice: applying sufficient levels of compression to address a venous problem, but allowing periods of reduced pressure so as not to significantly restrict arterial function on a continual basis. Nevertheless, the appropriateness of this type of bandage will depend on the degree of arterial disease present and the symptoms experienced by the patient (Hofman & Cherry, 1998). Inelastic bandaging may also be beneficial for those patients who predominantly experience pain at night (which may or may not relate to the presence of arterial disease) when, providing the patient is going to bed at night, less pressure is required to aid venous return.

From a theoretical perspective, inelastic bandages have generally been considered less effective than elastic regimes for immobile patients (Acton et al., 2006). However, a sub-group analysis, undertaken following a randomised control trial comparing a cohesive inelastic bandage with a multi-layer elastic system, demonstrated better healing rates for immobile patients with the inelastic system (Franks et al., 2004). This outcome is perhaps somewhat surprising, though when it comes to considering a patient's ability to mobilise, what is more significant is the mobility of the ankle joint. Being able to flex and rotate the ankle enables the patient to activate the calf muscle and foot pump, and thus benefit from the higher working pressures generated with regular ankle exercises.

Type 3 bandages

Bandages that fall in this group are elasticated (long stretch) and able to apply varying levels of sustained graduated compression (for periods up to a week). In comparison to inelastic bandages, the pressure applied to the limb is relatively constant, with less notable fluctuations in sub-bandage pressure according to whether the patient is active or resting. Likewise, there is a less pronounced loss of sub-bandage pressure over the course of wear-time with an elastic system as opposed to an inelastic system (Brouwer et al., 2005). On an individual basis these bandages are capable of reversing some of the effects of chronic venous hypertension, though they are frequently used in varying combinations, being dependent on the patient's ankle circumference to achieve a desired level of compression. This is referred to as 'multi-layer compression bandaging' – though this term also applies to inelastic systems or a combination of the two.

Elastic bandages are generally applied at 50–75% stretch. They are potentially hazardous if applied inexpertly or inappropriately (i.e. to patients with severe peripheral vascular disease).

Type 3 bandages are further divided into four different types according to the level of compression they are able to apply:

Type 3a: when applied in a spiral provides 12–14 mmHg; in a figure of eight, 14–17 mmHg. Can be used alone (with padding) to provide a reduced level of compression for patients with mixed venous/arterial disease or for those unable to tolerate high compression.
Examples: Elset (SSL); K-plus (Urgo); Litepress-Profore#3 (S&N).

Type 3b: Generally applied in a spiral as the final layer in a multi-layer system, provides approximately 18–24 mmHg. Because these bandages often contain latex, they should not come into contact with a patient's skin: latex-free bandages are available. Can also be used with padding and crepe to create a multi-layer system that provides reduced levels of compression.
Examples: Coban (3M); Coplus-Profore#4 (S&N); Ko-flex (Urgo); Ultra fast (Robinson).

Type 3c: High compression bandages that provide 25–35 mmHg. Applied in a spiral, with wool padding to protect the limb from potential pressure damage.
Examples: Setopress (SSL); Surepress (ConvaTec); Tensopress – Profore Plus (S&N).

Type 3d: Extra-high compression provides up to 60 mmHg at the ankle. These bandages are not routinely used in the management of clients with leg ulcers.
Examples: Blue line webbing (Seaton Healthcare Group).

> See the bandage application guide (Fig. 2.2b) for suggested bandage regimes to achieve full compression (using elastic and inelastic systems), reduced compression and support bandaging.

The need for a new bandage classification

In the future it is possible that instead of using terms such as 'reduced compression' and 'full compression', compression therapy will be prescribed more specifically in relation to the pressure that is applied and the stiffness within the bandage. Stiffness is important as the degree of stiffness influences the working and resting pressure. The stiffer the bandage, the higher the pressure during walking. This is thought to be one of the most important mechanisms that influence both the haemodynamic effect and ultimately ulcer healing. Traditional bandage systems, such as four-layer systems, have been shown to have a high level of stiffness, and therefore to act as both an elastic bandage (higher sustained resting pressure) and in a similar way to an inelastic bandage (providing a high working pressure). It is important that in future all bandages are tested for these properties within randomised controlled trials (Partsch, 2005a, b).

The reality is that it is not known what the ultimate working and resting pressures are or what different regimes may work best for individual patient groups. The real test is not what pressures are being found but the rate of ulcer healing.

Other unknown factors may influence the overall effectiveness of the varying compression systems, in particular the elasticity of the bandage and the amount of force used to apply the bandage (Partsch, 2005b).

The present situation of classifying bandages as either elastic or inelastic is increasingly becoming a problem with the development of new bandages and bandage systems, in addition to a greater understanding of the effects of compression therapy (Partsch, 2005a). Hence the need for a new means of categorising bandages.

LIMB ASSESSMENT AND THE CHALLENGE OF ACHIEVING GRADUATED COMPRESSION

Graduated compression refers to the variation in the sub-bandage pressure applied to different parts of the leg to enhance the flow of venous blood from the foot and ankle back towards the heart. In order to achieve this therapeutic effect the sub-bandage pressure needs to be greatest at the ankle, gradually reducing towards the knee (Thomas, 1998).

Therefore when referring to high compression therapy, the level of pressure we are aiming to achieve is around 40–50 mmHg at the ankle, reducing to 20–25 mmHg just below the knee.

By applying a bandage at the same tension from ankle to knee the bandage pressure will gradually reduce due to the principles explained by the law of Laplace, providing the leg is of a relatively normal shape. A normal shape being where the ankle circumference is (considerably) less than that of the calf (Fig. 14.1). The smaller surface area at the ankle results in relatively high pressures and as the surface area of the limb increases, particularly at the calf, the pressure will naturally reduce.

Problems arise when dealing with patients whose legs do not fit into the 'normal' category. This includes situations where limb shape is distorted – be it due to chronic oedema, injury, congenital abnormality or other disease process – or where legs are very thin or lack any natural gradient, i.e. the ankle and calf measurements are very similar (Fig. 14.2). It is likely that such patients will experience problems related to bandage application. This could result in excessive levels of pressure to vulnerable areas (see Fig.14.5) of the limb, which will result in increased pain and discomfort. Or there will be difficulty in achieving graduation and therefore in not obtaining the therapeutic effects considered necessary for healing to occur.

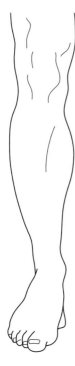

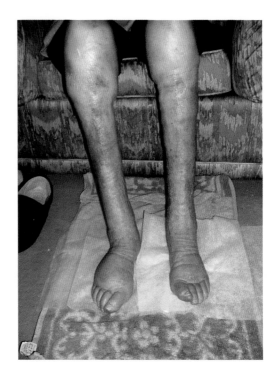

Fig. 14.1 The normal shaped leg.

Fig. 14.2 The thin or straight leg.

Alternatively, the problem of insufficient pressure often arises when the ulcer is located in the hollows behind the malleoli: because the bandage is somewhat elevated above the skin by the ankle bone, there is often little or no pressure to this area. This is why ulcers in this area can be so difficult to heal and require pads to increase the local pressure to these areas (Fig. 14.3).

The inverted 'champagne-bottle' shaped leg, which occurs following long-standing lipodermatosclerosis, often presents as a limb with a narrow ankle (and gaiter region) but with an abnormally large, oedematous calf. In some cases the lipodermatosclerosis can extend further, as seen in Fig. 14.4. When bandaging is

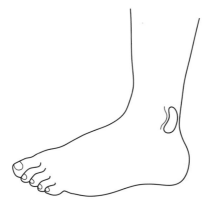

Fig. 14.3 Pressure pad to the retromalleoli area.

applied it may be possible to obtain the necessary high pressure at the ankle; however there is generally inadequate pressure at the calf to effectively reduce the oedema. Bandage slippage is often a common problem for patients with legs this shape, and ultimately this can lead to skin trauma and discomfort.

To achieve graduation in the awkward shaped leg, extra padding should be used to reshape the leg until it resembles a more normal shape. This may mean making an artificial calf (Fig. 14.5) or trying to reduce the difference between a narrow ankle and a large calf. Care must be taken not to apply too much padding, as a significant increase in the circumference of the limb will reduce the level of compression applied. The ankle circumference should be re-measured after application of padding.

Without appropriate reshaping, rather than enhancing the venous return the result is more akin to squeezing toothpaste out from the middle of the tube (Fig. 14.6).

Wool padding is the first layer of all multi-layer compression systems and is applied in a spiral technique. Cotton stockinette may be used beneath this layer for patients who find the wool hot or irritating. The padding serves several purposes: (i) it helps shape the limb; (ii) it protects the limb from excessive levels of pressure; and (iii) it absorbs exudate. Depending upon the size and

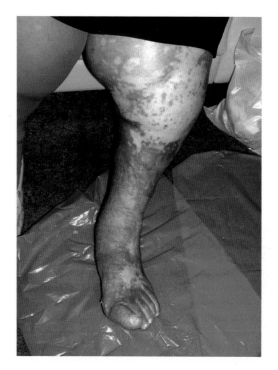

Fig. 14.4 The 'inverted champagne bottle' shape, in addition to severe knee swelling.

shape of the limb and the fragility of the skin, extra orthopaedic wool or padding can be applied, but always bear in mind how this will affect the application of the compression.

> When ordering or prescribing bandaging for the patient with an awkward shaped leg, make sure you have sufficient orthopaedic wool padding as more than one roll may be required. This is the cheapest component of multi-layer bandage regimes and will help to ensure the compression applied will stay in place and enhance healing rather than hamper it. Just remember that bulking up the limb is also likely to reduce the level of compression applied, so recheck the ankle circumference once the padding is in place.

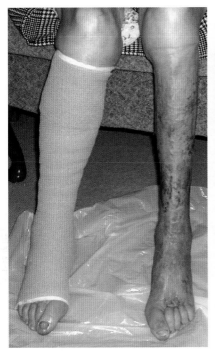 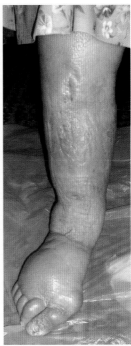

Fig. 14.5 (*Left*) Reshaping the thin leg (note pressure damage visible on the patient's left leg).

Fig. 14.6 (*Right*) Poor bandaging technique has contributed to forefoot and toe oedema.

Particular bony prominences and vulnerable areas of the leg, such as the tibial crest, dorsum of the foot and Achilles tendon, are more likely to be vulnerable to excessive levels of pressure and may require extra padding to prevent pressure necrosis. A variety of padding or wadding bandages is available. Synthetic types tend to maintain their loft better than natural products even when they become wet; however sensitivity and allergies are less likely to be a problem with natural fibres. New orthopaedic wools are being developed with improved cushioning ability and exudate management. Examples include: Flexiban (Activa); K-Soft (Urgo); Soffban/Profore #1(S&N).

> Using a cotton liner/stockinette (e.g. Actifast (Activa) or Tubifast (SSL)) may help to hold dressings in place and improve client comfort by reducing any friction beneath the bandages or sensitivity caused by the wool padding.
>
> Several sizes are available; order these on a 5- or 10-m roll rather than in 1-metre lengths in an attempt to reduce wastage.

BANDAGING TECHNIQUES

In the UK, the two most common means of bandage application include the simple spiral (Figs 14.7a–h) and a figure-of-eight technique (Figs 14.8a–f). More complex techniques are used on the continent, but these have not been widely adopted due to the specialist skills required in their application (Mear & Moffatt, 2002).

Regardless of whether a spiral or figure-of-eight technique is applied, some basic principles should be observed (Moffatt & Harper, 1997; Mear & Moffatt, 2002):

- The practitioner should always consider manual handling issues – think about the position of the patient and being able to get as close to the patient's leg as possible to avoid bending or over-extending.
- Always check and follow the manufacturer's instructions regarding bandage application.
- A 10-cm width bandage is appropriate for most adult lower limbs.
- After the bandage has been applied, encourage the patient to point and flex their ankle to remind them the bandage is not like a cast.
- Assist the patient into their shoes. Although a sock may seem to add more bulk to the layers (providing it is not too thick or too small), it can be helpful to aid sliding the foot into the shoe without disturbing the bandaging. An old pop-sock or nylon hosiery that can be cut to just cover the foot is ideal.

Bandage placement

- Ask the patient to flex their foot 'toes to nose' to help avoid excessive layers of bandage around the ankle.

- Bandages should always be applied from the base of the toes to just below the back of the knee (two finger-tip widths below the popliteal fossa).
- Consider any foot deformities, and work with the patient to find what is most comfortable for them in terms of avoiding excessive levels of pressure at vulnerable areas. Leaving the foot unbandaged to enable the patient to wear shoes will only lead to the foot becoming oedematous.
- The heel should be checked to ensure there are no gaps in the bandage.
- Toe bandaging may be required if the toes are very oedematous.
- Unless the patient's foot is particularly long it should be possible to enclose the foot with three bandage turns.
- If the forefoot is oedematous an extra bandage turn over this area will help to reduce the oedema.

Bandage overlap

- Bandage overlap must be consistent in order to ensure a constant number of layers and even pressure along the leg.
- Overlap should always be 50%, resulting in two (when applied as spiral) or four (when applied in a figure-of-eight) layers of bandage at any point along the leg.
- An overlap of more or less than 50% results in areas of inconsistent higher and lower pressures.
- Be aware if there is a lot of excess bandaging remaining when finishing off at the knee. Finishing off with several layers of bandage will only result in a tourniquet effect and will not enable venous return – instead, cut the bandage. The only exception to this is in the case of the non-cohesive inelastic bandages as the threads run from end to end – in this case, either bring the spiral back down the leg but with virtually no pressure, or use a smaller size bandage (i.e. 8 cm width).
- If the patient's limb is very long and a second bandage is required to reach the knee start the second layer where the first ended (try to avoid excessive overlap)

Fig. 14.7 The simple spiral technique.

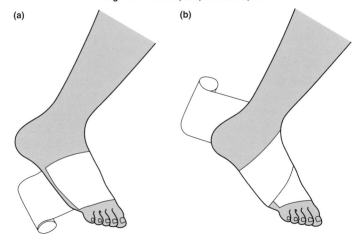

(a) Hold the bandage so the roll is on top, Start as near to the base of the toes, either medially or laterally. Use 2 turns of the forefoot if very oedematous.
(b) Once the bandage is secure take it across the foot towards the heel. Keep the bandage low on the heel, just taking in a little of the sole of the foot.

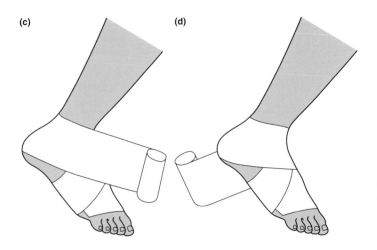

(c) Complete the turn around the heel, coming back towards the foot.
(d) Enclose the foot, sealing the gap at the base of the heel.

Fig. 14.7 *Continued*

(e)   **(f)**

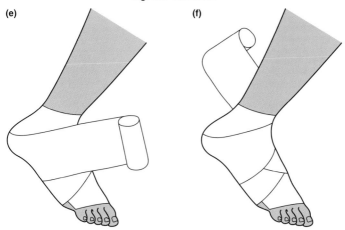

(e) Bring the bandage across the top of the foot to the ankle.
(f) Complete the turn around the ankle.

(g)   **(h)**

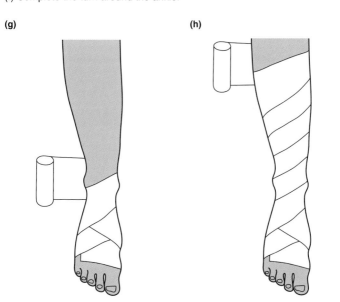

(g) Begin spiral technique around the leg, overlapping the previous turn by 50%.
(h) Continue up the leg, finishing 2 fingertips below the back of the knee.

Fig. 14.8 The figure-of-eight technique.

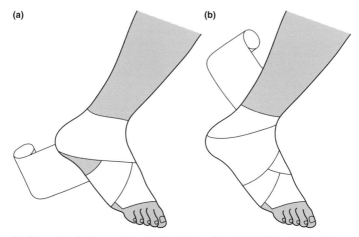

(a) Secure the foot as per the spiral technique (Fig 14.7ad). When taking the bandage to the ankle use a slightly larger angle (up the leg).
(b) From the ankle take the bandage around the leg, again at a slightly larger angle (up the leg).

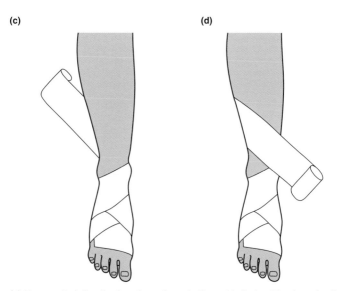

(c) Prepare to bring the bandage down to the ankle but not back under the foot.
(d) Bring the bandage back down the leg, turning around the Achilles region.

Fig. 14.8 *Continued*

(e)

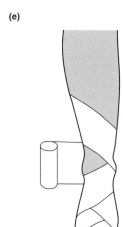

(f)

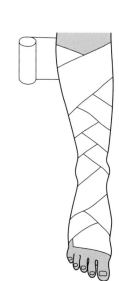

(e) Straighten the bandage around the back of the leg and prepare to take the bandage back up the leg on the next turn. A criss-cross pattern will emerge.

(f) Every time the bandage is passed around the back of the leg the turn will be either up or down (alternating). The bandage should overlap the second to last layer by 50%. Finish the bandage as per a spiral.

Bandage extension

- This varies according to the bandage being applied and individual manufacturer's recommendations for each of their products. Always consult the product information sheet that accompanies each bandage to ensure correct application.
- Keep the extension constant up the leg and only reduce this slightly above the calf. If the leg is well shaped (either naturally or by means of extra padding) the compression will be graduated without having to alter the extension or stretch applied to the bandage.

- Some bandages have symbols printed on them that aim to ensure the practitioner extends the bandage to the correct amount.

Examining the leg
- Always assess the effect of the bandaging on the patient's limb and make adjustments as necessary.
- Upon removal of the bandage consider the shape of the leg and foot; check for reduction of oedema (by measuring the ankle and calf) and ulcer size (wound mapping).
- Encourage the patient to express any problems or concerns regarding the bandage.
- Look for potential problems, such as puffy areas where oedema has formed. This indicates insufficient pressure in these areas either due to too few layers of bandage or insufficient bandage tension. Reddened, non-blanching areas indicate inappropriate high levels of pressure resulting in tissue damage. This can often be seen as a red line down the tibial crest (see Fig. 14.5). If this is not rectified, either by reducing the level of compression applied or increasing the amount of padding used, or both, tissue necrosis and pressure ulcers are likely to develop.
- If the leg ulcer is failing to show signs of healing always consider whether the level of compression is adequate for the size of the limb and whether the shape is enabling graduation of compression.

INTERMITTENT PNEUMATIC COMPRESSION THERAPY
Intermittent pneumatic compression (ICP) was originally developed for the prevention of deep vein thrombosis, but is now often used to treat venous ulceration, mixed arterial and venous ulceration and lymphoedema. The system consists of an inflatable boot connected to a pump. Compartments within the boot sequentially fill with air and thus apply pressure cyclically so assisting venous return, essentially mimicking the action of the foot and calf muscle pump.

A Cochrane review by Mani et al. (2001), evaluating the effectiveness of ICP for treating venous ulcers, concluded that while there is some evidence that ICP has some positive effect, the studies are too small to draw conclusions. Also, there is considerable variation in the ICP devices themselves and the way in which they are used (Gonsalkorale, 2002).

Nonetheless, the system is easy to use. Patients may apply this system at home over bandages and stockings. It may be particularly useful in patients who cannot tolerate high levels of compression, and is recommended as an adjunctive treatment in the international compression algorithm (Marston & Vowden, 2003).

CONTRAINDICATIONS TO COMPRESSION THERAPY

Even when there is evidence of venous disease there are some occasions where high compression therapy (30–40 mmHg) should not be used. These include when:

- There is significant arterial disease present, where the ABPI is below 0.8 (unless guided by a specialist practitioner) (see Box 14.1).
- Lower limb oedema is caused by cardiac, kidney or liver failure.
- Deep vein thrombosis is suspected or confirmed but anticoagulant treatment has not yet been commenced.

Special care should also be taken with those clients who:

- Have some form of sensory deficit, e.g. patients with diabetic neuropathy, are paralysed or have conditions such as multiple sclerosis.
- Are unable to communicate their needs effectively, such as those with learning disabilities, mental health issues and dementia or confusion.

Patients need to be able to let their nurse or other healthcare practitioner know if there are any problems with the treatment.

Box 14.1 What is the significance of an ABPI reading of 0.8?

In practice, this figure of 0.8 has become synonymous with the cut-off point for compression therapy and in determining ulcer aetiology.

The first point to clarify is the use of Doppler to determine ulcer aetiology (this is covered in much more depth in Chapter 5). It is a misconception to diagnose venous ulceration or mixed disease on the

Continued

---

basis of an ABPI reading. The ABPI will only inform the practitioner of the degree of peripheral arterial function. Venous disease is confirmed by the presence of other signs and symptoms (see Chapter 4).

In regards to deciding when compression is safe to apply, an ABPI of <0.8 has been routinely adopted as an exclusion criteria for compression therapy trials, though presently there is no clinical evidence to fully support or deny this approach (Vowden & Vowden, 2001; Partsch, 2003). Of course, it is important to take a considered approach to using compression therapy since the possibility of hindering arterial blood flow is a potential problem for some patients. However, as Vowden and Vowden (2001) point out, it is also incorrect to base the decision to apply or not to apply compression on just one figure. Rather, there are several factors that should be taken into consideration, such as:

- Any significant differences (15 mmHg or more) between the three main arteries at the ankle.
- The shape of the limb, presence of bony prominences and skin condition.
- The function of the microcirculatory vessels, which is likely to be affected by the presence of conditions such as diabetes mellitus and rheumatoid arthritis.
- How well the patient is likely to tolerate compression and the presence of any arterial symptoms.

Problems arise from a lack of understanding about what really are safe levels of compression to apply in the presence of arterial disease. These revolve around trying to provide guidance for practitioners to know when they can safely apply compression, and also to ensure that patients are protected from unsafe practice. Practitioners who consider themselves to be competent to apply compression therapy should be aware of this issue. However, in the authors' experience this level of understanding is not routinely witnessed, and the influence that this single 0.8 reading has over the decision-making process of ulcer diagnosis and choice of compression remains strong.

The way to challenge this blinkered approach to making decisions is to ensure education opportunities are available, so practitioners can develop their understanding of the effects of compression and know how to make treatment plans on the basis of a holistic assessment. In addition, education should be used to promote the importance of the multi-disciplinary team in the decision-making process when managing patients with complex multi-factorial or mixed ulceration.

If they cannot feel or explain that the bandaging is uncomfortable then there is the potential for complications, such as pressure damage, to occur.

Special considerations for the use of compression in patients with venous ulceration and diabetes mellitus are discussed in Chapter 6, and its use in mixed aetiology and rarer aetiologies in Chapter 7.

MANAGING VENOUS ULCERS

- Graduated, multi-layer, high compression systems are the recommended treatment for uncomplicated venous leg ulcers (Cullum et al., 2001; Marston & Vowden, 2003)
- Before applying any form of compression, every patient must have a full clinical assessment and a differential diagnosis made. Severe arterial insufficiency of the limb as well as cardiac/renal oedema and active DVT must be excluded.

The main cause of venous leg ulcers is chronic venous hypertension, resulting in high pressures being exerted on the superficial venous system (see Chapter 4). The consequent aim of venous ulcer management is to:

- Reduce blood pressure in the superficial venous system
- Aid venous return of blood to the heart
- Reduce oedema
- Promote ulcer healing

Compression therapy can be applied to the limb in a number of different ways. It can be in the form of bandaging, hosiery and intermittent pneumatic compression.

Other important actions that patients can perform themselves to aid venous return and reduce oedema are to exercise and elevate their legs.

When educating the patient about the best way to help heal their venous ulcer/s the advice given to the patient should include:

- When they are on their feet they need to be walking.
- When they are not walking they should be lying down or seated so that their legs are above the level of their heart.

- If possible, the foot of their beds could be raised to enhance venous return even further.
- Clients who are less mobile should be encouraged to perform ankle exercises.
- Periods spent standing or seated with the legs dependent need to be avoided or limited to short periods only.
- Compression bandaging is a therapy that has proven to be an effective treatment for healing venous leg ulcers, it is not just a dressing for the wound.

Choosing the right compression for your patient

In the UK the multi-layered bandage systems (e.g. Charing Cross 4-layer system, K-Four, Profore) are considered to be the 'gold standard' for the treatment of venous ulcers. They are commonly referred to as the 'four-layer bandage'. However, this term can be misleading as the number and type of bandages used varies according to a person's ankle circumference. Nor does this term tend to include inelastic systems, which are also proven to be effective for venous ulcer treatment but are more commonly used in mainland Europe.

The original four-layer bandage system was developed in the 1980s by a team of clinicians at Charing Cross Hospital, London. Utilising theoretical knowledge developed by Stemmer (1980) – relating to the levels of external compression required to enable healing of venous ulcers, combined with knowledge of the practical issues associated with managing leg ulceration on an outpatient basis – the concept of the four-layer bandage was born. The four-layer bandage was designed to (Moffatt, 2004b):

- Apply a pressure of 35–40 mmHg.
- Sustain these levels of compression for up to a week (so reducing the number of dressing changes and improving cost-effectiveness).
- Be tested to ensure it could achieve reproducible pressures on a wide range of patients and, with some adaptation, apply the required level of compression to significantly larger (over 25 cm) or smaller (under 18 cm) limbs.

Four-layer bandaging has been trialled on numerous occasions – it has been compared with single-layer elastic bandages, inelastic bandages and other multi-layer systems. The Cochrane systematic review (Cullum et al., 2001) of compression for venous leg ulcers states that:

- Compression aids ulcer healing rates when compared to not using compression.
- Multi-layered systems are more effective than single-layer systems.
- High compression is more effective than low compression.

Unfortunately, however, there is no clear guidance when it comes to choosing which high compression system is most effective.

In Wandsworth tPCT, both multi-layer elastic and inelastic bandages are recommended and used on a fairly equal basis. There have been several multi-centre, randomised controlled trials (RCTs) comparing the healing rates of ulcers with these two systems (Table 14.3). From a clinician's point of view, the results of these trials report similar healing rates regardless of the bandage used.

The availability of a number of good quality RCTs on compression bandaging has had a tremendous effect in ensuring a large number of patients receive treatments based on the best available evidence. However, it is worth bearing in mind that RCTs are performed on patients who are very different from those treated in routine practice, and who are likely to have more complex health needs and reduced levels of mobility. Appropriate, consistent, high quality compression that is well applied is the factor that leads to fast healing. While complex patients may take longer to heal, compression therapy is no less beneficial.

Both elastic and inelastic bandages have been trialled in numerous RCTs, and both have proven to be equally successful at healing ulcers. This means that patients have a wider choice of effective bandage treatments, each with varying features that may make one type of bandage more suitable than another according to the patient's needs.

The only problem is that the research has not helped us to know when one type of material may be beneficial over another. This choice is still based on clinical opinion and experience, which is very variable.

Table 14.3 Multicentre randomised control trials comparing the healing rates of ulcers with four-layer and inelastic bandaging.

Study	Total no. of patients	Patient and ulcer details	Trial duration (weeks)	Total no. of healed ulcers	Trial investigators conclusions
Partsch et al., 2001 Four-layer bandage – Profore (4LB) vs short-stretch bandage – Rosidal K (SSB)	112: 4LB 53 SSB 59	Mean age: 4LB 68; SSB 71 Mean ulcer duration (weeks): 4LB 5; SSB 4 Median ulcer size(cm^2): 4LB 1.5; SSB 1.9	16	76: 4LB 33 SSB 43	There was no significant difference between ulcer healing rate and the median time to healing with either bandage system
Ukat et al., 2003 Profore (P) vs. Comprilan (C)	89: P 44 C 45	Mean age: P 67; C 70 No. of ulcers >6 months old: P 23; C 25 Median ulcer size (cm^2): P 6.5; C 6.6	12	23: P 13 C 10	Patients treated with Profore healed quicker than those with Comprilan, and there may be associated cost and time savings

Franks et al., 2004 Comparison of generic four-layer bandage system (4LB) with a cohesive short-stretch bandage (CSSB)	159*: 4LB 74 CSSB 82	Mean age: 4LB 67.5; CSSB 70.9 Mean ulcer duration (weeks): 4LB 8; CSSB 8 Median ulcer size (cm^2): 4LB 5; CSSB 3.5	24	111: 4LB 51 CSSB 60	The healing rates were similar for the two bandage systems
Nelson et al., 2004 Trial of four-layer bandage (4LB) and short-stretch compression bandage (SSCB)	387: 4LB 195 SSCB 192	Mean age: 4LB 71.9; SSCB 71.3 Median ulcer duration (months): 4LB 3; SSCB 3 Median ulcer size (cm^2): 4LB 3.81; SSCB 3.82	Follow-up continued until healing of reference limb or for a minimum of 12 months	Median time to healing (days): 4LB 92 SSCB 126	Four-layer bandages were more likely to result in the healing of venous leg ulcers than short-stretch bandages

*Three patients did not achieve pre-randomisation selection so were excluded from the study.

The available options

Inelastic bandaging
Pros:

- As these bandages do not tend to provide sustained levels of high compression, they can offer some potential for use with clients with mixed venous and arterial disease (under the supervision of specialist practitioner) or to aid management of painful venous ulceration.
- Non-cohesive bandages can be washed and re-used many times.
- Easy for practitioners to learn to apply.
- Also a relatively easy option for those clients wishing to apply their own bandages.
- Fewer layers of bandaging are required for an ankle circumference under 25 cm.
- Cohesive type bandages tend to stay in place for longer periods and can be left in situ for up to a week, providing there are no significant fluctuations in the size of the limb due to oedema.

Cons:

- Less able to provide sustained compression over the course of a week and may require more frequent reapplication, especially at the beginning of treatment.
- There are some suggestions that these bandages may have lower resting pressures than elastic bandages, which may make them less effective for immobile patients; however good ankle function may help to overcome this issue.

Elastic bandaging
Pros:

- Applies sustained levels of compression (for periods up to a week).
- Less slippage.
- Applies relatively constant levels of compression, regardless of whether the client is active or resting.
- Varying combinations of bandages can be used to obtain more specific levels of compression as desired.

- Multi-layer systems may have similar properties to inelastic bandages in terms of increased levels of pressure during activity.

Cons:

- Applies constant levels of compression, which may make them less tolerable for some clients.
- Bandages are less suitable for washing and re-use.
- Requires a more complex application technique in regards to the correct tension to be applied to the bandage, allowing a greater potential for too much or too little pressure.
- Bandaging may be perceived as bulky and affect footwear.

Hosiery
Pros:

- Washable and reusable.
- Less bulky than bandages, minimising problems with footwear.
- Relatively easy for practitioners to apply.
- The correct levels of compression are more likely to be consistently applied.
- Patients can manage their leg ulceration more independently.
- Different classes of hosiery can be layered to achieve different levels of compression.
- Several variations of hosiery kits are available, allowing for even greater patient choice.

Cons:

- As the hosiery applies high levels of sustained compression without the use of padding, patients must be able to remove stronger hosiery at night.
- Hosiery may be inappropriate for very large or wet wounds, due to the need for larger, more bulky dressings.
- May be inappropriate for very painful ulcers, due to the physical action of pulling hosiery over the wound.
- Any oedema in a limb needs to be reduced prior to fitting with hosiery.

A small range of hosiery kits designed to apply the correct amount of pressure required for venous ulcer healing are presently available in the UK. Each has some useful variation, potentially making one type more suitable for a patient than another:

- Activa leg ulcer hosiery kits come with two liners and are also available in an XXL size.
- Jobst Ulcercare (BSN) has a zipper in the stronger hosiery to enable easier application and removal.
- SurPress ComfortPro (Convatec) is latex-free, and applies a slightly reduced level of pressure at 35 mmHg.
- Venotrain (Ulcertec) comes in a choice of short or longer length styles.

Vari-stretch bandaging

This is a new type of compression bandage called Proguide (trade-name of Smith & Nephew) that comes as a two-layer system (padding plus one compression bandage). The Proguide system applies high levels of compression (40 mmHg) even when applied at a reduced tension (< 50%), making it an unsuitable choice for any client with even mild arterial disease (ABPI < 0.8). This bandage regime is best suited for those clients able to tolerate high levels of pressure on a weekly basis.

Using an application guide (markings on the bandages, which, in an unstretched state, appear as an oval enclosing two crossing lines) and new elastomer technology, the bandage is designed to be easier to apply and less sensitive to changes of the limb due to increasing or decreasing amounts of oedema. These features help to minimise potential problems such as variations of pressure levels applied by different practitioners, reduce the risk of pressure damage and yet ensure sufficient levels of compression to reverse the effects of venous hypertension (Thomas, 2003b).

The bandage is applied at 50% stretch (until the oval becomes a circle and the two crossed lines are at 90-degree angles) with a 50% overlap using a spiral technique.

The bandage is designed to apply a high level of compression, at least 40 mmHg (full compression) at the ankle. The smart elastomeric fibres ensure that, as long as the bandage is applied within a 30–70% stretch range, the sub-bandage pressure should remain around 40 mmHg. The bandage can remain in place for up to 7 days.

There are three different kits available, depending upon the patient's ankle size. The bandaging is latex-, colophony- and thiuram-free so is suitable for clients with sensitive skin (Thomas, 2003b).

> Regardless of what form of external compression is decided to be the most appropriate, if the correct size or bandage regime is not used then the pressure applied is likely to be too little or too much.
>
> Inadequate pressure levels will delay wound healing. Too high a pressure could lead to pressure necrosis.
>
> It is recommended that ankle and calf measurements are taken as a part of the patient's ongoing assessment. Not only will this help to ensure the correct bandage or hosiery is in use in order to achieve the necessary or desired pressures, it will enable more accurate assessment and monitoring of any oedema changes.

Benchmarks for compression therapy

The International Leg Ulcer Advisory Board (Marston & Vowden, 2003) has suggested some general points for consideration when choosing the most suitable system for a patient. These include:

- Clinical effectiveness – is there evidence to support its use?
- The ability to provide sustained compression – can it stay in place for up to a week?
- Will it enhance the calf-muscle pump?
- Is it non-allergenic?
- Is it easy to apply (easy to learn to apply)?
- Is it conformable and comfortable?
- Is it durable?

While the benchmarks offer a starting point, practitioners need to consider which of these are most important from the patient's perspective. Sustainability, for example, helps in saving time and money with less frequent visits required and application of bandaging. However, if exudate levels are heavy and/or the patient is unable or too uncomfortable keeping a bandage on for a week at a time, then it is not a useful criterion. Something that is comfortable and resolves the problem is more likely to be chosen. As Dowsett (2004) concluded, we can base treatments on the best evidence available to us but if it is not acceptable to the patient, then it will never get the chance to work.

Patient concordance is an important issue in choosing the right bandage for that patient, and as such is covered in much more depth in Chapter 11. Patients are frequently blamed for not complying with treatments such as compression bandaging. While there is little evidence to suggest how big an issue concordance actually is, in practice the perception (expressed by practitioners) appears to be that concordance is a common problem. On the other hand, patients frequently express another point of view, reporting that they have not been informed about the purpose of the bandage or that they had not been given any choice in the type of bandage used.

Our approach needs to be considerate of our patients' individual needs. We will only understand these through careful assessment and open discussion.

Patients who have had a previously bad experience with compression may be reluctant to try this therapy again, so it is important to consider all the options and discuss these with the patient before commencing any treatment. An initial bad experience with compression may damage the practitioner–patient relationship, and can result in severe deterioration of the ulcer. Moffatt (2004a) suggests slowly introducing compression over the course of a number of weeks, to give the patient time to adjust.

If your patient is experiencing moderate to severe levels of pain they are unlikely to be able to tolerate high levels of compression initially, even if the compression should help in the long run.

Assess the patient's current analgesia and develop a plan with them to:

- Start taking regular analgesia, **or**
- Increase their present dose, **or**
- Review their present analgesia and consider a different type or an adjuvant.

Then over the course of a week or two start introducing the compression.

Remember, some compression is better than no compression. The important thing is that you and your patient are working together towards a common goal.

Case study

You be the judge – is compliance the real issue? Rose, a 98-year-old woman, is referred to you by her district nurses with an ulcer history of 6 weeks' duration, which occurred following a trauma to the leg. There are some small varicosities and venous oedema, she has an ABPI of 0.71. There are no other significant health problems. Rose is referred to you because of her mixed disease and because she is non-compliant with her treatment.

You arrive at Rose's house before the community nurse and she begins to tell you about her leg ulcer. The first thing she asks you is if you'll be able to 'make the bandages less'. She presently has a three-layer system (padding, crepe and a 3A bandage) in place, as applied by the community nurse. Rose tells you that since the wound became a problem and she has needed bandages she has been unable to leave her house as she feels more unsteady with the bandage on. She now only gets to go out when her daughter is around to push her in the wheelchair. Rose goes on to tell you that she would rather have the swelling and wound than the bandage, and for the first time in her life she has felt so fed up that she could actually contemplate taking a pill to end it all. What other options could Rose be offered?

MANAGING ARTERIAL ULCERS

Where arterial disease is the primary cause of the ulcer, the prognosis of wound healing is often poor with conservative treatment alone – even if the most effective and expensive dressings are chosen. The only way to improve the potential for healing arterial ulceration is to improve the blood supply to the limb and thus enhance tissue perfusion (Moffatt, 2001). Therefore further assessment and intervention by a vascular team is vital for the management of clients with these ulcers; this is covered in more detail in Chapter 12.

Compression therapy is contraindicated for the management of arterial ulcers. An ABPI reading under 0.92 signifies the presence of arterial disease, with 0.8 generally being regarded as the cut-off point for *full* compression therapy. In practice, however, actual arterial ulceration is less likely to present where the ABPI is over 0.5 (Vowden & Vowden, 2001).

The options for treatment (while the patient is awaiting vascular review) include retention and some light support bandages.

The lightest form of bandages are referred to as type 1. These are often highly elastic but only apply minimal pressure to the limb (Thomas, 1998). They will help to hold dressings in place and contain the exudate.

If a little more support is required, to help reduce oedema for example, and can be tolerated by the patient then a type 2 bandage may be considered. Bandages falling into this category range in their ability to provide very light, to moderate, to high levels of support. Depending upon the degree of arterial disease and the amount of oedema present, it would be advisable to apply light or moderate levels of support only, unless advised otherwise under the guidance of a vascular team or specialist practitioner. Examples of light support include Soffcrepe – Profore #2 (S&N) and K-lite (Urgo). For more moderate support (approximately 12 mmHg) or for larger limbs (ankle circumference greater than 25 cm), Elasto-crepe (BSN) may be a suitable option.

Controlling or attempting to reduce oedema in a limb is difficult when trying to manage it in conjunction with arterial disease. However, it is an important management tactic in terms of attempting to optimise tissue perfusion. Where oedema is present it is usually due to limb dependency related to ischaemic pain, thus analgesia is imperative. The presence of oedema can result in increased exudate and skin maceration, not to mention additional pain and discomfort. Other potential causes of oedema should also be considered and investigated prior to the application of any support bandaging. While elevation of the legs will help to resolve the oedema, this may not be suitable advice for patients with severe ischaemia: elevation is likely to exacerbate the level of pain experienced due to reducing the effect of gravity on tissue perfusion, and may exacerbate the ischaemia.

> Regardless of the bandage type, it should always be applied toe to knee and with a layer of padding.

MANAGING MIXED ARTERIAL AND VENOUS ULCERS
There is the potential for both venous and arterial disease to be present and contributing to the underlying pathology of a leg ulcer, although there is some controversy, however, as to whether

the term 'mixed ulcer' is a correct one. Vowden & Vowden (2001) suggest that this term implies the ulcer has a dual aetiology, whereas what is more likely is that the ulcer is essentially of venous origin but the degree of arterial insufficiency present prevents the use of high levels of compression.

The development of both venous disease and peripheral arterial disease are strongly age-related, therefore the potential for this problem becomes more prevalent in the older person. The concept of mixed ulceration also demonstrates that ulcer aetiology is not entirely static, and explains why patients whose ulcers are slow to heal should be reassessed on a regular basis (3-monthly).

When managing any complex ulcer, which is essentially all of them except an uncomplicated venous ulcer, it is important to ensure the multi-disciplinary team (MDT) is utilised. The vascular team and leg ulcer specialists should be involved in the management of patients with mixed arterial and venous ulceration. See Chapter 12 for further discussion on managing these patients.

In the case of mixed arterial and venous disease the guiding factors will be:

- The degree of peripheral arterial occlusive disease (PAOD)
- The degree of venous disease
- The options for surgical intervention

For patients with an ABPI between 0.5 and 0.8 and depending on signs present (skin changes) and the symptoms experienced, a reduced level of compression between 15 and 25 mmHg may be appropriate (Marston & Vowden, 2003). Use of inelastic bandages or intermittent pneumatic compression may also prove to be useful systems because high pressures are not applied for extended periods. Likewise for some patients with only a mild degree of venous disease, high levels of compression may not actually be necessary to achieve healing, albeit over a slightly longer time frame. An ABPI under 0.5 and/or a history of ischaemic rest pain is a contraindication to compression therapy. However, if surgical intervention is appropriate and successful the arterial disease may be able to be corrected and then compression applied (Vowden & Vowden, 2001); although it can not be overstated that this decision should be made in conjunction with all members of the MDT.

MANAGING OTHER ULCER TYPES AND MULTI-FACTORIAL ULCERATION

When managing some of the other rarer types of leg ulcers (e.g. vasculitic, skin cancers, infectious disease-related), treatment will need to be guided by the appropriate medical team and will primarily rely on other forms of medical or surgical interventions. If venous disease and or oedema (remembering this may also require medical attention/intervention) are additional problems then compression therapy may be beneficial. However, the patient should be carefully screened for any contraindications to compression therapy. Furthermore, and as is the case in the management of mixed arterial and venous ulcers, the level of compression applied should be guided by the absence or presence of PAOD and in context of the holistic assessment (Marston & Vowden, 2003).

Indications for reduced compression

Conditions where high compression is not appropriate but reduced levels of compression therapy (15–25 mmHg) could be used include (Marston & Vowden, 2003):

- The management of an ulcer where both arterial (ABPI is over 0.5 but under 0.8) and venous disease are present.
- Following arterial reconstruction surgery (in consultation with the client's vascular team).
- Patients with active phlebitis.
- Patients with diabetes mellitus or rheumatoid arthritis (where microcirculatory function may be affected, or neuropathy is an issue).
- Where a patient has diminished sensation affecting the lower leg (e.g. paralysis, stroke, multiple sclerosis, diabetic neuropathy).
- When a patient is unable to tolerate full compression.

The bandage regimes recommended to achieve reduced levels of compression are set out in the bandage application guide (see Fig. 2.2b).

The principle (Laplace's law) which enables the application of high levels of pressure is also utilised to apply reduced levels. Practitioners may struggle to remember Laplace's law and its association to compression therapy, but it is by being aware of and being able to apply this concept to the practical activity of bandaging that enables the practitioner to know how to increase or decrease the level of compression applied.

CONCLUSION

The variety of products or means of applying compression presently available offers practitioners and patients many possible treatment options. Some practitioners might take the view that compression only comes in one type – or rather one amount of pressure. However, this is not true. The amount of support or compression applied to the limb needs to be carefully tailored to the individual according to the presence of venous disease, arterial disease, oedema, other underlying medical conditions and what the patient feels able to tolerate. By having a good understanding of your patient, the type of bandages available and an understanding of Laplace's law, it is possible to find a level of compression that enhances the venous blood return without reducing the arterial blood supply or compromising other conditions – and ultimately aid healing.

REFERENCES

Acton, C., Charles, H. & Hopkins, A. (2006) Are short-stretch bandages better than long-stretch? *Wounds UK* **2**(2): 90–92.

Brouwer, E.R., Damstra, R.J. & Partsch, H. (2005) Why does pressure decrease with short stretch bandages? In: *European Wound Management Association (EWMA): Free Paper Session* V51–55 (17/09/05). (EWMA Stuttgart Meeting program and abstracts document) http://www.stuttgart2005.org/documents/oral_presentations/Sa_1030_12.pdf

Charles, H. (2001) Using compression bandages in the treatment of venous leg ulceration. *Professional Nurse* **17**(2): 123–125.

Clark, M. (2003) Compression bandages: principles and definitions. In: *European Wound Management Association (EWMA) Position Document: Understanding Compression Therapy*. London, MEP Ltd, pp. 5–7.

Coull, A. & Clark, M. (on behalf of the Steering Group) (2005) Best practice statement for compression hosiery. *Wounds UK* **1**(1): 70–78.

Cullum, N., Nelson, E.A., Fletcher, A.W. & Sheldon, T.A. (2001) Compression for venous leg ulcers. Cochrane Database of Systematic Reviews 2001, Issue 2. Art. No.: CD000265. DOI: 10.1002/14651858. CD000265 http://www.mrw.interscience.wiley.com/cochrane/clsysrev/articles/CD000265/frame.html

Dowsett, C. (2004) Our agenda is to raise the standard of venous leg ulcer care. *Journal of Wound Care* **13**(5): 181–185.

Franks, P.J., Moody, M., Moffatt, C.J., Martin, R., Blewett, R., Seymour, E., Hildreth, A., Hourican, C., Collins, J., Heron, A. & Wound Healing Research Group (2004) Randomized trial of cohesive short-stretch versus four-layer bandaging in the management of venous ulceration. *Wound Repair and Regeneration* **12**(2): 157–162.

Gonsalkorale, M. (2002) External intermittent pneumatic compression. *Journal of Tissue Viability* **12**(2): 40–41. [Editorial]

Hofman, D. & Cherry, G. (1998) The use of short-stretch bandaging to control oedema. *Journal of Wound Care* **7**(1): 10–12.

Mani, R., Vowden, K. & Nelson, E.A (2001) Intermittent pneumatic compression for treating venous leg ulcers. Cochrane Database of Systematic Reviews 2001, Issue 4. Art. No.: CD001899. DOI: 10.1002/14651858.CD001899 http://www.mrw.interscience.wiley.com/cochrane/clsysrev/articles/CD001899/frame.html

Marston, W. & Vowden, K. (2003). Compression therapy: a guide to safe practice. In: *European Wound Management Association (EWMA) Position Document Understanding Compression Therapy*. London, MEP Ltd, pp. 11–17.

Mear, J. & Moffatt, C. (2002) Bandaging technique in the treatment of venous ulcers. *Nursing Times* **98**(44) (*NT* Plus Wound Care Supplement).

Moffatt, C. (2001) Leg ulcers. In: *Vascular Disease Nursing and Management* (S. Murray, ed.). London, Whurr Ltd, pp. 200–237.

Moffatt, C. (2004a) Factors that affect concordance with compression therapy. *Journal of Wound Care* **13**(7): 291–294.

Moffatt, C. (2004b) Four-layer bandaging: from concept to practice. Part 1: The development of the four-layer system. *World Wide Wounds* (Online): http://www.worldwidewounds.com/2004/december/Moffatt/Developing-Four-Layer-Bandaging.html

Moffatt, C. & Harper, P. (1997) *Leg Ulcers*. Edinburgh, Churchill Livingstone.

Nelson, E.A., Iglesias, C.P. Cullum, N. & Torgerson, D.J. on behalf of the VenUS 1 collaborators (2004) Randomized clinical trial of four-layer and short-stretch compression bandages for venous leg ulcers (VenUS 1). *British Journal of Surgery* **91**: 1292–1299.

Partsch, H. (2003) Understanding the patho physiological effects of compression. In: *European Wound Management Association (EWMA) Position Document Understanding Compression Therapy*. London, MEP Ltd, pp. 2–4.

Partsch, H. (2005a) The use of pressure change on standing as a surrogate measure of the stiffness of a compression bandage. *European Journal of Vascular and Endovascular Surgery* **30**: 415–421.

Partsch, H. (2005b) The Static Stiffness Index: a simple method to assess the elastic property of compression material in vivo. *Dermatologic Surgery* **31**: 625–630.

Partsch, H., Damstra, R.J., Tazelaar, D.J., Schuller-Petrovic, S., Velders, A.J., de Rooij, M.J.M., Tjon Lim Sang, R.R.M. & Quinlan, D. (2001)

Multicentre, randomised controlled trial of four-layer bandaging versus short-stretch bandaging in the treatment of venous leg ulcers. *VASA Zeitschrift für Gefässkrankheiten (Journal for Vascular Diseases)* **30**: 108–113.

RCN Institute (1998) *Clinical Practice Guidelines: The Management of Patients with Venous Leg Ulcers.* London, Royal College of Nursing.

SIGN (1998) *The Care of Patients with Chronic Leg Ulcer.* Edinburgh, Scottish Intercollegiate Guidelines Network, SIGN Publication No. 26.

Stemmer, R., Marescaux, J. & Furderer, C. (1980) Compression therapy of the lower extremities particularly with compression stockings. *Hautarzt*, **31**(7):355–65.

Thomas, S. (1998) Compression bandaging in the treatment of venous leg ulcers. *World Wide Wounds* (Online): http://worldwidewounds. com/1997/september/Thomas-Bandaging/bandage-paper.html

Thomas, S. (2003a) The use of the Laplace equation in the calculation of sub-bandage pressure. *World Wide Wounds* (online): http://www. worldwidewounds.com/2003/june/Thomas/Laplace-Bandages. html

Thomas, S. (2003b) An evaluation of a new type of compression bandaging system. *World Wide Wounds* (Online): http://www. worldwidewounds.com/2003/september/Thomas/New-Compression-Bondage.html/

Ukat, A., Konig, M., Vanscheidt, W. & Munter, K.C. (2003) Short-stretch versus multilayer compression for venous leg ulcers: a comparison of healing rates. *Journal of Wound Care* **12**(4): 139–143.

Vowden, P. & Vowden, K. (2001) Doppler assessment and ABPI: Interpretation in the management of leg ulceration. *World Wide Wounds* (Online): http://www.worldwidewounds.com/2001/march/ Vowden/Doppler-assessment-and-ABPI.htm

Part V
Evaluating Outcomes

This section covers the vital aspect of evaluation. Chapter 15 addresses the complex issues of how to evaluate the effects of a leg ulcer service. This is one of the most difficult challenges faced by nurse specialists who may have had no training or experience of this kind. The chapter describes some of the approaches that may be taken, as well as guidance on how to interpret the information from such evaluations.

The final chapter of this book is dedicated to the important issue of prevention of ulcer recurrence and evaluation of care. These are very important aspects, as without attention to issues such as reducing risk factors and use of compression hosiery, the majority of patients will experience a further leg ulcer. This chapter addresses the practical strategies that can be employed in the different clinical situations seen within a leg ulcer service.

Continuous, reflective evaluation of care is the single most important factor in helping ensure that patients can 'live well' with an ulcer and heal in the least amount of time.

Evaluating Outcomes of a Leg Ulcer Service

LEARNING OBJECTIVES

Nurses involved in leg ulcer management should be able to demonstrate:

❏ An understanding of the importance of service evaluation in ensuring the long-term viability of leg ulcer services.
❏ An understanding of the different approaches to service evaluation and when these are required.
❏ The ability to describe those outcomes that can be evaluated within a service evaluation and how these must be interpreted within different patient populations.
❏ An understanding of how the risk factors within the patient population influence outcomes such as healing rates and recurrence rates.
❏ The ability to describe the difficulties in developing outcomes of care for patients with ulceration that fails to heal.
❏ The ability to describe the range of other factors that can be measured in service evaluations.

INTRODUCTION

Evaluation should be an integral part of all nursing care. Historically, nurses have been very poor at evaluating the care of patients with leg ulceration. The literature frequently reports that patients remain unhealed for years and even decades without referral for a specialist opinion (Callam et al., 1985; Moffatt et al., 1992). Over the last few years there has been a shift in emphasis towards measuring outcomes of care; and the field of leg ulceration has been an excellent example of how this can influence decision makers in the healthcare system (Bosanquet, 1992; Franks & Posnett, 2003). Leg ulceration is now on the healthcare agenda within the NHS, although there is still much room for improvement. Practice is increasingly supported by clinical guidelines based on rigorous systematic reviews of the evidence, although these struggle to keep up with the increasing complexity of patients (RCN, 1998, 2006; SIGN, 1998).

APPROACHING SERVICE EVALUATION

In addition to the individual responsibility of nurses to evaluate their care, there is also a growing requirement for tissue viability specialists, leg ulcer specialists and nurse consultants to provide evidence of the effectiveness of their service. This type of information is required to assist with resource allocation and is increasingly important within an NHS that is driven by priority areas of care, with decreasing amounts of money available for investment in new services. Leg ulcer care must compete with many other areas of chronic disease management.

The approach to care laid out in this book is a real-life service model. Central to the effectiveness of this approach is the continuous process of service evaluation. Service evaluation can be a complex task and a full exploration of the subject lies outside the brief for this book; however, some of the main aspects are explored in this chapter.

> Nurses should seek advice if they are required to undertake a full service evaluation. Clinical audit and clinical governance units are useful sources of help.

Many different methods of evaluation exist, from simple questionnaires to complex clinical and cost-effectiveness studies. It is vital that the scope of the evaluation is carefully planned. Attention should be placed on deciding the aims and objectives of the evaluation and the methods required. Evaluation can be resource-intensive and this should be considered when planning such a project. It is much better to undertake a simple evaluation well than to be over-ambitious and fail to capture the information required.

Every attempt should be made to standardise the approach to data collection, for variations can lead to problems in analysis and interpretation. An example of this is the way in which the type of ulcer aetiology is confirmed. It is often useful to examine published studies to gather ideas about the most useful data to collect; this will then allow for benchmarking between similar services (Thomsom et al., 1996; Vowden et al., 1997).

The literature highlights the numerous factors that have been evaluated in leg ulcer studies (Phillips et al., 1994; Dodds, 2002; Adam et al., 2003; Morgan et al., 2004). The greatest information relates to healing rates. However, there is a growing awareness of the need to explore other factors that may be more important to patients such as symptom control and psychosocial elements, including health-related quality of life (HRQoL) issues (Franks et al., 1994; Bowling, 1995).

> Analysis of quality-of-life tools is complex due to the confounding effects of age and sex; advice from a statistician should always be sought.

Table 15.1 outlines some of the key factors that may be included in such a project. It is always useful to establish a team approach to evaluation and to draw on the expertise from audit departments or service development units who have greater experience in these areas.

HEALING RATES AS AN OUTCOME MEASURE

Over the last 15 years there has been growing emphasis on healing rates as the primary outcome measure in leg ulcer studies (Moffatt et al., 1992; Lambourne et al., 1996). While they appear to be simple to measure there are many factors that complicate their use as an outcome measure.

The literature indicates a huge variation in outcomes of compression therapy in trials and population studies. A number of factors influence this:

- The composition of the patient population
- The maturity of the service
- Familiarity with the bandage system
- Differences in length of time to evaluate healing
- Differences in application of bandages
- How quickly compression therapy is commenced

Table 15.1 Factors to include in evaluation of leg ulcer services.

	Comment	Methodology issues
Demographic factors		
Age	Complex ulcer aetiology is likely to increase with age (Moffatt et al., 2004)	Consider using a structured approach to describing ulcer aetiology (Nelzen et al., 1991)
Gender	Male patients may have reduced healing (Franks et al., 1995a)	Related issues such as living alone may affect outcome
Social class/financial status	Limited evidence that delayed healing occurs in lower social classes (Franks et al., 1995b)	Standardised methods of describing social class/financial status are available (OPCS, 1991)
Living status	Ulcers in men living alone have the greatest impact on HRQoL (Franks & Moffatt, 1998)	May be linked to levels of social isolation and access to social support
Housing status	Patients living in nursing/residential settings may have poor healing (Franks et al., 2002)	May indicate a higher risk of depression and social deprivation. Ulceration may lead to patient being admitted to residential care
General mobility status	Bed/chair-bound patients have the poorest outcome for healing (Franks et al., 1995a)	A simple classification of general and ankle mobility has been used in research (Franks et al., 1995a)
Ankle function	Fixed ankle joint affects ulcer healing, probably due to reduced venous return (Sochart & Hardinge, 1999)	Progressive reduced ankle function occurs with each year of failed ulcer healing
Accessing services	Low prevalence reported in South Asians and increased risk in Afro-Caribbeans (Franks et al., 1997; Moffatt et al., 2004)	Cultural issues may be influencing whether certain patient groups are accessing services or the prevalence may be different

Employment status	Little known about its impact on ulcer healing (Phillips et al., 1994)	Standardised methods of assessing financial status according to job profile are available (OPCS, 1991)
Clinical factors		
Ulcer aetiology*	Use standardised format for describing aetiology (Nelzen et al., 1991)	All practitioners should use a common method of describing patients
Deep vein thrombosis/popliteal reflux	Associated with delayed healing (Skene et al., 1992; Brittenden et al., 1998)	Patients may be unaware they have experienced a DVT
Cardiovascular risk factors	Predictor of concurrent PAOD	Including smoking, hypertension, MI, TIA and high cholesterol levels
Arterial status***	ABPI levels fall with increasing age	More complex investigations will be required to determine the site and severity of arterial occlusion
Venous status**	Often described using clinical signs and symptoms	Venous Duplex considered the 'gold standard'
Ulcer size: >10cm or <10cm	Small ulcers associated with faster total healing than large ulcers	Can be used to predict healing (Tallman et al., 1997)
Ulcer duration: <6 months, >6 months, >18 months	Increasing duration of ulcer associated with delayed healing	Can be used to predict healing (Franks et al., 1995a; Tallman et al., 1997)
Treatment	Prospective evaluation of treatment may require a 6-month period. Retrospective evaluation can also be used if time prevents long-term follow-up	Useful for evaluating whether appropriate care is being prescribed as well as estimates of healing and changes in prevalence
Dressings	Frequently required for monitoring of prescribing budgets	Dressing costs should not be used to predict quality of services

Table 15.1 *Continued.*

	Comment	Methodology issues
Antimicrobial agents	Important to ensure these are used in the correct clinical situation	Expensive products that should be appropriately used
Compression therapy	Careful description of use of bandages is required	See discussion on healing rate analysis
Other treatments including drug therapy	Medical devices, e.g. VAC therapy, intermittent pneumatic compression, should be evaluated	Evaluation requires that estimates of cost be matched to outcomes of intervention
Recurrence rates	Large variations occur. Every attempt should be made to examine how the service meets the needs of patients whose ulcers recur	A number of factors have been found to be associated with increased recurrence: previous large ulcer, history of DVT, low use of hosiery (Moffatt & Dorman, 1995)
Resource usage****	Generally falls outside the scope of clinical audits	Requires specialist statistical expertise
Nurse time****	Most expensive component of care	Reduction in nurse time is the main factor in the cost-effective argument of leg ulcer care (Franks & Posnett 2003)
Use of resources****	Requires careful analysis of all resources used in both acute and community settings	Cost-effectiveness analysis provides evidence on both clinical and cost outcomes of care (Franks & Posnett 2003)

*Ulcer aetiology – consider using a framework.
**Venous status – should be defined by venous Duplex scan where possible.
***Arterial status – ABPI may be supplemented by arterial Duplex, angiograms, etc.
****Evaluation of use of resources will require expert advice.

Differences in randomised controlled trials of compression therapy

To avoid confounding results, many randomised controlled trials of compression therapy select patients with new venous ulceration and without other health problems. In such trials it is often possible to achieve healing rates well over 70% at 12 weeks (Moffatt et al., 2003). Other studies using patients with more chronic ulcers of longer duration often report lower healing rates, although the compression systems are the same (Morrell et al., 1998). In some studies the difference in expected outcome may relate to the choice of bandage, its application, or the number of patients experiencing an adverse event (Callam et al., 1992). Some studies report variations in healing rates according to the centres involved (Partsh et al., 2001). This may be due to an inherent bias towards a familiar bandage system or variations in the effectiveness of application, particularly if the system is new. Systematic reviews synthesise the results from trials and provide an estimate of the results as a whole (Fletcher et al., 1997).

Risk factors that influence healing rates

Randomised controlled trials are designed to test the efficacy of treatments, often in a best-case scenario situation. When treatments are used within routine clinical practice the outcome may be very different. For example, multi-layer bandaging studies within services report healing rates as low as 30% and as high as 70% at 12 weeks, there are a number of reasons for this (Moffatt et al., 1992; Morrell et al., 1998). A number of independent risk factors for delayed healing have been identified, which include:

* The duration of the ulcer
* The size of the wound

Ulcers that have been present for more than six months and are larger than $10\,cm^2$ have reduced healing rates compared to newer, smaller ulcers (Franks et al., 1995a; Tallman et al., 1997). These factors have now been incorporated into a model that can predict the chance of healing (Tallman et al., 1997). Failure to heal can be predicted as early as four weeks after treatment commences, which means that other interventions can then be initiated at a much earlier stage.

The increasing duration of an unhealed ulcer appears to be a very important factor; however it tells us nothing about the reason why the ulcer is not healing. This may simply be due to a lack of appropriate treatment. However, it may also indicate important issues such as chronic infection or poor wound bed preparation (see Chapters 8 and 13). It is often very difficult in clinical practice to identify and influence all the factors causing delayed healing in this complex group.

Other independent risk factors
Other important risk factors for delayed healing include:

- Poor general mobility (particularly being chair/bed-bound)
- Fixed ankle joint
- History of deep vein thrombosis

More recently, psychological factors such as social support and levels of ulcer pain have been shown to influence healing (Morgan et al., 2004) (see Chapters 9 and 10). While the risk-factor profile of a population affects the outcome of care, research has shown that it does not account for all the differences seen in the healing rates in similar studies undertaken in different geographical areas using similar service models (Franks & Moffatt, 1996). It is likely that many other, as yet unknown, factors influence the healing rates of these complex patients. The length and maturity of the service as well as the demographic characteristics of the patients may be fundamentally different, so care should be taken in drawing too much inference from services that appear to be similar but in fact are very different.

TIME FRAME FOR EVALUATION
Studies frequently report healing rates at 12 or 24 weeks of treatment (Moffatt et al., 1992; Morrell et al., 1998). However, these are arbitrary time points. Follow-up must always be long enough to determine the major changes that will occur as a result of treatment. Adhering to similar healing rate time-scales from published studies allows for some comparison of results.

It is also important to identify patients who fail to respond to treatment and the reasons for this. Statistical analysis using life table analysis will take account of patients who stop treatment for whatever reason and those lost to follow-up. This will provide a more comprehensive evaluation of all patients, not just those who have completed the treatment or who have healed.

THE CHALLENGE OF DEVELOPING AND MEASURING OUTCOMES FOR NON-HEALING PATIENTS

With the changes in patient profile, there is a growing awareness of the challenges required in evaluating success in the patients who do not heal, where the priorities of care may be very different (Hofman et al., 1997; Moffatt et al., 2004). Healing is still a key outcome of care, since it has a major impact on resource usage. However, reduction in the size of the wound or improvements in symptom management may have profound benefits for patients which cannot be captured by measuring healing alone (Ebbeskog & Ekman, 2001).

PATIENT INVOLVEMENT IN OUTCOMES

Previous studies have relied on outcomes for patients that have been predetermined by health professionals. Patients with leg ulceration are viewed as passive towards the care they receive, with little professional expectation that they would wish to be involved in determining what factors are important to them in the evaluation process (Cullum & Roe, 1995). There is a move towards much greater involvement in decision making in healthcare. Patients are being asked about what services should be provided, where they should be based and increasingly offered choices about how they wish their illness to be managed (McIvor, 1991).

USING MIXED METHODS IN EVALUATION

Evaluation may require a range of methodologies, including:

- Observation of care
- Examination of documentation
- Interviews with a range of healthcare providers and patients

Qualitative interviews may provide useful information about the patient journey, and the multiple methods' approach may provide a richer picture of how the service is operating. Table 15.2 outlines some of the wider factors that may be considered.

Table 15.2 Other dimensions to assess in service evaluation.

Correct assessment	Patient evaluation of care
Appropriateness and timeliness of referrals	Uptake of training/improvement in skills
Quality of assessment	Access and equity of care (vulnerable groups)
Treatment decision-making	Communication pathways
Correct choice of dressings	Process of care delivery
Correct choice of compression/therapy	Organisational views of the service
Application of bandages	Patient views on service
Assessment of pain	Discharge planning
Control of pain	Recurrence programmes/recurrence rates
Referral to specialist team(s) and appropriateness of those referrals	Specialist intervention and outcome

EVALUATING PATIENT SATISFACTION

Researchers have struggled to develop appropriate methodologies to evaluate patient satisfaction (Roberts & Tugwell, 1987). Few attempts have been made within the leg ulcer literature, and there are many complexities that make evaluation of satisfaction difficult to interpret. Key amongst these is the dependent relationship between patient and professional in a predominantly elderly group unused to expressing an opinion on health matters (Bowling, 1995).

EVALUATION OF PATIENTS WITH COMPLEX NEEDS

One of the major challenges that researchers have faced is in determining the contribution that leg ulceration makes to patients who may be suffering from a number of concurrent conditions that are influencing their lives (Franks & Moffatt, 1998). We are only just beginning to understand the significance of leg ulceration in relation to the psychosocial status of patients, because of the focus on clinical parameters alone (Morgan et al., 2004). Research has identified a number of social factors that are associated with poor clinical outcomes (Franks et al., 1995b). Factors such as low social class, lack of central heating, being male and living alone were all found to be associated with poor healing of venous ulceration (see Table 15.1). Further work has highlighted that perceived social support is linked to outcome, with those with lowest social support having the poorest outcomes (Moffatt et al., 2002).

There is still much work to be undertaken to confirm these results and to try and explain these relationships. The quality-of-life literature has identified the importance of depression in ulcer healing, yet relatively little is still known about how patients' psychological status affects healing (Moffatt et al., 2002) (see Chapter 10).

CONCLUSION

The approach to evaluation presented in this chapter requires the involvement of the multi-disciplinary team. Specialist nursing roles are increasingly requiring audit and evaluation of services. The principles laid out in this chapter have been successfully used in a large number of service evaluations. If access to expert support is poor, simple evaluation can still be useful to demonstrate the value of services. The value of evaluation cannot be overstated as the problem of leg ulceration competes with finite resources and ever increasing healthcare demands.

REFERENCES

Adam, D.J., Naik, J., Hartshorne, T., Bello, M. & London, N.J. (2003) The diagnosis and management of 689 chronic leg ulcers in a single-visit assessment clinic. *European Journal of Vascular and Endovascular Surgery* **25**(5): 462–468.

Bosanquet, N. (1992) Cost of venous ulcers: from maintenance therapy to investment programmes. *Phlebology* (Suppl. 1): 44–46.

Bowling, A. (1995) *Measuring Disease.* Buckingham, Open University Press.

Brittenden, J., Bradbury, A.W., Allan, P.L., Prescott, R.J., Harper, D.R. & Ruckley, C.V. (1998) Popliteal vein reflux reduces the healing of chronic venous ulcers. *British Journal of Surgery* **85**(1): 60–62.

Callam, M.J., Ruckley, C.V., Harper, D.R. & Dale, J.J. (1985) Chronic ulceration of the leg: extent of the problem and provision of care. *British Medical Journal* **290**: 1855–1856.

Callam, M.J., Harper, D.R., Dale, J.J., Brown, D., Gibson, B., Prescott, R.J. & Ruckley, C.V. (1992) Lothian and Forth Valley leg ulcer healing trial. Part 1: Elastic versus non-elastic bandaging in the treatment of chronic leg ulceration. *Phlebology* **7**(4): 136–141.

Cullum, N. & Roe, B. (eds) (1995) *Leg Ulcers: Nursing Management: A Research Based Guide.* London, Scutari.

Dodds, S.R. (2002) Shared community-hospital care of leg ulcers using an electronic record and telemedicine. *International Journal of Lower Extremity Wounds* **1**(4): 260–270.

Ebbeskog, B. & Ekman, E.L. (2001) Elderly people's experiences: the meaning of living with venous leg ulcers. *European Wound Management Association Journal* **1**: 21–23.

Fletcher, A., Cullum, N. & Sheldon, T.A. (1997) A systematic review of compression treatment for venous leg ulcers. *British Medical Journal* **315**(7108): 576–580.

Franks, P.J. & Moffatt, C.J. (1996) Leg ulcer healing rates: multivariate models to adjust for risk factors for healing. *British Journal of Dermatology* **136**: 28. (Abstract)

Franks, P.J. & Moffatt, C.J. (1998) Who suffers most from leg ulceration? *Journal of Wound Care* **7**: 383–385.

Franks, P.J. & Posnett, J. (2003) Cost effectiveness of compression therapy. In: *EWMA Position Document. Understanding Compression Therapy.* London, MEP Ltd, pp. 8–10.

Franks, P.J., Moffatt, C.J., Oldroyd, M., Bosanquet, N., Connolly, M., Greenhalgh, R.M. & McCollum, C.N. (1994) Community leg ulcer clinics: effect on quality of life. *Phlebology* **9**(2): 83–86.

Franks, P.J., Moffatt, C.J., Connolly, M., Bosanquet, N., Oldroyd, M.I., Greenhalgh, R.M. & McCollum, C.N. (1995a) Factors associated with healing leg ulceration with high compression. *Age & Ageing* **24**: 407–410.

Franks, P.J., Bosanquet, N., Connolly, M., Oldroyd, M.I., Moffatt, C.J., Greenhalgh, R.M. & McCollum, C.N. (1995b) Venous ulcer healing: effect of socio-economic factors in London. *Journal of Epidemiology and Community Health* **49**(4): 385–388.

Franks, P.J., Morton, N., Campbell, A. & Moffatt, C.J. (1997) Leg ulceration and ethnicity. A study in west London. *Public Health* **111**(5): 327–329.

Franks, P.J., Doherty, D.C. & Moffatt, C.J. (2002) Are socio-demographic factors important in the development of chronic leg ulceration? *Ostomy/Wound Management* **48**: 73–74.

Hofman, D., Ryan, T.J., Arnold, F., Cherry, G.W., Lindholm, C., Bjellerup, M. & Glynn, C. (1997) Pain in venous leg ulcers. *Journal of Wound Care* **6**(5): 222–224.

Lambourne, L.A., Moffatt, C.J., Jones, A.C., Dorman, M.C. & Franks, P.J. (1996) Clinical audit and effective change in leg ulcer services. *Journal of Wound Care* **5**: 348–351.

McIvor, S. (1991) *Obtaining the Views of the Users of the Health Service.* London, King's Fund Centre for Health Service Development.

Moffatt, C.J. & Dorman, M.C. (1995) Recurrence of leg ulcers within a community ulcer service. *Journal of Wound Care* **4**(2): 57–61.

Moffatt, C.J., Franks, P.J., Oldroyd, M., Bosanquet, N., Brown, P., Greenhalgh, R.M. & McCollum, C.N. (1992) Community leg ulcer clinics and impact on ulcer healing. *British Medical Journal* **305**: 1389–1392.

Moffatt, C.J., Doherty, D. & Franks, P.J. (2002) Professional dilemmas of non-healing. *Ostomy/Wound Management* **48**: 73–74.

Moffatt, C.J., McCullagh, L., O'Connor, T., Doherty, D.C., Hourican, C., Stevens, J. & Mole Franks, P.J. (2003) Randomized trial of four layer and two-layer bandage systems in the management of chronic venous ulceration. *Wound Repair and Regeneration* **11**: 166–171.

Moffatt, C.J., Franks, P.J., Doherty, D.C., Martin, R., Blewett, R. & Ross, F. (2004) Prevalence of leg ulceration in a London population. *Quarterly Journal of Medicine* **97**(7): 431–437.

Morgan, P.A., Franks, P.J., Moffatt, C.J., Doherty, D.C., O'Connor, T., McCullagh, L. & Hourican, C. (2004) Illness behaviour and social support in patients with chronic venous ulcers. *Ostomy/Wound Management* **50**: 25–32.

Morrell, C.J., Walters, S.J., Dixon, S., Collins, K.A., Brereton, L.M.L., Peters, J. & Brooker, C.G.D. (1998) Cost effectiveness of community leg ulcer clinics: randomised controlled trial. *British Medical Journal* **316**: 1487–1491.

Nelzen, O., Bergqvist, D. & Lindhagen, A. (1991) Leg ulcer etiology – a cross sectional population study. *Journal of Vascular Surgery* **14**: 557–564.

OPCS (Office of Population Censuses and Surveys) (1991) *Standard Occupational Classification. Volume 3. Social Classifications and Coding Methodology.* London, HMSO.

Partsch, H., Damstra, R.J., Tazelaar, D.J., Schuller-Petrovic, S., Velders, A.J., de Rooij, M.J., Sang, R.R. & Quinlan, D. (2001) Multicentre, randomised controlled trial of four-layer bandaging versus short-stretch bandaging in the treatment of venous leg ulcers. *VASA Zeitschrift für Gefässkrankheiten (Journal for Vascular Diseases)* **30**(2): 108–113.

Phillips, T., Stanton, B., Provan, A. & Lew, R. (1994) A study of the impact of leg ulcers on quality of life: financial, social and psychologic implications. *Journal of the American Academy of Dermatology* **31**: 49–53.

Roberts, J.G. & Tugwell, P. (1987) Comparison of questionnaires determining patient satisfaction with medical care. *Health Services Research* **22**: 637–654.

Royal College of Nursing (1998, 2006) *Clinical Practice Guidelines. The Management of Patients with Venous Leg Ulcers.* London, Royal College of Nursing.

SIGN (Scottish Intercollegiate Guidelines Network) (1998) *The Care of Patients with Chronic Leg Ulcer.* Edinburgh, SIGN, SIGN Publication No 26.

Skene, A.I., Smith, J.M., Dore, C.J., Charlett, A. & Lewis, J.D. (1992) Venous leg ulcers: a prognostic index to predict time to healing. *British Medical Journal* **305**: 1119–1121.

Sochart, D.H. & Hardinge, K. (1999) The relationship of foot and ankle movements to venous return in the lower limb. *Journal of Bone and Joint Surgery (British volume)* **81**(4): 700–704.

Tallman, P., Muscare, E., Carson, P., Eaglstein, W.H. & Falanga, V. (1997) Initial rate of healing predicts complete healing of venous ulcers. *Archives of Dermatology* **133**(10): 1231–1234.

Thomson, B., Hooper, P., Powell, R. & Warin, A.P. (1996) Four-layer bandaging and healing rates of venous leg ulcers. *Journal of Wound Care* **5**(5): 213–216.

Vowden, K.R., Barker, A. & Vowden, P. (1997) Leg ulcer management in a nurse-led, hospital-based clinic. *Journal of Wound Care* **6**(5): 233–236.

Prevention of Recurrence and Patient Evaluation

LEARNING OBJECTIVES

Nurses involved in leg ulcer management should be able to demonstrate:

❏ An understanding that leg ulcer recurrence is a common problem.

❏ An understanding of the importance of regular assessment to identify those patients who are failing to make progress.

❏ An understanding of the use of compression hosiery in preventing recurrence.

❏ An understanding that the patient's attitude and commitment to treatment will influence recurrence.

❏ An understanding of the importance of monitoring the patient with established peripheral arterial occlusive disease.

INTRODUCTION

The leg ulcer pathway described in this book encourages continuous patient evaluation. This is important for a number of reasons:

• To ensure those patients who are failing to progress are identified early and referred for specialist opinion.

• To prevent prolonged patient suffering with treatment that is failing.

• To identify complex patients who require input from the multi-disciplinary team.

• To encourage a professional climate that fosters continuous high quality care through constant evaluation of practice.

ONE-MONTH REVIEW

The pathway requires that patients who are failing to show a reduction in the size of their ulcer within one month are referred to the specialist leg ulcer team. The decision to encourage early referral is research-based. This has shown that ulcers that fail to make progress within the first four weeks of treatment will frequently fail to heal or take a protracted time with conventional treatment, and therefore early intervention with other therapies may be required (Margolis et al., 2000). At this evaluation time-point the specialist team can check for the following:

- Has the aetiology of the ulcer been correctly defined?
- Is the treatment being delivered appropriate and correctly applied?
- Are symptoms such as pain being effectively controlled?
- Have other concurrent health problems been identified and controlled where possible?
- Are other leg ulcer treatments or health interventions required?
- Does the patient require urgent referral to the multi-disciplinary team?

THREE-MONTH EVALUATION

Nurses are required to evaluate the progress of their patients regularly every 3 months to check that progress is being made, and to return to the first phase of the pathway (assessment) to ensure that all issues relating to assessment, treatment and referral have been considered. When the service in Wandsworth was last evaluated, over 80% of patients in the service had been referred for specialist opinion (Moffatt et al., 2004). This is very important for a number of reasons:

- Approximately 40% of patients with an ulcer have a correctable vascular abnormality, such as varicose veins or peripheral arterial occlusive disease (PAOD) (Nelzén, 1999). Studies have shown that corrective vein surgery significantly reduces the rate of ulcer recurrence (Barwell et al., 2000). It is essential that nurses refer patients for specialist opinion or request the general practitioner to do so.
- Failed healing is frequently associated with poor symptom control, and this has a significant impact on the patient's life (Franks & Moffatt, 1998).

- Delayed healing can lead to professional disillusionment, which can ultimately affect the relationship between nurse and patient (Moffatt, 2004)
- Failed treatment is associated with a huge use of health resources (Bosanquet et al., 1993)

SUDDEN DETERIORATION

The pathway requires that any sudden deterioration in the ulcer triggers an evaluation. Common problems include the development of infection or a deterioration in the patient's general health that affects their progress. The integration of the specialist and community aspects of the pathway attempts to provide ready access to advice for all patients within the area, irrespective of where they are receiving their leg ulcer treatment.

ASSESSMENT OF THE PATIENT'S ARTERIAL STATUS

The pathway recommends that all patients with a healed ulcer have their ABPI recorded every 3–6 months, in conjunction with renewal of their hosiery. The optimum time for Doppler reassessment has not been established through research, but this recommendation is based on expert clinical opinion and an appreciation that increasing age is associated with a fall in ABPI (Vowden & Vowden, 2006). Patients with an established arterial component to their ulcer require regular assessment every 3 months, or more frequently if a change in symptoms indicates that the peripheral circulation is deteriorating.

OTHER REASONS FOR SPECIALIST REFERRAL

A number of other reasons for referral are included in the pathway, these include:

- Support and advice
- Ulcers that remain unhealed for more than 3 months
- Ulcers that enlarge without an obvious cause
- Persistent or unexplained pain
- Patients unable to tolerate compression
- Persistent skin problems
- Resistant cellulitis
- Recurrent ulceration

These criteria encourage nurses to seek advice when they are facing difficulty with individual patients. The specialist leg ulcer nurses can then decide whether referral to the hospital ulcer clinic or the wider multi-disciplinary team is required. Specification of the types of problems associated with ulceration has helped to prompt earlier referral for assistance, rather than continuing with ineffective care or poor symptom control.

FACTORS INFLUENCING VENOUS ULCER RECURRENCE

While research relating to the recurrence of ulceration remains sparse, studies suggest that the rate of recurrence is high (Erickson et al., 1995; Moffatt & Dorman, 1995; McDaniel et al., 2002). Concordance with wearing compression hosiery has been shown to affect the rate of ulcer recurrence (Erickson et al., 1995).

In many cases, ulcer recurrence occurs spontaneously or in response to minor trauma. Professionals should avoid blaming the patient for re-ulceration: tampering with the skin is rare and usually indicates psychological dependence on professional care or social isolation and loneliness (Muir Gray, 1983). Uncontrolled varicose eczema causing skin irritation is a frequent cause of re-ulceration. Patients with urinary incontinence may develop severe dermatitis leading to ulceration.

Professional attitudes to ulcer recurrence

Professionals may be fatalistic in their attitudes to ulcer recurrence and delegate this task to less qualified staff (Flanagan et al., 2001). Effective recurrence programmes should be an integral part of all leg ulcer services. Creative approaches to this include the development of leg clubs that encourage patient participation and long-term follow-up in a relaxed environment (Fassiadis et al., 2002). Programmes involving carers and healthcare assistants can be useful, particularly in the frail-immobile group. The patients should also be regularly assessed by a trained healthcare professional to ensure that any changes in the patients' medical condition or arterial status are identified. Any change in symptoms, such as pain or numbness, should be reported immediately. Effective patient education should emphasise the importance of seeking medical advice immediately there is an ulcer, as the longer the ulcer is present the greater the chance of delayed healing (Franks et al., 1995).

Patient assessment

A detailed patient history can identify whether the patient is at an increased risk of ulcer recurrence. In addition to a clinical history, the practitioner should assess factors that may influence their adherence to hosiery (Table 16.1). These will include:

- The patient's attitude to their health
- The 'ownership' they have of their condition
- Level of motivation

An account of the patient's knowledge and understanding of their treatment will assist in the development of an individualised patient education programme. Many of the problems with hosiery can be overcome by knowledgeable and imaginative clinical management (Moffatt & Dorman, 1995).

Oedema and ulceration

Oedema, irrespective of the underlying cause, is significantly associated with re-ulceration. Sudden development of oedema may be caused by heart failure, liver and renal disease. Bilateral oedema can be a presenting symptom in patients with abdominal tumours who are otherwise asymptomatic.

A change in diuretics or a cessation of therapy in patients with chronic heart failure may lead to oedema. Certain drugs are associated with fluid retention, resulting in ankle oedema. Deterioration in the patient's health status or uncontrolled pain may mean that patients do not go to bed at night but sleep in a chair with their legs in a dependent position. This causes severe dependency oedema with a high risk of ulcer recurrence.

A randomised controlled trial of compression hosiery (18–24 mmHg) identified a number of factors associated with an increased risk of venous ulcer recurrence. These were:

- Previous size of the ulcer (>10 cm)
- History of deep vein thrombosis
- Unsuitable for stockings (Franks et al., 1995)

Table 16.1 Assessment issues and their solutions.

	Problems to consider	Possible solutions
General health status	Check for concurrent health problems such as cardiac failure	Use lower compression levels in vulnerable patients
Patient preference and comfort	Problems with concordance are significantly influenced by these issues	Consider the wide range of products and materials available. Offer patients some choice and allow them to make final decision
Skin integrity	Allow a few weeks following healing to ensure the epithelium is robust	Note potential skin problems such as varicose eczema, skin sensitivity, contact dermatitis. Treat these conditions accordingly
Arterial circulation	Regularly monitor and record the ABPI	See Chapter 14 on the criteria for the level of compression
Allergies	Dyes, latex or elastane found in hosiery are common allergens	Use a cotton tubular under-layer
Level of compression	Consider risk factors for recurrence	High levels of compression can be difficult to apply. Consider layering hosiery to achieve a higher level of compression or provide the patient with a hosiery aid or information to obtain one (some are available on prescription, others the patient will have to purchase)

Foot and leg deformities/shape distortion	Use protection over vulnerable sites	Ensure deformities do not require a custom-made stocking
Measurement for hosiery	Follow agreed protocol to decide whether circular/flat knit and off-the-shelf/made-to-measure hosiery is required	Consider range of hosiery available for individual patient needs – consider garments with zippers if dexterity is a problem
Disproportionate limb shape	Follow custom-made protocol to ensure a correct fit	Consider whether garment should have an open or closed toe. Maintain any compression bandaging currently in use until custom-made hosiery is received to ensure limb shape remains stable
Patient understanding	This process should begin at the time of the first assessment	Patients need to understand that they are a potential ulcer patient for life
Manual dexterity	Ensure you observe that the patient or their carer can correctly apply and remove the hosiery	Use the adaptive aids available and consider the role of family and carers
Footwear	Check that shoes fit well	Check the patient after one week to ensure that no problems have emerged

Other authors have also found increased recurrence rates in those who have had a previous deep vein thrombosis (Stacey et al., 1991). These factors indicate that the severity of the underlying disease may be an important factor associated with recurrence.

Patient attitudes towards and experience of wearing compression hosiery

Johnson identified that patients reported difficulties in the use of compression hosiery (Johnson, 1988), and Travers found that of 32 women, 17 did not wear their stockings at all, while 60% found the cosmetic appearance unacceptable (Travers et al., 1990). Other factors influencing their use included:

- Friable skin
- Difficulty in applying and removing stockings
- Skin irritation

A large randomised controlled trial of 18–24 mmHg and 25–35 mmHg hosiery found that the recurrence rates were lowest in the higher compression group but concordance was problematic (Harper et al., 1995).

A systematic review of randomised controlled trials into ulcer recurrence found weak evidence that compression hosiery reduced recurrence and recommended further research in this area (Nelson, 2001).

Current recommendations based on the limited research available and expert opinion suggest that patients should be fitted with the highest level of compression they can tolerate, provided that concordance is good.

COMPRESSION HOSIERY AND ITS CORRECT USE
Hosiery classification

In order for recurrence to be reduced to a minimum it is essential that the practitioner understands the current classifications of compression hosiery. Patients with a healed venous ulcer should be fitted with the highest level of compression they can tolerate and safely apply. A pressure of at least 18–24 mmHg is recommended, while a higher pressure of 25–35 mmHg is preferable (see Chapter 14). Research has not yet been undertaken to determine the exact range of pressure that may be most beneficial in preventing recurrence in the different groups of patients.

> It is important to remember that applying a low level of compression is better than none.

If patients have problems with the application and removal of hosiery, two lower level compression stockings can be used to apply an accumulative pressure (the second layer applies approximately 70% of the pressure applied by the first layer of stocking).

The development of new technologies has led to considerable advances in the production of compression hosiery. There are two methods for making compression garments, and it is important to understand how these manufacturing processes affect the choice of garments.

Circular knit garments

These are knitted on a cylinder and have no seam. They may be particularly useful for patients at low risk of ulcer recurrence or the development of oedema. The use of thin microfibres within these garments allows for the production of sheer, silky materials that are very attractive to patients who are concerned with their appearance. They are less suitable for patients with a distorted limb shape (such as the inverted 'champagne bottle' shape) or in those with arthritic limbs. The circular nature of the knitting process may cause the development of tight bands and rolling of the material, causing pain and tissue trauma.

Flat knit garments

Stockings produced by a flat knit machine are knitted row by row using a knitting pattern, and when the garment is complete the two edges are sewn together. These garments can be made in unlimited shapes and sizes. They are particularly used in the management of patients with venous ulceration and lymphoedema who often have gross limb deformities. Many of these garments have an inelastic component and are particularly useful at controlling oedema reduction due to the increased stiffness within the garment.

Custom-made hosiery

Custom-made garments are required for patients with extreme limb distortion. When measured and fitted correctly they can give an almost perfect fit to each individual limb. Flat knit hosiery is also available in a wide range of ready-made garments. The Department of Health drug tariff in the UK recently included these types of garments on prescription. They are now available in the community as well as through specialist hospital centres.

Measuring the limb

Accurate measurement is important to achieve a correctly fitting garment. Some basic circumferential measurements are required when fitting ready-to-wear garments. The following principles should be used:

- Take measurements when the area is largely free of oedema, i.e. immediately after removal of compression bandages or in the morning before any swelling can develop.
- Do not pull the tape tight enough to make an indentation in the skin, as this will be too restrictive.
- Precise measurements are required for custom-made garments. Most manufacturers provide measuring forms to assist the fitter.

The accurate measurement of the limb should always be carefully recorded. When two limbs are involved, both limbs should be measured separately (Lymphoedema Framework, 2006). Many of the reported problems with hosiery relate to inaccurate measurement or the wrong prescription. While many patients' limbs will be adequately accommodated by the standard sizes available, a custom-made stocking should be prescribed if the measurements fall outside those recommended.

Correct choice of garment

Care should be taken to ensure the hosiery is of sufficient length for tall patients, and not too long for short patients. When using open-toed stockings it is important to check they are long enough, otherwise bands of oedema may develop over the forefoot. It is generally accepted that below-knee stockings are adequate in venous ulcer prevention (Lawrence & Kakkar, 1980), although thigh-length stockings may be required in a number of clinical situations:

- When oedema extends to the thigh
- When varicosities are present in the thigh region
- Where oedema accumulates around the knee joint
- When arthritic changes make below-knee stockings uncomfortable for the patient to wear

When to apply hosiery

The limb is ready for the application of hosiery once the ulcer has completely healed (epithelialised) and gained some of its tensile strength. Often the trauma of application and removal of a stocking can damage friable skin, so it is advisable to wait a few weeks after the ulcer has healed before commencing with hosiery. A measuring board can be used to measure the limb, whereby the patient stands with their foot flat on the floor but against the board. If this is unavailable the patient can be measured in the standing position with their calf muscle contracted. In immobile patients who are unable to stand two people should undertake the procedure to ensure accuracy of the measurement. Fig. 16.1 shows the different points on the limb that should be measured, using a tape-measure, for a ready-made garment.

Problem solving

For very immobile patients, garments containing zippers can be considered. Patients who complain of slippage may benefit from a garment with a siliconised band, although this is only available in thigh-length garments. Adhesive skin glue may be helpful in extreme cases. However, glue should be used with caution in patients who are prone to skin irritation or those with known contact allergy. Patients who develop oedema and repeated ulcer recurrence in the retromalleolar region may benefit from hosiery containing silicone padding in this area. This applies pressure to the perforating veins and by increasing local pressure to the area reduces oedema. The decision to prescribe open- or closed-toe garments is often a matter of patient preference. Care should be taken in those with hallux valgus as bands of pressure over this area may cause tissue necrosis. Open- rather than closed-toe garments

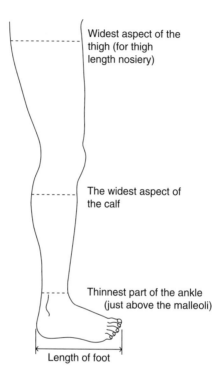

Widest aspect of the thigh (for thigh length nosiery)

The widest aspect of the calf

Thinnest part of the ankle (just above the malleoli)

Length of foot

Fig. 16.1 Positions used for measuring ready-made compression hosiery.

may be preferred when using the very high levels of compression. While removal of compression hosiery at night is the preferred option, it may be left in place for a week in those who are unable to do so. The leg can then be washed and creamed and a clean stocking applied.

Fitting the stocking

After the initial prescription the practitioner should fit the garment to ensure there are no problems. Patients must be carefully instructed on how to take care of their leg and thus reduce the chance of ulcer recurrence. This must include the daily application of emollients and avoidance of products that may cause an allergic reaction, or ones containing paraffin, which may cause the garment to deteriorate. A cotton tubular liner may be useful if the skin is friable or the stocking causes local erythema or irritation. If this situation persists a stocking with a high cotton content may be used. Managing the transition from high compression bandaging to hosiery may be difficult and may involve some degree of trial and error in finding the right garment for some patients. Oedema may occur if the pressure applied by the stocking is considerably less than that applied by the bandage. Regular follow-up is required during this important phase.

Application and removal techniques
Application and removal techniques should be observed to ensure the patient will be able to manage on their return home; information leaflets can be provided to give instructions. The patient should be given the following advice:

- Remove all wrinkles. This can be assisted by wearing household rubber gloves to smooth the compression garments by stroking gently upwards.
- Wash the garments frequently and according to the manufacturer's instructions. Durability is impaired by not washing them often enough.

Application aids
The following aids may make the application of compression garments easier for patients:

- Rubber gloves
- Easi-slides
- Stocking applicators
- Silk slipper
- Mat
- Frames

NB. There are several stocking removal aids that can assist those who have difficulty removing their compression garment.

Common problems associated with wearing compression garments

Common problems observed in these patients include:

- Over-stretching the stocking over the calf.
- Turning down the top of the stocking causing a ridge.
- Pressure damage over the dorsum of the foot due to ridges in the stocking.
- Tourniquet effect due to a rolled stocking that could not be removed.
- Poor care of the stocking causing damage or shrinkage.

The patient should be informed about the care of the stocking and that it will need to be replaced at least every 6 months. Tears, ladders or holes will affect the overall performance. Patients who have heavy jobs may require more frequent renewal of the garment.

Particular care should be taken with patients who are mentally frail and who may push the stocking down. In some cases, these vulnerable patients may be best managed with a multi-layer bandage system with a cohesive outer layer that prevents patient tampering, while providing sustained compression.

Allergy and compression garments

Allergy to compression garments is relatively rare. Before fitting it is important to identify whether the patient has experienced a previous allergy or a skin reaction to compression. Allergens include fabric dye, latex and nylon. The combination of emollients and compression can cause skin reactions.

If an allergy is suspected, the recommendations are to:

- Treat the contact dermatitis appropriately (see Chapter 8).
- Use garments without latex.
- Consider garments with linings that can eliminate the problem.
- Apply cotton tubular bandage as an under-layer.

RECURRENCE OF ULCERATION IN PATIENTS WITH A HISTORY OF PERIPHERAL ARTERIAL OCCLUSIVE DISEASE (PAOD)

Patients with established PAOD are at high risk of re-ulceration. This is influenced by the following factors:

- Deterioration in the overall health status of the patient.
- Increased stenosis or occlusion of the arteries reducing tissue perfusion.
- Failure of previous interventions, e.g. angioplasty or arterial surgery.
- Patient's inability to modify risk factors, e.g. smoking.
- Development of concurrent diabetes.
- Presence of other systemic conditions, e.g. rheumatoid arthritis.

It is essential that any patient presenting with a new episode of ulceration is assessed and that an ankle to brachial pressure index is recorded.

Patients whose arterial status deteriorates should be urgently referred for specialist opinion. An ulcer is unlikely to heal in the presence of severe disease unless the peripheral perfusion to the limb is improved. Critical limb ischaemia may lead to amputation and possible death.

> The aetiology of the ulcer may change over time. In those aged over 80 years, 50% have concurrent peripheral vascular disease that may affect their treatment programme.

Many patients with ulceration suffer with PAOD in conjunction with venous disease. The arterial status of the patient governs the priorities of treatment. Improvement in peripheral perfusion through interventions such as angioplasty can allow the introduction of low levels of compression to treat the venous component of the ulcer. This should be carried out under the supervision of the specialist leg ulcer team. While long-term follow-up is essential for all patients with healed leg ulceration, it is particularly critical for this patient group.

ULCER RECURRENCE ASSOCIATED WITH SYSTEMIC DISEASE

A number of systemic diseases are associated with leg ulceration (see Chapter 7). Recurrence of leg ulceration in these patients may be due to a number of reasons:

- Deterioration in the systemic condition
- Poor overall health
- Poor nutritional status
- Increased risk of infection
- Reduced mobility
- Long-term effects of steroid therapy causing susceptibility to trauma and slow wound healing

Recurrence of ulceration may indicate a resurgence of the underlying condition and should prompt reassessment and urgent referral.

Patients with these types of ulceration are challenging because of the difficulties of controlling the underlying condition. It is often impossible to predict how long healing will take, and in some patients whether healing will occur. In conditions such as sickle cell ulceration, improvement in healing may be linked to other systemic treatment such as blood transfusions that increase the overall haemoglobin level. Patients with clotting disorders may find that episodes of ulceration are reduced following anticoagulation therapy.

THE PATIENT AS EXPERT IN THEIR CONDITION

Successful prevention of ulcer recurrence requires engagement of the patient and/or carer. The patient must be taught about their ulcer and what strategies are required to reduce the risk of recurrence. They should receive appropriate information that is easily understood.

There is increasing awareness that patients become experts in their own condition, and the electronic era is leading to greater access to information. However, not all available information is correct and the nurse must ensure the patient has a clear understanding of their condition and its treatment.

SUMMARY

- Patients who fail to make any progress within 1 month should be reassessed and specialist referral considered.
- Approximately 40% of patients have a vascular abnormality that may be amenable to surgical or radiological correction, thus helping to prevent recurrence. Referral to a vascular surgeon should be considered.
- If the ulcer fails to heal within 3 months the patient should be reassessed and referral for specialist opinion sought.
- Comprehensive assessment will help to identify patients at an increased risk of recurrence.
- Any sudden deterioration in the ulcer or increase in symptoms requires reassessment, including repeating an ABPI using Doppler.
- Formation of oedema, irrespective of the cause, will lead to rapid ulcer recurrence.
- The patient's attitude and commitment to using compression hosiery will influence recurrence.
- Professionals frequently fail to provide ongoing monitoring and recurrence programmes. These must be an integral part of service delivery.
- Practitioners must understand the way in which compression hosiery is classified in order that the correct garments are selected and fitted.
- Hosiery is made using two different knitting techniques: circular and flat knit. Practitioners must understand how the type of construction and the yarn used influences the correct choice of garments.
- Correct measurement and fitting of hosiery are required to encourage patient adherence to therapy.
- Patients with established PAOD should be regularly monitored to detect changes in their clinical status.
- Patients become experts in their own condition and should be respected for their knowledge and given choices about their treatment.

REFERENCES

Barwell, J.R., Taylor, M., Deacon, J. & Ghauri, A.S. (2000) Surgical correction of isolated venous reflux reduces long term recurrence rate in chronic venous leg ulcers. *European Journal of Vascular and Endovascular Surgery* **20**(4): 263–268.

Bosanquet, N., Franks, P., Moffatt, C., Connolly, M., Oldroyd, M., Brown, P., Greenhalgh, R. & McCollum, C. (1993) Community leg ulcer clinics: cost effectiveness. *Health Trends* **25**: 146–148.

Erickson, C.A., Lanza, D.J., Karp, D.L. & Edwards, J.W. (1995) Healing of venous ulcers in an ambulatory care programme: the roles of chronic insufficiency and patient compliance. *Journal of Vascular Surgery* **22**: 629–636.

Fassiadis, N., Godby, C., Agland, L. & Law, N. (2002) Preventing venous ulcer recurrence: the impact of the well leg clinic. *Phlebology* **17**(3–4): 134–136.

Flanagan, M., Rotchell, L., Fletcher, J. & Scofield, J. (2001) Community nurses', home carers' and patients' perceptions of factors affecting venous leg ulcer recurrence and management of services. *Journal of Nursing Management* **9**(3): 153–159.

Franks, P.J. & Moffatt, C.J. (1998) Who suffers most from leg ulceration? *Journal of Wound Care* **7**: 383–385.

Franks, P.J., Oldroyd, M.I., Dickson, D., Sharp, E.J. & Moffatt, C.J. (1995) Risk factors for leg ulcer recurrence: a randomised trial of two types of compression stocking. *Age and Ageing* **24**: 407–410.

Harper, D.R., Nelson, E.A., Gibson, B., Prescott, R.J. & Ruckley, C.V. (1995) A prospective randomised controlled trial of Class 2 and Class 3 elastic compression in the prevention of venous ulceration. *Phlebology* (Suppl. 1): 872–873.

Johnson, G.V. (1988). Elastic stockings. *British Medical Journal* **296**: 720.

Lawrence, D. & Kakkar, V.V. (1980) Graduated static external compression of the lower limb: a physiological assessment. *British Journal of Surgery* **67**: 119–121.

Lymphoedema Framework (2006) *Template for Practice: Compression Hosiery in Lymphoedema*. London, MEP Ltd.

Margolis, D.J., Berlin, J.A. & Strom, B.L. (2000) Which venous ulcers will heal with limb compression bandaging? *American Journal of Medicine* **109**(1): 15–19.

McDaniel, H.B., Marston, W.A., Farber, M.A. & Mendes, R.R. (2002) Recurrence of chronic venous ulcers on the basis of clinical, etiologic, anatomic, and pathophysiologic criteria and air plethysmography. *Journal of Vascular Surgery* **35**: 723–728.

Moffatt, C.J. (2004) Perspectives on concordance in leg ulcer management. *Journal of Wound Care* **13**(6): 243–248.

Moffatt, C.J. & Dorman, M.C. (1995) Recurrence of leg ulcers within a community ulcer service. *Journal of Wound Care* **4**(2): 57–61.

Moffatt, C.J., Franks, P.J., Doherty, D.C., Martin, R., Blewett, R. & Ross, F. (2004) Prevalence of leg ulceration in a London population. *Quarterly Journal of Medicine* **97**(7): 431–437.

Muir Gray, J.A. (1983) Social aspects of peripheral vascular disease in the elderly. In: *Peripheral Vascular Disease in the Elderly* (S. McCarthy, ed.). London, Churchill Livingstone, pp. 191–199.

Nelson, E.A. (2001) Systematic reviews of prevention of venous ulcer recurrence. *Phlebology* **16**(1): 20–23.

Nelzén, O. (1999) How can we improve outcomes for leg ulcer patients? In: *Venous Disease: Epidemiology, Management and Delivery of Care* (V. Ruckley & A. Bradbury, eds). London, Springer Verlag, pp. 246–253.

Stacey, M.C., Burnand, K.G., Lea Thomas, M. & Pattison, M. (1991) The influence of phlebographic abnormalities on the natural history of venous ulceration. *British Journal of Surgery* **78**: 868–871.

Travers, J.P., Harrison, J.D. & Makin, D.S. (1990) Post operative use of compression stockings in preventing recurrence of varicose veins. *Paper presented to the Venous Forum of the Royal Society of Medicine.* London, Vol. **7**(8): 383–385.

Vowden, K. & Vowden, P. (2006) Doppler and ABPI or LOI in screening for arterial disease. *Wounds UK* **2**(1): 13–16.

Index